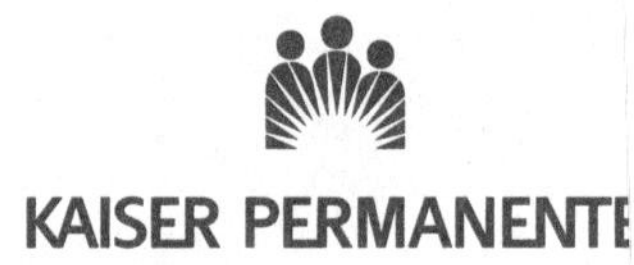

Dear Health Plan Member,

We are delighted to give you this *Kaiser Permanente Healthwise® Handbook* as an additional benefit of membership. Members who use this book tell us that it is an extremely useful tool in helping them care for themselves and their families.

The *Kaiser Permanente Healthwise® Handbook* is designed to help you increase your confidence in managing your health in partnership with us. It is a comprehensive, easy-to-understand guide that has been reviewed and revised by hundreds of Kaiser Permanente physicians and other health professionals. The book provides information on over 200 health topics, including everything from headaches to ingrown toenails. For helpful hints on convenient home treatment or sound advice on when to call for professional help, check out the book. It also has the answers to many questions you might have about how to stay healthy, including how to start an exercise program, how to eat healthfully, and how to manage stress. So whether it's allergies or arthritis, backache or burns, rashes or relaxation, runny nose or ringing in the ears—you'll find a wealth of good information right at your fingertips in this home health guide.

Take a few minutes now to glance through it. We think you will find it of interest even when you are well. And, when you are sick, knowing what's in the book can help you quickly decide on the most appropriate care for yourself and your family. Keep the book handy—perhaps by your telephone along with your local Kaiser Permanente member guide to services.

Your Kaiser Permanente health care team will always be there when you need them. We value our role as your "partner in health" and look forward to helping you and your family stay healthy.

Francis J. Crosson, M.D.
Executive Director
The Permanente Federation

George C. Halvorson
Chairman and Chief Executive Officer
Kaiser Foundation Health Plan and Hospitals

KAISER PERMANENTE

HEALTHWISE® HANDBOOK

A Self-Care Guide for You and Your Family

- *Over 200 Health Care Problems*
- *Prevention*
- *Home Treatment*
- *When to Call Kaiser Permanente*

Donald W. Kemper, MPH

The Healthwise Staff

The Physicians and Staff of Kaiser Permanente

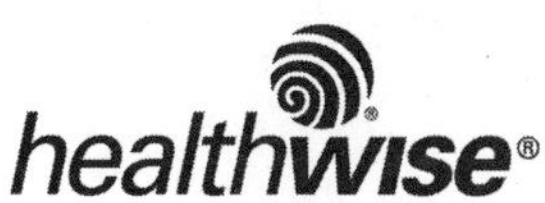

Healthwise, Incorporated, Boise, Idaho
(A nonprofit organization)

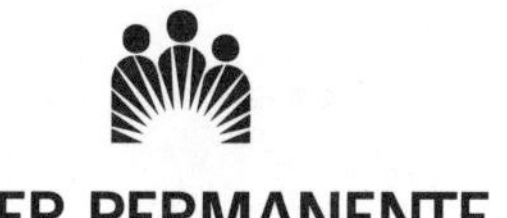

Kaiser Permanente cover concept by Seventeenth Street Studios, current Kaiser Permanente cover design and illustrations by Kathy Locke of Locke Veach Communications Group

Illustrations by Nucleus Communications, Inc.

First edition published 1994.
Revised editions 1999, 2000, 2001, 2002, 2003.

15hwhb/Kaiser 3rd national/2nd/9-03
ISBN:1-877930-96-2

Printed in the United States of America.

Table of Contents

To Our Readers viii
About Healthwise ix
Acknowledgements x
The Healthwise® Self-Care Checklist 1
Ask-the-Physician Checklist 2

Chapter 1: Making Wise Health Decisions 3
Skills for Making Wise Health Decisions 3
Advance Health Care Directives 9

Chapter 2: Living a Healthy Life 15
Immunizations 15
Screening and Early Detection 20
Be Physically Active 21
Eat Right 22
Maintain a Healthful Body Weight 22
Be Tobacco-Free 24
Avoid Drugs and Excess Alcohol 27
Manage Stress 27
Take Care of Your Teeth 27
Practice Safety 29
Pursue Healthy Pleasures 30
Help to Make a Healthier World 30

Chapter 3: First Aid and Emergencies 31
Dealing With Emergencies 31
Accidental Tooth Loss 32
Animal and Human Bites 33
Blood Under a Nail 34
Blunt Abdominal Wounds 35
Breathing Emergencies 36
Rescue Breathing and CPR 36
Bruises 40
Burns 41

Chemical Burns .43
Choking .44
Choking Rescue Procedure (Heimlich Maneuver) .45
Cuts .46
Electrical Burns .49
Fishhook Removal .50
Freeing Trapped Limbs .51
Frostbite .51
Head Injuries .52
Heart Attack .54
Heat Exhaustion and Heat Stroke .55
Hyperventilation .56
Hypothermia .57
Insect and Spider Bites and Stings .59
Nosebleeds .60
Objects in the Ear .61
Objects in the Eye .62
Objects in the Nose .63
Poisoning .63
Puncture Wounds .65
Scrapes .66
Shock .67
Snake Bites .68
Spinal Injuries .69
Stroke .70
Tick Bites .71
Unconsciousness .73

Chapter 4: Abdominal Problems 75

Abdominal Pain .75
Constipation .78
Dehydration .80
Diarrhea .82
Heartburn .83
Hernia .85
Irritable Bowel Syndrome .87

Nausea and Vomiting 90
Rectal Problems 91
Stomach Flu and Food Poisoning 93
Ulcers 95
Urinary Incontinence 98
Urinary Tract Infections 100

Chapter 5: Back and Neck Problems 103
Back Problems 103
Neck Problems 113

Chapter 6: Bone, Muscle, and Joint Problems 117
Arthritis 117
Bunions and Hammer Toes 119
Bursitis and Tendinitis 120
Carpal Tunnel Syndrome 124
Knee Problems 126
Muscle Cramps and Leg Pain 127
Osteoporosis 129
Plantar Fasciitis 130
Sports Injuries 132
Strains, Sprains, and Fractures 134
Temporomandibular (TM) Disorder 136
Weakness and Fatigue 138

Chapter 7: Chest and Respiratory Problems 141
Allergies 141
Asthma 146
Bronchitis (Chest Cold) 150
Chest Pain 151
Colds 154
Coughs 157
Fever 158
Heart Palpitations 160
Influenza (Flu) 161
Laryngitis 163
Pneumonia 163

Sinusitis 165
Sore Throat and Strep Throat 167
Swollen Lymph Nodes 169
Tonsillitis 170

Chapter 8: Eye and Ear Problems 173
Dry Eyes 174
Eye Infections 175
Styes 177
Dizziness and Vertigo 178
Ear Infections 180
Earwax 183
Hearing Loss 184
Swimmer's Ear 186
Tinnitus 188

Chapter 9: Headaches 189
Headaches in Children 191
Migraine Headaches 192
Tension Headaches 194

Chapter 10: Skin, Hair, and Nail Problems 197
Acne 197
Atopic Dermatitis 200
Blisters 201
Boils 202
Canker Sores 203
Cold Sores 204
Dandruff 205
Dry Skin 206
Fungal Infections 207
Hives 209
Ingrown Toenails 209
Lice and Scabies 210
Rashes 211
Skin Cancer 212
Sunburn 214
Warts 215

Chapter 11: Infant and Child Health. 217
Facts About Infants and Young Children 217
Bed-Wetting 221
Chickenpox 222
Colic 224
Cradle Cap 225
Croup 226
Diaper Rash 227
Diarrhea and Vomiting 228
Fever 231
Fever Convulsions 233
Impetigo 235
Pinworms 236
Prickly Heat (Sweat Rash) 237
Roseola 238

Chapter 12: Chronic Conditions. 239
Diabetes 239
High Cholesterol 242
High Blood Pressure 245

Chapter 13: Women's Health 249
Breast Health 249
Gynecological Health 253
Pregnancy: How to Make a Healthy Baby 255
Bleeding Between Periods 258
Menopause 259
Menstrual Cramps 262
Missed or Irregular Periods 263
Premenstrual Syndrome 264
Vaginitis 266
Yeast Infections 268

Chapter 14: Men's Health 271
Genital Health 271
Erection Problems 271
Prostate Infection (Prostatitis) 273

Prostate Enlargement .274
Prostate Cancer .275
Testicular Problems .276

Chapter 15: Sexual Health 279
Birth Control .279
Sexually Transmitted Diseases .283
HIV Infection and AIDS .286

Chapter 16: Fitness and Physical Activity 291
The Benefits of Exercise .291
Your Personal Fitness Plan .292
Overcome Barriers to Exercise .294
Setting Your Fitness Goals .294

Chapter 17: Nutrition 297
10 Simple Guidelines for Eating Well .297
Eating Well: A Basic Plan .298
Nutrition for Children .306

Chapter 18: Mental Health Problems and Mind-Body Wellness 307
Mental Health Problems .307
Alcohol and Drug Problems .308
Anger and Hostility .311
Anxiety .312
Depression .313
Eating Disorders .316
Sleep Problems .317
Suicide .319
Violent Behavior and Abuse .321
The Mind-Body Connection .323
Dealing With Chronic Pain .325
Stress and Distress .326

Chapter 19: Complementary Medicine 331
General Risks and Benefits of Complementary Medicine .333
Choosing the Right Therapy for You .334

Chapter 20: Your Home Health Center 339
Self-Care Tools 339
Nonprescription Medications and Products 343
Prescription Medications 351
Medication Problems 353
Save Money on Medications 354
Home Medical Tests 355
Home Medical Records 356
Health Information at Home 356
Index 359

To Our Readers

A book shut tight is but a block of paper.
Chinese proverb

No book can replace the need for physicians—and no physician can replace the need for people to care for themselves. The purpose of the *Kaiser Permanente Healthwise® Handbook* is to help you and your physicians work together to manage your health problems.

The *Kaiser Permanente Healthwise Handbook* includes basic guidelines on how to recognize and cope with more than 200 of the most common health problems. These guidelines are based on sound medical information from leading medical and consumer publications that has been reviewed by physicians, nurses, pharmacists, physical therapists, and other health professionals. We have made every effort to present the information in a way that is easy to read and easy to use.

We recommend that you review pages 1 and 2 right away. Page 1, the Healthwise® Self-Care Checklist, is a process you can follow every time a health problem arises. Page 2, the Ask-the-Physician Checklist, will help you get the most out of every physician visit.

You may also wish to read Chapters 1 and 2 before using the rest of the book. Chapter 1, Making Wise Health Decisions, presents a process you can use when you need to make a health decision; ways to develop a partnership with your physician; and skills you can use to reduce your health care costs. Chapter 2, Living a Healthy Life, presents information about lifestyle choices that are important to staying healthy and detecting health problems early. The rest of the book is designed to be used on a topic-by-topic basis whenever a problem or interest develops.

If you receive professional advice in conflict with this book, please follow your physician's advice. Because your physician is able to take your specific history and needs into consideration, his or her recommendations may prove to be the best. Likewise, if any self-care advice fails to provide positive results within a reasonable period, you should consult a health professional.

This book is as good as we can make it, but we cannot guarantee that it will work for you in every case. Nor will the authors or publishers accept responsibility for any problems that may develop from following its guidelines. This book is only a guide; your common sense and good judgment are also needed.

We wish you the best of health!

About Healthwise

Healthwise is a nonprofit organization whose mission is to help people make better health decisions. We create consumer health information that is based on the most current and reliable medical studies available. Expert writers and editors put this medical evidence into user-friendly terms, and a team of nationally recognized medical specialists from key centers of excellence reviews every word.

Healthwise information reaches more than 20 million families worldwide each year through our self-care handbooks, online content, and nurse call center resources. Health plans, employers, hospitals, physician groups, community organizations, government agencies, and e-health care companies trust Healthwise to support successful self-care, shared decision making, and Information Therapy™ programs. Healthwise products and consulting services have been shown to improve health and satisfaction while reducing unnecessary costs.

We publish the *Healthwise® Handbook, La salud en casa: Guía práctica de Healthwise* (a Spanish translation of the *Healthwise Handbook*), and *Healthwise® for Life* (a medical self-care guide for adults over 50).

The online content of the Healthwise® Knowledgebase is recognized by many as the most comprehensive and reliable source of consumer health information on the Web. The "More Info" icons in this handbook link the basic self-care information in the handbook to in-depth medical information in the Healthwise Knowledgebase. People trust the Healthwise Knowledgebase for evidence-based, commercially unbiased, and referenced information on thousands of health problems, surgeries, medical tests, treatments, medications, and support groups.

Our readers often provide the best ideas for improving this book. If you have a suggestion that will make this book better, please write us at *Healthwise Handbook* Suggestions, c/o Healthwise, P.O. Box 1989, Boise, ID 83701, or e-mail us at moreinfo@healthwise.org. To learn more about our health information programs, products, and services, visit our Web site at www.healthwise.org.

Acknowledgements

This Kaiser Permanente version of the *Healthwise® Handbook* has been produced as a partnership between two nonprofit organizations. Healthwise, Incorporated, founded in 1975, has been a pioneer in empowering medical care consumers through education. Kaiser Permanente has been dedicated to improving the health of its members by providing high-quality, group-practice, prepaid medical care since 1945. Kaiser Permanente includes a rich collaboration between Kaiser Foundation Health Plan and Hospitals and the Permanente Medical Groups, as well as an affiliation with Group Health Co-operative, based in Seattle, Washington. Kaiser Permanente is now America's leading integrated health care organization with over 8.4 million members in 9 states and the District of Columbia, with its headquarters in Oakland, California.

Healthwise and Kaiser Permanente are both committed to helping patients become true partners with their team of health care professionals. The shared goals are to improve health, prevent disease, and promote the wise use of medical care. The *Kaiser Permanente Healthwise® Handbook* is an integral part of a larger effort to educate members, patients, and professionals through print, electronic media, and face-to-face interactions.

Healthwise, Incorporated

The first edition of the *Healthwise Handbook,* published in 1976, was written and edited with major contributions from Kathleen McIntosh and Toni Roberts. Funding for the original development of the handbook was provided by the W. K. Kellogg Foundation of Battle Creek, Michigan. Since then, scores of people have helped to improve and update the book. The 15th edition, published in 2002, was edited by Katy Magee. Jo-Ann Kachigian provided invaluable project coordination, editing, and proofreading assistance for this Kaiser Permanente edition, while layout and production were provided by Terrie Britton and John Kubisiak. The principal medical reviewers for the 15th edition were Steven L. Schneider, MD, and A. Patrice Burgess, MD.

Kaiser Permanente

The first Kaiser Permanente edition of the *Healthwise Handbook* was published in 1994, under the leadership of Steven M. Freedman, MD, who coordinated the book's medical review by more than 300 Kaiser Permanente physicians and other health professionals. The handbook is the cornerstone for the Kaiser Permanente Self-Care Program, with its goal to support member self-care and integration within all aspects of medical care delivery and patient education. Leadership for this effort was provided by Dr. Freedman as well as by Pamela J. Larson, MPH; David S. Sobel, MD, MPH; and Joyce O. Arango, DrPH. Many other individuals provided valuable assistance as well, with cover customization, design of promotional materials, and with efforts to support dissemination in the medical centers and other Kaiser Permanente regions.

This is the third national edition of the *Kaiser Permanente Healthwise Handbook.* The principal medical reviewers were David S. Sobel, MD, MPH, and Gary H. Wong, MD. Coordination of the book revision process was provided by Frayne B. Rosenfield, MPH, and Kimberly A. West, MS.

We would like to especially thank the Kaiser Permanente health care professionals across the country who contributed their time and expertise in the medical review of this book, including:

Physicians

Travis Abbott, MD
Vernon Ansdell, MD
Mark Binstock MD, MPH
John Charde, MD
Mark Clark, MD
Nancy Cohen, MD
Jong Davis, MD
Catherine Dragstedt, MD
Alan T. Elliott, MD
Kenneth M. Ellner, MD
Kitty Evers, MD
Nathan Fujimoto, MD
Carole Gardner, MD
Scott Gee, MD
Harley Goldberg, DO
Howard Gould, MD
Bev Green, MD
Jeffrey Hoffman, MD
Tim McAfee, MD, MPH
Harry Miller, MD
Adrienne Mims, MD, MPH
Jeffrey Palmer, MD
David Preskill, MD
Willie Rainey, MD
Paul Reiss, MD
Jerry Salkowe, MD
Larry Scherzer, MD
Robert Schreiner, MD
David S. Sobel, MD, MPH
Ken Spiegelman, MD
David Starr, MD
Thomas Syltebo, MD
Robert van der Meer, MD
Winkler Weinberg, MD
Martha Wilber, MD
Gary H. Wong, MD
David Zelman, MD
Les Zendle, MD

Dentist

Don Prasnikar, DDS

Nurses

Betty Dennis, RN, BSN
Catherine Futch, RN, MN, CNAA
Judith Griffith, RN, MS
Leanne Johnston, RN, BSN
Jennifer Miller, RN, BSN
JoAnn Somers, RN, BSN
Crystal Stokes, RN, BSN

Health Education Staff for Kaiser Permanente

Joyce O. Arango, DrPH
Ron Blidar, CHES
Sally Butler, LCSW
Amy Conway, MPH
Lisa Cruz
Joyce Cusack, MHS
Judy Derman, MHS
Joanne Ferguson, RN
Lynda Garrett, MPH, RN
Ann Gordon, MPH

Joy R. Gray, MPH
Patricia Greenfield, RN, DNSc
Lorinda Sheets Hartwell, DrPH
Mary Hobbs, MPH
Jamie Hunter-Mitchell
Susan Kayman, DrPH, RD
Suzanne Kordesh, MPH, RD
Judith Krowley, RN, BSN
Jean Kumamoto, MPH
Pamela J. Larson, MPH
Kecia Leatherwood, MS
Linda Madsen, MSW
Lisa Morgan, PT, MPH
Ron B. Nakamura, MPH
Denise Portello, MPH, RD
Becky Reid
Linda Rieder, MPH
Sandra M. Roberts, RN
Devara Rodriguez, MPH
Frayne B. Rosenfield, MPH
Victoria Samper, MS
Carol Shenise, MS, RN
Scott Thomas, PhD
Janet Tobacman, MPA
Dennis Tolsma, MPH
Jennifer Torreson, MPH
Kimberly A. West, MS
Carol Whitman, MPH, RN
Amanda Wylie, BA
Deborah Zahn, MPH

Proofreader

Lisa Killen, MBA

We also wish to thank the many other health professionals and consumers whose review, suggestions, and input on previous editions were the foundation for the current book.

Most of all, we would like to thank the millions of Kaiser Permanente members who use the *Kaiser Permanente Healthwise Handbook*. It is your actions that reward us the most and inspire us to constantly look for ways to improve this self-care guide and other patient education resources.

The Healthwise® Self-Care Checklist

Step 1. Observe the problem.

- When did it start? What are the symptoms? ______________________

____

____

____

____

- Where is the pain? Dull ache or stabbing pain? ______________________

____

- Measure your vital signs:

Temperature: __________ Pulse: __________/minute

Breaths: _______/minute Blood Pressure: ______/________

- Think back:

Have you had this problem before? Yes ______ No ______

What did you do for it? ______________________

____

Any changes in your life (stress, medications, food, exercise, etc.)?

____

____

Does anyone else at home or work have these symptoms?

____

Step 2. Learn more about it.

- *Kaiser Permanente Healthwise® Handbook* (note page number): ___________
- Other books or articles: ______________________
- Advice or opinions of others (lay or professional): ______________________

____

____

Step 3. Make an action plan.

- What do you think is wrong? ______________________
- What have you decided to do about it? ______________________

____

____

____

Step 4. Evaluate your progress.

- Are you getting better or worse? ______________________

____

____

____

Ask-the-Physician Checklist

Before the visit:

- Complete the Healthwise® Self-Care Checklist on page 1 and take it with you.
- Take a list of any medications you are currently taking. If you have seen a physician before for a similar problem, take the record from the visit with you.

During the visit:

- State your main problem first.
- Describe your symptoms (use page 1).
- Describe past experiences with the same problem.

After the visit:

Write down:

- What's wrong: ______________________________
- What might happen next: ______________________________
- What you can do at home: ______________________________

____

For drugs, tests, and treatments, you may want to ask:

- What's its name? ______________________________
- Why is it needed? ______________________________
- What are the risks? ______________________________
- Are there alternatives? ______________________________
- What if I do nothing? ______________________________
- (For drugs) How do I take this? ______________________________
- (For tests) How do I prepare? ______________________________

At the end of the visit, ask:

- Am I to return for another visit? ______________________________
- Am I to phone in for test results? ______________________________
- What danger signs should I look for? ______________________________
- When do I need to report back? ______________________________
- What else do I need to know? ______________________________

____

____

You, the individual, can do more for your health and well-being than any doctor, any hospital, any drug, and any exotic medical device.
Joseph Califano

1

Making Wise Health Decisions

Throughout your life you will have to make health decisions for yourself and your family. The decisions you make will influence your overall well-being as well as the quality and cost of your care. In general, people who work with their physicians to make health decisions are happier with the care they receive and the results they achieve.

Why should you help make decisions with your physician? Aren't you paying him or her to know what to do? Well, the choices aren't always black and white. There are often several approaches to diagnosing and treating a health problem, and you are more likely to feel better about the chosen approach if it is the one best suited to your needs and values.

The best way to make health decisions is to combine the most reliable medical facts with your personal values. Among your personal values are your beliefs, fears, lifestyle, and experiences. They all play a role in helping you make decisions about your health. Put more simply:

Medical Information + Your Information =
Wise Health Decisions

Skills for Making Wise Health Decisions

The following are some simple steps for you to follow when you have a health decision to make. Depending on the decision, the process may take a few minutes or hours, or as long as several weeks. Take as much time as you need to make the decision that is right for you.

1. What are you trying to decide? Tell your physician that you want to share in making a decision. Ask your physician to clearly state the decision that needs to be made and what your choices are.

2. Get the facts. Learn all about each option by using resources like the library, the Internet, and your physician. Make sure the information you collect is based on sound medical research, not the results of a single study or facts published by a company that will profit by your using their product.

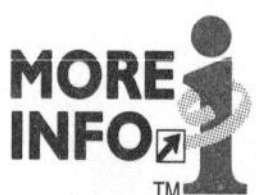

In this book, a special icon marks some of the health problems for which more information will help you make better decisions about your care. Read the inside front cover of this book to learn more about where you can find reliable health information.

3. What do you think? Think about your own needs and values and what you hope for as the best possible outcome. Then sort out the information you've gathered into a list of pros and cons as you see them for each option. You may want to share your list with your physician to make sure you have all the information you need.

4. Try on a decision. Write down what you expect will happen if you choose a particular option. Ask your physician if what you expect is reasonable. Ask again about the side effects, pain, recovery time, or long-term outcomes of that option. Then see if you still feel it's the best choice for you.

5. Make an action plan. Once you and your physician have made a decision, find out what you can do to make sure that you will have the best possible outcome. Write down the steps that you need to take next. Think positively about your decision, and do your part to ensure success by following your physician's advice. Remember, when you share in making a decision, you share the responsibility for the outcome.

Work in Partnership With Your Physician

Your relationship with your physician greatly influences your ability to make wise health decisions and the outcome of your care. Tell your physician that you want to be a partner in making decisions about your health. Chances are, your physician will be happy to know that you are interested in taking an active role in your health. Common goals, shared effort, and good communication are the basis of good physician-patient partnerships.

MORE INFO For more information, see the inside front cover.

Skills for Becoming a Good Partner

You can hold up your end of the partnership bargain with your physician by doing the following:

1. Take good care of yourself. Many health problems can be prevented if you protect yourself and your family by getting immunizations, being screened for health problems, and making healthful lifestyle choices. Don't put off needed services. If your symptoms and the guidelines in this book suggest that you should see a physician, don't put it off. Ignoring problems often leads to complications. See Chapter 2, Living a Healthy Life, for more information about how you can have more control over your health.

2. Practice medical self-care. You can manage a lot of minor problems on your own. All it takes is for you to trust your common sense and monitor how well your efforts are working. Use this book, your own experience, and advice from others to create a self-care plan.

- Use the Healthwise Self-Care Checklist on page 1 to record your self-care plan. Note whether home treatment seems to help. If you do end up calling your physician or advice nurse, he or she will want to know what your symptoms are; what you've tried to do for the problem; and how well what you tried to do worked.

The Advice Nurse

At Kaiser Permanente you have the option of speaking to an advice nurse. Advice nurses are registered nurses who have special training to answer your questions about health problems and help you decide how to manage minor illnesses.

A call to the advice nurse can often save you a physician visit or help you decide if you need an urgent or routine appointment.

Advice nurses can also help when your physician diagnoses a health problem or recommends a test or treatment that you don't fully understand. Sometimes the advice nurse can answer your questions. Other times, he or she may help you come up with questions you can ask your physician at your next visit.

- Plan a time to call a health professional if the problem continues. If the problem seems to be getting more severe, don't wait too long before calling for help.

3. Prepare for office visits. Most medical appointments are scheduled to last only 10 to 15 minutes. The better prepared you are, the more value you can get from the visit.

- Prepare an Ask-the-Physician Checklist like the one on page 2 and take it with you.

- Complete a self-care checklist like the one on page 1 and take it with you.
- Write down your hunches or fears about what is wrong. These are often helpful to your physician.
- Write down the 3 questions that you most want to have answered. There may not be time to ask a long list of questions.
- When your primary care physician refers you to a specialist, a little preparation and good communication can help you have a good visit. Before you go see a specialist:
    - Know your diagnosis or expected diagnosis.
    - Learn about your basic treatment options.
    - Know what your primary care physician would like the specialist to do (take over the case, confirm the diagnosis, conduct tests, etc.).
    - Ask your primary care physician to remain involved in your care. Ask the specialist to send new test results or recommendations to both you and your regular physician.

4. Be an active participant in every medical visit.

- Be honest and straightforward. If you don't intend to take a prescribed medication, say so. If you are getting complementary treatment, such as acupuncture or chiropractic treatments, let your physician know. To be a good partner, your physician has to know what's going on.
- If your physician recommends a drug, test, or treatment, get more information about the risks and benefits, costs, other alternatives, and the likely outcomes before agreeing to go through with it.
- Take notes. Write down the diagnosis, treatment and follow-up plan, and what you can do at home. Then read your notes back to the physician to make sure you have it right. If you think it will help, take a friend along to write down what the physician says while you listen.

5. Learn all you can about your health problem. Throughout this book, special icons mark topics for which more information will help you make better decisions about your care. The information at your disposal—whether you get it from your physician, the library, or the Internet—is a powerful tool for helping you make wise health decisions.

If you have a complicated problem or want to know more about your health options:

- Start by asking your physician if he or she has information about your problem that you could take home. Some physicians offer video- or audiotapes, brochures, or reprints from medical journals.

Calling Kaiser Permanente

Often a phone call to Kaiser Permanente is all you need to manage a problem at home or determine if an appointment is needed. Here's how to get the most from every call:

Prepare for your call.
Write down a 1-sentence description of your problem. Then list 2 to 3 questions you have about the problem.

Have your symptom list handy.

Have your calendar handy in case you need to schedule an appointment.

- Call the Kaiser Permanente advice line, and ask if they can help you get more information.
- If you use the Internet to find health information, start by searching sources such as the Agency for Health Care Policy Research (AHCPR), the Centers for Disease Control and Prevention, or a national organization that represents a particular disease. These sources present information that is based on the analysis of a large body of medical evidence.
- For information on a variety of health topics and links to many other quality sites, use Kaiser Permanente Online at www.kaiserpermanente.org, an interactive Web site on the Internet that is available to Kaiser Permanente members only.
- The inside front cover of this book offers tips to help you get more information about health problems and your testing and treatment choices.
- If you have questions or concerns about the information you find, discuss them with your physician.
- Also, please refer to your Kaiser Permanente member guide to services for more information on Kaiser Permanente facilities available in your area and how best to use services.

Finding a Physician Who Will Be a Partner

An important part of your health care experience is building a relationship with your personal physician or nurse practitioner, who will coordinate and oversee your medical care. We encourage you to select a primary care physician or nurse practitioner early in your relationship with Kaiser Permanente. You may choose from the following departments:

- Adult or Internal Medicine—treats adults (specializes in diagnosis and treatment of nonsurgical diseases)
- Family Practice—treats people of all ages
- Pediatrics—treats children

Contact your local facility or refer to your Kaiser Permanente member guide to services for more information on how to connect with a personal physician or nurse practitioner.

You Have the Right to:

- Receive information about your Health Plan.
- Participate in a candid discussion of all available treatment options.
- Express your wishes about future care.
- Receive personal medical records and/or information so you can participate in your health care.
- Receive information about the people who provide your health care.
- Request an interpreter in your primary language.
- Receive care with dignity and respect.
- Have impartial access to treatment.
- Be assured of privacy and confidentiality.
- Have a safe, secure, clean, and accessible health care environment.
- Participate in physician selection.
- Know and use member satisfaction resources.

Partner Potential

During your first visit, tell your physician that you would like to share in making treatment decisions.

Pay attention to how you feel during the visit.

- Does the physician listen well?
- Does the physician speak to you in terms you can understand?
- Does the physician spend enough time with you?
- Do you think you could build a good working relationship with the physician?

If the answers are "no," look for another physician. It may take more than one visit for you to decide if you will be able to work with a physician.

Is It Time for a Change?

If you are unhappy with how your physician treats you, it may be time for a change. Before you start looking for a new physician, tell your current physician how you would like to be treated. Your physician would probably be pleased to work with you as a partner if only you would tell him or her that's what you want. Otherwise, your physician may think that you, like many people, want him or her to do all the work.

Skills to Use in the Hospital

When you need to be in the hospital, there are things you can do to improve the quality of the care you receive. However, if you are very sick, ask your spouse or a friend to help watch out for your best interests.

- Ask "why?" Don't agree to anything unless you have a good reason. Agree only to those procedures that make sense for you.
- Provide an extra level of quality control. Check medications, tests, injections, and other treatments to see if they are correct. Your diligence can improve the quality of the care that you receive.

Advance Health Care Directives

What is an advance health care directive (AHCD)?
An AHCD is a way to make your health care wishes known if you are unable to speak for yourself or prefer someone else to speak for you. An AHCD can serve one or both of these functions:

- Power of attorney for health care (to appoint a health care agent)
- Instructions for health care treatment and preferences (to indicate your wishes), in some states called a living will

The legal requirements and terminology may vary from state to state.

I've never completed an advance health care directive before. Why should I?
An accident or serious illness can put you in a position where you cannot speak for yourself. In these situations, having an advance health care directive assures that your physician knows your wishes about the kind of care you want and/or who the person is that you want to make decisions on your behalf.

Does this mean only *one* person can decide for me? What if I want others involved too?
Often many family members *are* involved in decision making. And most of the time, that works well. But occasionally, people will disagree about the best course of action, so it is usually best to name just one person as the agent (with a backup, if you want).

Don't the physicians make all those life-and-death decisions anyway?
Actually, physicians tell you about your medical condition, the different treatment options that are available to you, and what may happen with each type of treatment. Though physicians provide guidance, the decision to accept, refuse, or stop a treatment is yours.

What if something happens to me and no form has been completed?
If you are not able to speak for yourself, the physician and health care team will turn to family members or

friends. The most appropriate decision maker is someone with a close, caring relationship with you, who is aware of your values and beliefs, and is willing and able to make the necessary decisions.

My values and beliefs? But I haven't talked with anyone about these!
That's why it is a good idea to talk with family or close friends about the things that are important to you regarding quality of life and how you would want to spend your last days and weeks. Knowing the things that are most important to you will help your loved ones make the best decisions possible on your behalf. If your wishes are not known to others, then your agent will decide based on what he or she thinks is in your best interest.

What if I don't want to appoint an agent or don't have one to appoint?
You do not have to appoint an agent. You can still complete the instructions for health care treatment and preferences, which will provide your physicians with information to guide your care.

What kinds of things can I write in my instructions for health care treatments and preferences?
You can, if you wish, write your preferences about accepting or refusing certain treatments that may be life-sustaining (like IV hydration, antibiotics, dialysis, feeding tubes, breathing machines, and CPR), receiving pain medication, making organ donations, indicating your main physician for providing your care, or other things that express your wishes and values.

If I appoint an agent, what can that person do?
Your agent will make all decisions for you, just like you would if you could. Your agent can choose your physician and where you will receive your care, speak with your health care team, review your medical record and authorize its release, accept or refuse all medical treatments, and make arrangements for you if you die. You should instruct your agent on these matters so he or she knows how to decide for you. The more information you share, the better your agent will be able to make those decisions on your behalf.

When does my agent make decisions for me?
Usually the agent makes decisions only if you are unable to make them yourself, such as if you've lost the ability to understand things or communicate clearly. In California, however, if you want, your agent can speak on your behalf at any time, even when you are still capable of making your own decisions. You can also appoint a "temporary" agent. For example, if you suddenly become ill, you can tell your physician that there is someone else you want to make decisions for you. This spoken instruction is as legally binding as a written one!

Are there other spoken instructions that don't involve a written form?
In some states, you can make a legally binding individual health care treatment and preferences instruction by speaking to any health care provider at any time. All health care providers must document your wishes in your medical record. But it is often easier to follow your instructions if you have written them down in advance.

Do I need an attorney to help with this?
No. Completing an advance health care directive isn't difficult, and an attorney is not necessary. Actually, the most important part of this is talking to your loved ones. Without that conversation, the best form in the world may not be helpful!

Okay, I'll talk to them. But what should I do with the form after I complete it?
Make copies for all those who are close to you. Take one to your physician to discuss and ask that it be included in your medical record. Photocopied forms are just as valid as the original. And be sure to keep a copy for yourself in a visible, easy-to-find location—not locked up in a drawer.

What if I change my mind?
You can revoke your form (or your verbal instructions) at any time. It's a good idea to retrieve old forms and replace them with new ones.

Do physicians or hospitals require a patient to have an advance health care directive form?
No, they cannot require you to complete one. But physicians and hospitals should have information about the form and your right to make health care decisions available to you and your family.

Resources

- You may obtain the most current advance health care directive forms for your state by contacting the Member Services, Patient Assistance, or Health Education Departments at your local Kaiser Permanente medical center.
- Partnership for Caring offers state-specific forms that you may download from its Web site at www.partnershipforcaring.org. You may call 1-800-989-9455 to order a printed copy.
- *Finding Your Way: A Guide for End-of-Life Medical Decisions* is a 13-page discussion-starter booklet written for consumers by Sacramento Healthcare Decisions. For a single copy, visit www.sachealthdecisions.org.

(Adapted from Advance Health Care Directive Fact Sheet for Consumers, December 2001, California Coalition for Compassionate Care)

Shared Decisions About Medical Tests

Medical tests are important tools, but they have limits. Informed consumers know that medical tests have costs and risks as well as benefits.

Learn the facts:

- What is the name of the test, and why do you need it?
- If the test is positive, what will the physician do differently?
- What could happen if you don't have the test?

Consider the risks and benefits:

- How accurate is the test? How often does it indicate a problem exists when there is none (false positive)? How often does it indicate there is no problem when there is one (false negative)?
- Is the test painful? What can go wrong?
- How will you feel afterward?
- Are there less risky alternatives?

If a test seems risky or not likely to change the recommended treatment, ask your physician if you can avoid it. Try to agree on the best approach. No test can be done without your permission, and you have the right to refuse to have a test.

Let your physician know:

- Your concerns about the test.
- What you expect the test will do for you. Ask if that is realistic.
- Any medications you are taking (prescription and nonprescription).
- Whether you have other medical conditions.
- Whether you prefer to accept or decline the test.

If you agree to a test, ask what you can do to reduce the risk of errors. Should you restrict food, alcohol, exercise, or medication before the test? After the test, ask to review the results. Take notes for your home records. If the results of the test are unexpected and the error rate of the test is high, consider redoing the test before basing further treatment on the results.

Shared Decisions About Medications

The first rule of medications is to know why you need each drug before you use it.

Learn the facts:

- What is the name of the medication and why do you need it?
- How long does it take to work?
- How long will you need to take it?
- How and when do you take it (with food, on an empty stomach, etc.)?
- Are there nondrug alternatives?

Consider the risks and benefits:

- How much will this medication help?
- Are there side effects or other risks?
- Could this medication interact with other medications that you currently take?
- Is a generic form of the medication that will work as well available and appropriate for you?

Let your physician know:

- If you have ever had an allergic reaction to any medications.
- Your concerns about the medication.
- What you expect it will do. Ask if that is realistic.
- About all other medications you are taking (prescription and non-prescription).
- Whether you prefer to take the medication or try other ways of treating the problem.
- About any herbal or alternative therapies you are using.

See Chapter 20 for more information about how to manage medications.

Shared Decisions About Surgery

Every surgery has risks. Only you can decide if the benefits are worth the risks.

Learn the facts:

- What is the name of the surgery? Get a description of the surgery.
- Why does your physician think you need the surgery?
- Are there other options besides surgery?
- Is this surgery the most common one for this problem? Are there other types of surgery?
- Is the surgery a covered benefit or is there a charge?
- Can it be done on an outpatient basis?

Consider the risks and benefits:

- How many similar surgeries has the surgeon performed? How many surgeries like this are done at this hospital?
- What is the success rate? What does success mean to your physician? What would success mean to you?
- What can go wrong? How often does this happen?
- How will you feel afterward? How long will it be until you're fully recovered?
- How can you best prepare for the surgery and the recovery period?

Let your physician know:

- How much the problem really bothers you. Are you willing to put up with symptoms to avoid surgery?
- Your concerns about the surgery.
- Whether or not you want to have the surgery at this time.
- If you want a second opinion. Second opinions are helpful if you have any doubt that the proposed surgery is the best option for your problem. If you want a second opinion, ask your primary care physician or your surgeon to recommend another specialist. Ask that your test results be sent to the second physician. Consider getting an opinion from a physician who isn't a surgeon and who treats similar problems.

If I'd known I was going to live this long, I'd have taken better care of myself.
Eubie Blake

2

Living a Healthy Life

Most of this book focuses on helping you deal with health problems. This chapter is meant to be used as a guide to help you prevent illness and injury by making wise health and lifestyle choices.

These basic health habits are the foundation of lifelong health and well-being:

- Stay up to date with immunizations and health screenings.
- Be physically active.
- Eat right.
- Maintain a healthful body weight.
- Be tobacco-free.
- Avoid drugs and excess alcohol.
- Manage stress.
- Take care of your teeth.
- Practice safety.
- Pursue healthy pleasures.
- Help to make a healthier world.

Maintaining these health habits will give you the best chance of staying healthy and active and feeling good about yourself throughout your life. If you have health problems, good health habits are even more important. It's never too late to make lifestyle changes that may help you recover faster or make living with a chronic disease easier.

Immunizations

Immunizations work by helping your immune system recognize and quickly attack diseases before they can cause problems. Some immunizations are given in a single shot while others require several shots over a period of time.

Childhood immunizations protect against pertussis (whooping cough), polio, measles, mumps, rubella, *Haemophilus influenzae* type b, varicella zoster (chickenpox), hepatitis A, hepatitis B, and pneumococcal infection.

Immunizations also protect against tetanus and diphtheria, although booster shots are needed every 10 years to maintain lifelong protection.

If your children are immunized, these serious illnesses will not be a problem. Schedule your child's immunizations according to the Kaiser Permanente preventive care guidelines for your area. There is no need to delay immunizations because of colds or other minor illnesses. Be sure to keep good records. Children often need to show immunization records at school.

The need for immunizations does not end with childhood. Thousands of people are hospitalized, and many die, as the result of influenza and other diseases that can be prevented by immunization. If you are in one of the high-risk groups for whom the influenza or pneumococcal vaccine is recommended (see page 19), make sure you get immunized.

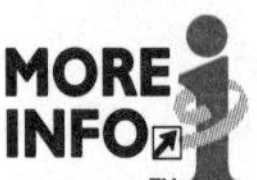

Medical experts are constantly reviewing the effectiveness of immunization programs. Therefore, immunization recommendations change periodically. Your primary care physician or public health department can provide the most up-to-date information about immunizations.

Diphtheria, Pertussis, and Tetanus (DTaP)

Infectious diseases like diphtheria and pertussis were major killers before the vaccine was developed. This vaccine also protects against tetanus ("lockjaw"), a bacterial infection that can result when a wound is contaminated. The bacteria enter the body through cuts and thrive only in the absence of oxygen. So the deeper and narrower the wound, the greater the possibility of tetanus. With proper immunization, these diseases are rare.

Childhood immunizations for these diseases are given together, with a series of shots starting at age 2 months. Follow the DTaP guidelines provided by Kaiser Permanente. The first booster is given during the preteen or teen years. After that, get a Td (tetanus and diphtheria) booster every 10 years.

Keeping up to date with Td boosters is important because tetanus can be fatal. If it has been at least 5 years since your last shot, and you have a wound (especially a puncture wound) that is very dirty or that you suspect may be contaminated, get a Td booster.

Otherwise, there is no need for more frequent vaccinations because this increases the risk of an uncomfortable local reaction.

Polio

Polio is a viral illness that can lead to paralysis. It is rare today because of the polio vaccine. A series of 4 doses by the age of 6 gives lifelong immunity. Nonimmunized adults need immunization only if they have a high risk of polio exposure.

There are 2 types of polio vaccine:

IPV (Inactivated Polio Vaccine): This shot is the recommended polio vaccine for almost everyone in the United States.

OPV (Oral Polio Vaccine): This form of the vaccine is in drops taken by mouth. Until recently, OPV was recommended for most children. However, OPV is no longer used except in limited circumstances.

Measles, Mumps, and Rubella (MMR)

Measles (rubeola), mumps, and rubella (German measles) were once common childhood illnesses. Today they are quite rare, thanks to the MMR vaccine. Two shots, one given at age 12 to 15 months and one at age 4 to 6 years, provide lifelong protection (immunity).

If there is a measles outbreak in your area and your baby has not been immunized, call your physician or health department to discuss an early MMR shot. If your child receives the vaccine before he or she is 12 months old, another dose should be given at 15 months of age.

Reactions to Childhood Immunizations

Temporary, mild reactions to immunizations are common. Babies often develop a fever after the DTaP shot, and the location of the shot may feel hard. A mild rash or fever may develop 10 to 14 days after the MMR vaccine is given. The rash will go away without treatment. The hepatitis B vaccines have caused nausea, low-grade fever, rash, and joint pain in some adults.

- Acetaminophen drops may soothe the discomfort and relieve fever. Some physicians recommend giving acetaminophen before the shot. See Fever on page 231.
- Keep written notes on any reactions you observe.

Tell your health professional if you think reactions are excessive.

If you don't have records showing that you received 2 doses of MMR vaccine and you did not have these illnesses as a child, discuss your need for immunization with your physician.

Chickenpox (Varicella)

It is recommended that all children receive the chickenpox vaccine at 12 to 18 months of age. Because the chickenpox vaccine is relatively new, it is not known how long the vaccine protects a person against chickenpox. However, some people who have had the vaccine appear to be protected for as long as 20 years.

Chickenpox is more serious in newborns, teens, and adults. The varicella vaccine is required by many states before a child can enter school or childcare. People older than 11 or 12 years who have never had chickenpox or have not received the chickenpox vaccine should be vaccinated. Teens and adults need 2 doses of the vaccine. People older than 12 who aren't sure whether they have had chickenpox should discuss their need for testing and/or immunization with their physician.

Hepatitis A Virus (HAV)

Unlike other types of hepatitis, infection with the hepatitis A virus (HAV) usually does not cause long-term problems. However, it is very contagious and can cause serious illness in some cases. The vaccine consists of two shots and is extremely effective.

Vaccination against hepatitis A is recommended for:

- Anyone 2 years of age or older who lives in or is traveling to an area where HAV infection is common. This includes parts of the United States.
- People who use drugs.
- Men who have sex with men.
- People who have liver disease.
- People who have a blood-clotting disorder, such as hemophilia.

Food handlers should consider getting the hepatitis A vaccine.

Hepatitis B Virus (HBV)

The hepatitis B virus (HBV) infects liver cells and can destroy them. Over time, chronic HBV infection can lead to serious, sometimes fatal liver disease. Vaccination prevents HBV infection and its possible complications. See page 97.

It is recommended that all babies be vaccinated against HBV. Three shots provide long-term immunity. Immunization is also recommended for:

- All people under age 25 years who were not previously vaccinated, especially if they are at high risk for exposure to HBV.
- People who use drugs.
- Health care workers.
- People planning extended travel to China, Southeast Asia, Africa, and other areas where HBV infection rates are high.
- People who have more than one sex partner.
- Men who have sex with men.

Haemophilus influenzae Type b (Hib)

Haemophilus influenzae type b does not cause the flu. This bacterial infection can cause meningitis, pneumonia, skin and bone infections, and other serious illnesses in young children. Every child between 2 months and 5 years of age should be immunized against Hib. Children over 5 and adults need immunization only if they have sickle cell anemia or problems involving the spleen or immune system.

Influenza Virus

Annual influenza vaccinations are recommended for everyone age 50 and older, for younger people who have chronic diseases, and for pregnant women. Health care workers and others who are likely to be exposed to the flu virus may also wish to get the vaccine every year. The vaccine can be given to anyone older than 6 months of age. The vaccine is most effective when it is given in the autumn, well before the start of the flu season.

Pneumococcal Infection

In addition to infecting the lungs (pneumonia), pneumococcal bacteria can infect the blood (bacteremia) or the covering of the brain (meningitis). In children, pneumococcal bacteria cause ear infections as well. A new form of the pneumococcal vaccine is recommended for all children less than 2 years old. Some children ages 2 to 5 years old may also benefit from receiving this vaccine.

For adults, a one-time-only dose of the pneumococcal vaccine is recommended for people age 65 and older. If you received the vaccine before age 65, and it has been more than 5 years since you received the vaccine, ask your physician if you need a booster shot. Younger people who have chronic diseases, especially respiratory illnesses or diabetes, should also consider getting the pneumococcal vaccine.

Other Immunizations

If you are in close contact with people who have contagious diseases or you are planning travel to areas where illnesses such as hepatitis A, malaria, typhoid, and yellow fever are common, contact your local health department to find out if you need other immunizations.

Be Wise, Immunize

It's wise to immunize.

Immunizations:

- Prevent disease.
- Cost much less than treating the diseases they prevent.
- Are safe and effective.
- Reduce the risk of epidemics.
- Are the law. Children must be immunized (or parents must sign a certificate of exemption) before children can begin public school.

Screening and Early Detection

Another way to protect your health is to detect an illness early, while it is still easy to treat. You can do this in 2 ways: by getting periodic medical exams from health professionals and by becoming a good observer of your own body and health.

Periodic Medical Exams

Many physicians used to recommend a complete physical every year. Now, most physicians recommend specific medical exams based on age, sex, and risk factors. These exams are more effective than the annual physical in detecting treatable illness.

See the recommended schedule for preventive exams provided by your local Kaiser Permanente facility. The most appropriate schedule of preventive exams is one you and your physician agree upon, based upon your health conditions, values, and risk factors.

The recommendations apply to healthy people in each age category. You may be at a higher risk for certain diseases. Family history (whether your relatives have or had the disease), other health problems, or behaviors such as smoking all increase your risk. Talk with your physician about whether you need more frequent exams.

Periodic self-exams are also an important part of staying healthy. See the breast self-exam on page 251 and the testicular exam on page 278. If you have high blood pressure, see page 245.

For more information on cholesterol screening, see page 243.

Flexible Sigmoidoscopy

Flexible sigmoidoscopy is a screening test for precancerous polyps and cancers of the colon and rectum. The sigmoidoscope is a flexible viewing instrument that is inserted into the rectum to examine the lower bowel. The exam takes about 10 to 15 minutes, is only mildly uncomfortable, and is very safe.

Having flexible sigmoidoscopy exams reduces your risk of dying from colorectal cancer. Most experts recommend that you have a flexible sigmoidoscopy exam around age 50. In addition to screening, physicians sometimes wish to examine the colon for the cause of rectal bleeding, diarrhea, or constipation.

Tuberculin Test

A tuberculin test is a skin test for tuberculosis (see page 164), not an immunization. A positive result does not necessarily mean that you have tuberculosis, but it does mean that the bacteria have probably entered your body. Whether you should be tested depends on the prevalence of tuberculosis in your area and your risk of exposure. Once you have had a positive skin test, the test should not be repeated. Subsequent tests will always be positive and may cause more severe reactions.

Other Recommended Tests and Exams

Infants

Well-baby visits are recommended at birth to 1 week, 2 to 4 weeks, and at 2, 4, 6, 9 to 10, 12, 14 to 15, 18, and 21 to 24 months of age. Your physician may recommend a different schedule. Babies at high risk for hearing problems may be tested during this time. Immunizations are given at many visits.

Children Age 2 to 10 Years

Well-child visits are recommended at 2 to 3 years, 4 to 6 years, 8 years, and 10 years. A vision test is recommended at age 3 to 4 years, and some childhood immunizations are given at age 4 to 6 years. Regular blood pressure checks are recommended and may be done at any visit.

Children/Teens Age 10 to 18 Years

Preteens and teens should be seen at least every 2 years. Regular blood pressure checks are recommended and may be done during any visit. Pap tests and chlamydia tests are recommended starting when a female becomes sexually active. See pages 254 and 283.

Pregnant Women

Discuss the frequency of visits and testing with your physician. During the first prenatal visit, blood tests, urinalysis, blood pressure, and screening for hepatitis B are recommended. Additional tests are needed during the pregnancy.

Be Physically Active

Every body needs regular physical activity. Along with a positive attitude and a healthful diet, your fitness level plays a major role in how well you feel, what illnesses you avoid, and how much you enjoy life. Regular physical activity:

- Lowers your risk of premature death and death caused by heart disease.
- Reduces your risk of developing diabetes, high blood pressure, colon cancer, and osteoporosis.
- Helps lower high cholesterol and blood pressure levels.
- Improves your mood, relieves stress, and promotes a sense of well-being.
- Helps build and maintain healthy bones, muscles, and joints.
- Helps you maintain a healthful body weight.

If you already make regular physical activity a part of your life, keep up the good work. If you aren't physically active, there is good news. The latest research shows that exercise doesn't have to be vigorous to improve your health. Many everyday activities raise your heart rate and, if done regularly, will keep your heart and lungs healthy, make your muscles stronger, and improve your flexibility. For more specific information about designing your personal fitness plan and staying motivated, see Chapter 16.

Eat Right

How and what you choose to eat affects many aspects of your health. Your diet plays an important role in helping you:

- Meet your nutritional needs and maintain a healthful weight.
- Have regular bowel movements.
- Prevent diseases such as heart disease, diabetes, and certain cancers.
- Treat diseases such as diabetes and high blood pressure.

Another important aspect of your diet is how carefully you prepare and handle foods. You need good food preparation and food handling habits in order to avoid food-borne illnesses. For more information about food safety, see Stomach Flu and Food Poisoning on page 93.

For more information about how you can evaluate and improve your diet, see Chapter 17.

Maintain a Healthful Body Weight

Healthy bodies come in a variety of shapes and sizes. Weight is not the only measurement of health. In fact, your weight may say very little about your health. No matter what your shape or body size, you can improve your health by eating a balanced diet, getting regular physical activity, and learning to feel good about your body.

Heredity plays a big role in your body shape and what you weigh. It would be impossible for most of us to look like fashion models or world-class athletes, but we can all learn to appreciate our bodies and treat them well to maximize our health and self-esteem.

What Is a Healthful Weight?

Your health is determined by more than just your weight. Other measurements of health include:

- Your fitness level.
- The quality of your diet and your eating habits.
- The presence of disease indicators such as high cholesterol.
- The presence or family history of diseases such as high blood pressure, heart disease, and diabetes.
- How fat is distributed on your body.
- Your self-esteem and body image.

You can improve your health without changing your weight. The amount you weigh now could be, or could become, a healthful weight for you.

If you think that your current weight puts you at risk for health problems, talk to your health professional about different ways you can manage your weight. Most people are concerned about being overweight, but for some people being underweight is a health concern. Being **obese** can increase your risk of developing high blood pressure, high cholesterol, heart disease, type 2 diabetes, sleep apnea, some cancers, and other long-term illnesses. Losing as little as 5 percent to 10 percent of your body weight can lower your blood pressure, reduce other risk factors for heart disease, and improve your blood sugar levels.

Set Realistic Goals

Before you start a weight management program, think about your goals, your expectations, and your readiness to make lifestyle changes. A realistic weight management program should focus on the following:

- Reducing your risk of health problems.
- Increasing your fitness level by becoming more physically active.
- Making positive lifestyle changes that will become lifelong habits.
- Coming to accept the size and shape of your body.

Tools for Change

Set your body in motion

Regular physical activity makes you feel stronger and more energetic. It also improves your overall health. Physical activity makes your body burn more calories, not just while you're physically active, but throughout the day. So if you get physically active and eat a healthful diet, you will find it easier to manage your weight. In addition, regular physical activity builds muscle. Increasing the amount of muscle in your body (lean muscle mass) is healthier for you and will make your body look more toned. For tips on making regular physical activity a part of your healthful lifestyle, see Chapter 16.

Plan your meals

People who eat regular meals find it easier to maintain a healthful weight than do people who overeat, skip meals, or snack. Meals that are planned are usually more nutritious than those that are grabbed at the last minute. Taking time to plan what you will eat will improve your diet and can help you control your weight. Skipping meals usually leads to feelings of deprivation, which can lead to overeating at the next meal or eating a less-than-nutritious snack.

Focus on reducing fat and added sugars
Eat a variety of nutritious foods that are low in fats and added sugars. Eating mainly fruits, vegetables, and grains helps you feel full, achieve good health, and manage your weight (see page 302).

Enjoy your food
You can enjoy all the foods you love and still control your weight. The key is to be sensible about how much you eat and to balance calorie intake with calorie burn-off (physical activity). Here are some tips:

- Enjoy your occasional steak (or cake) twice as much: eat half in the restaurant and take the rest home to enjoy the next day.
- Have 1 helping of your favorite food and enjoy every bite.
- Craving an ice cream cone? Walk to the ice cream shop, have a single dip, and walk home.

All foods can fit into a healthful diet; the proper balance of those foods is what's most important.

Be Tobacco-Free

It's never too late to quit using tobacco, even if you've been doing it for 20 or 30 years. Quitting smoking or chewing tobacco is the most important thing you can do to improve your own health and the health of those around you. Quitting is not easy. If you have already tried to quit, you know how difficult it is. But don't give up—with the right attitude and enough help, you will eventually succeed.

Tobacco use increases your risk for many health problems, including cancer, heart disease, and stroke. Your tobacco use also puts others at risk. Children who are exposed to cigarette smoke in the home have more ear infections and are prone to other health problems such as asthma. Perhaps the greatest risk to your children is that they will learn from you. Children whose parents use tobacco are more likely to use tobacco themselves.

When you stop using tobacco, it doesn't take long for your body to start to heal and for your risk of developing other health problems to decrease.

- When you quit smoking, your risk of heart attack is cut in half within 1 year after quitting. Five years after quitting, your risk is about the same as that of a person who never smoked.
- While the lung damage that smoking causes is not reversible, quitting smoking prevents more lung damage from occurring. Shortness of breath and cough will decrease.
- When you give up tobacco products, damage to your lips, tongue, mouth, and throat is reduced. Your risk for mouth and throat cancer decreases.

- If you have asthma, you will have fewer and less severe attacks after you quit smoking.
- After quitting smoking, a man may have fewer problems getting and maintaining erections.

Cigars and Smokeless Tobacco

Cigars have become popular in recent years. Many people who smoke cigars feel it is safe because they do not inhale the cigar smoke. However, holding cigars and cigar smoke in your mouth increases your risk for cancers of the mouth, tongue, throat, and larynx.

Smokeless tobacco, or snuff, can be chewed, inhaled, or held in your cheek. There is a direct link between using these products and developing mouth and throat cancer.

Facts you should know about cigars and smokeless tobacco:

- They contain nitrosamines, which cause cancer.
- They contain nicotine, which raises your heart rate and blood pressure.
- They may produce leukoplakias (wrinkled, thick, white patches) on the inside of the mouth. Leukoplakias can develop into mouth cancer.

Smoking Cessation Aids

Nicotine replacement products can help you break the habit of using tobacco and prevent nicotine withdrawal symptoms. The products deliver nicotine to the bloodstream without the dangerous tars, carbon monoxide, and other chemicals released by tobacco and smoke. You gradually reduce the amount of nicotine you give yourself until your body is no longer dependent on nicotine.

Nicotine replacement treatment comes in 4 forms: chewing gum, skin patches, nasal spray, and inhaler.

All nicotine replacement products can cause side effects. You may need to try more than one product before you find the one that works best for you.

Using a nicotine replacement product works best if you also enroll in a tobacco cessation program. Such programs help you deal with the habit of smoking or chewing tobacco, while the replacement product helps you overcome your addiction to nicotine.

A medication that does not contain nicotine is now available to help control irritability and cravings when you quit using tobacco. The medication is available only with a physician's prescription. First try to stop using tobacco without the medication. Many people succeed without it.

Tips for Quitting

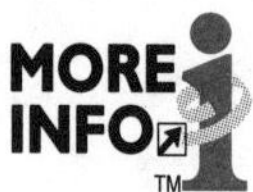

No one can tell you when or how to quit smoking or chewing tobacco. Only you know why you use tobacco and what will be most difficult as you try to stop. The important thing is that you try. Believe that you will succeed, if not the first time, then the second time, or twenty-second time.

Preparation

- List your reasons for quitting: for your own health and your family's health, to save money, to prevent wrinkles, or whatever. Read through your list daily for 1 month, and your chances of success will increase.
- Figure out why you smoke. Do you use tobacco to pep yourself up? To relax? Do you like the ritual of smoking or chewing? Do you use tobacco out of habit, often without knowing why you are doing it? If specific situations trigger your desire to smoke or chew tobacco, changing your routine may help you stop.
- Decide how and when you will quit. About half of ex-tobacco users quit "cold turkey." The other half cut down more slowly.
- Find a healthful alternative that can replace what smoking or chewing does for you. For example, if you like to have something to do with your hands, pick up something else: a coin, worry beads, pen, or pencil. If you like to have something in your mouth, substitute sugarless gum or minted toothpicks.
- Plan a healthful reward for yourself for when you have stopped using tobacco. Take the money you save by not buying tobacco and spend it on yourself.
- Plan things to do for when you get the urge to smoke or chew. Urges don't last that long: take a walk, brush your teeth, have a mint, drink a glass of water, or chew gum.
- Choose a reliable tobacco cessation program. Good programs have at least a 20 percent success rate after 1 year. Great programs have a 50 percent success rate. A higher success rate may be too good to be true.

Action

- Set a quit date and stick to it. Choose a time that will be busy but not stressful.
- Remove ashtrays and all other reminders of using tobacco. Choose nonsmoking sections in restaurants. Avoid alcohol. Do things that reduce the likelihood of using tobacco, like taking a walk or going to a movie.
- Ask for help and support. Choose a trusted friend, preferably another former tobacco user, to give you a helping hand over the rough spots.

MORE INFO For more information, see the inside front cover.

- Know what to expect. The worst will be over in just a few days, but physical withdrawal symptoms may last 1 to 3 weeks. After that, it is all psychological. See Chapter 18 for relaxation tips.
- Keep low-calorie snacks handy for when the urge to munch hits. Your appetite may perk up, but most people gain fewer than 10 pounds when they quit using tobacco. The health benefits of quitting outweigh a few extra pounds. The information in Chapter 17 can help you plan healthful meals and snacks.
- Get out and exercise. It will distract you, help keep off unwanted pounds, and release tension. See Chapter 16.
- Don't be discouraged by slip-ups. It often takes several tries to quit using tobacco for good. If you do slip up and smoke or chew, forgive yourself and learn from the experience. You will not fail as long as you keep trying.
- Good luck!

Avoid Drugs and Excess Alcohol

When you say "no" to drugs and limit the amount of alcohol that you drink, you prevent accidents and several diseases and avoid a lot of other problems for yourself and your family. If drug or alcohol abuse is a problem for you or someone close to you, now is the time to seek help. For more information about drug and alcohol problems, see page 308.

Manage Stress

Stress is practically unavoidable, but it doesn't have to have a negative impact on your health and well-being. By learning how to deal with stress in ways that make you feel more in control, you may be able to improve your health, your relationships, your job or school performance, and your outlook on life.

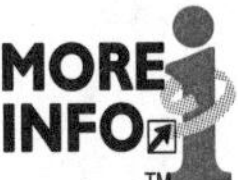

It shouldn't surprise you that some of the key factors in helping you manage stress are eating a healthful diet, getting regular exercise and enough sleep, avoiding drugs and tobacco, and drinking alcohol only in moderation. All these lifestyle factors work together.

For more information about how stress can affect your health and how you can identify and deal with the sources of stress in your life, see Chapter 18.

Take Care of Your Teeth

Your teeth will last a lifetime if you care for them properly. Brushing and flossing regularly, eating a mouth-healthy diet, and visiting your dentist for regular checkups will help keep your teeth healthy.

Brushing

- Brush at least twice a day for 3 to 5 minutes each time.
- Use a fluoride toothpaste (young children should use only a pea-sized dab). Tartar-control toothpastes may help slow the formation of hard mineral build-up (tartar) on the teeth.
- Brush your tongue. Plaque build-up (a sticky film made of bacteria) on the tongue can cause bad breath.

Start brushing your child's teeth as soon as they come in. Brush your child's teeth for the first 4 to 5 years, until your child seems able to do it alone. A good teaching method is to have your child brush in the morning and you brush at night until your child masters the skill.

If your local water supply does not contain enough fluoride, your child may need a fluoride supplement. Discuss this with your dentist.

Flossing

Flossing properly once a day is the best way to remove plaque from below the gums and between the teeth.

Start flossing your child's teeth as soon as they touch each other. As with brushing, you will have to help with flossing until the child is old enough to manage it alone.

Diet

- Avoid high-sugar foods, especially sticky, sweet foods like taffy and raisins. The longer sugar stays in touch with your teeth, the more damage it will do.
- Brush after between-meal snacks.
- Don't snack before bedtime. Food is more likely to cause cavities at night because saliva doesn't clean the mouth as well at night.
- Mozzarella and other cheeses, peanuts, yogurt, milk, and sugar-free chewing gum (especially gum that contains xylitol) are good for your teeth. They help clear the mouth of harmful sugars and reduce plaque formation.

Dental Checkups

Most people who do not have serious problems with their teeth need to visit the dentist twice a year. During a dental checkup the dentist will examine your teeth and gums for signs of tooth decay and gum disease. X-rays of your teeth are usually taken once a year. If you don't have any active tooth decay or gum disease, changes in your brushing and flossing habits probably won't be necessary.

A dentist or dental hygienist will clean your teeth. He or she will scrape hard mineral buildup (tartar) off of your teeth with a small metal tool; floss your teeth thoroughly; and use a polishing compound to help clean and polish your teeth. Cleanings may be uncomfortable but usually aren't painful. Other procedures (application of sealants to prevent cavities or fluoride treatments) may be done during a routine office visit if needed.

The Academy of Pediatric Dentistry recommends that your child see a dentist either by 1 year of age or within 6 months after his or her first tooth comes in.

Practice Safety

Taking safety precautions is one of the most important things you can do to protect yourself and your family from accidents and injuries. Let common sense and these partial lists be your guides.

At Home

- Post emergency telephone numbers near telephones.
- Have an emergency plan in case of accidents, fire, or injury. Practice the plan with your family.
- Install smoke and carbon monoxide detectors in your home, and check them twice a year to make sure they work.
- Keep a working fire extinguisher in your home. Make sure everyone in the house (including the babysitter) knows how to use it.
- Keep all medications, cleaning and automotive supplies, and other hazardous products securely stored and out of the reach of children.
- Turn off appliances after use. Unplug small appliances and put them away after they have cooled.
- Store firearms unloaded and securely, out of the reach of children. Store ammunition separately.
- Prevent falls by securing rugs that slip, keeping stairs and hallways clear of clutter, and turning on lights.
- Practice safer sex. See page 287.

When on the Move

- Don't drink and drive.
- Make sure everyone in your car is wearing a safety belt. See "Automobile Seat Restraints" on page 30.
- Obey traffic laws and speed limits.
- Keep your car, bike, skateboard, skis, and other recreational gear in good operating condition.
- Wear helmets and sport-specific padding when bicycling, in-line skating, playing baseball, etc. Wear eye protection when playing racquet sports.
- Never let children play unattended near water.

At Work

- Follow your employer's safety guidelines.
- Wear clothing and protective equipment that is appropriate for your job (hard hat, gloves, goggles, earplugs, etc.).

- Protect yourself against smoke, dangerous fumes, and exposure to chemicals.
- Know the location of fire extinguishers and emergency exits nearest your workstation.

Pursue Healthy Pleasures

Give yourself permission to make yourself happy. The good things in life make it easier to deal with the things that aren't so good. If it's been a while since you've indulged yourself in something pleasurable, try this exercise:

- Make a list of 10 (or more) things that give you pleasure.
- Do at least 1 of the things on your list every day for 1 week.
- Enjoy and repeat!

Help to Make a Healthier World

Do what you can to make your home, your community, and your world a better place. Support a cause that is working to make positive changes. Recycle. Mentor. Tutor. Volunteer. And remember, peace on Earth begins at home: seek nonviolent ways to resolve conflicts at home, at school, at work, and in your community. See pages 311 and 321.

Automobile Seat Restraints

Wearing seat belts saves lives and prevents injuries. No one is strong enough to brace themselves against a sudden impact in a motor vehicle, even at very low speeds. Seat belts reduce the risk of serious injury and death.

- Wear your seat belt every time you are in a vehicle. Keep the belt snug and close to your body. Always use both the lap and shoulder belts.
- Seat belts are necessary even if your car is equipped with air bags. Air bags inflate from the steering wheel or dashboard of your car in the event of sudden impact. They are very effective in protecting front-seat riders, but they must be used with seat belts.
- Children younger than 12 years of age should sit in the back seat. Use child safety seats for infants, children under 4, and those weighing less than 40 pounds. See page 228.

Most folks don't know what can be done with a little will and their own hands.
Gloria Naylor

3

First Aid and Emergencies

This chapter covers both serious medical emergencies and minor first aid situations. Review this chapter before you need it. Then, when you are faced with an emergency or injury, you will know where to turn. Your confidence in dealing with both major and minor emergencies will be reassuring to an injured person.

Some of the medical emergencies covered in this chapter include:

- Bleeding, see Cuts on page 46.
- Breathing emergencies, page 36.
- Head injuries, page 52.
- Heart attack, page 54.
- Poisoning, page 63.
- Shock, page 67.
- Stroke, page 70.
- Unconsciousness, page 73.

Medical Emergencies

If you think you have an emergency medical condition, call 911 or go to the nearest hospital.

An emergency medical condition is a medical or psychiatric condition that manifests itself by acute symptoms of sufficient severity (including severe pain) such that you could reasonably expect the absence of immediate medical attention to result in serious jeopardy to your health, serious impairment to your bodily functions, or serious dysfunction of any bodily organ or part.

Dealing With Emergencies

Take a deep breath. Count to 10. Tell yourself you can handle the situation.

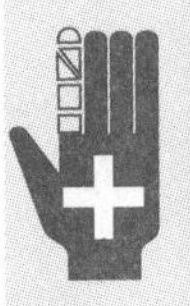

Assess the danger. Protect yourself and the injured person from fire, explosions, or other hazards. If you suspect a spinal injury, do not move the person unless the danger is great.

Prepare for the Emergency Room

- If possible, call ahead to let emergency room staff know you are coming.
- Call your physician, if possible. He or she may meet you at the emergency room or call in important information.
- If you think you may have to wait to be seen by a physician, take this book and your medical records with you. While you are waiting you can:
  - Use page 1, the Healthwise Self-Care Checklist, to help you think through the problem and report symptoms to the physician.
  - Use page 2, the Ask-the-Physician Checklist, to organize questions for the physician.
  - Review the medical test checklist on page 12.
  - Use your home medical records to prepare to discuss your medications, past test results, or treatments. Information about your allergies, medications, and health conditions may be critical.

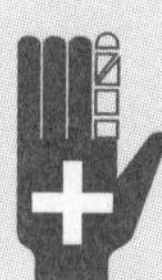

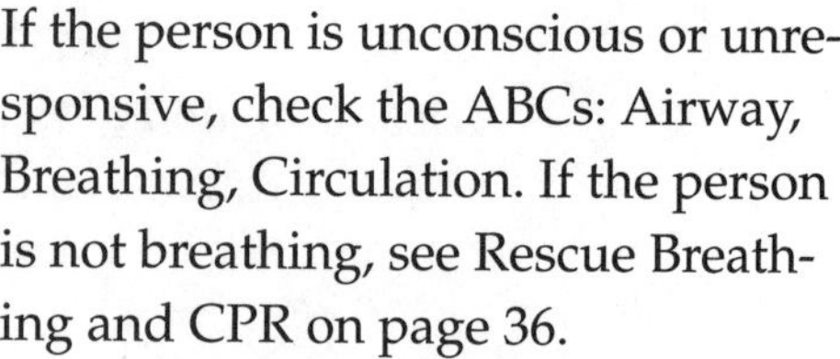

If the person is unconscious or unresponsive, check the ABCs: Airway, Breathing, Circulation. If the person is not breathing, see Rescue Breathing and CPR on page 36.

Identify and prioritize the injuries. Treat the most life-threatening problems (bleeding, shock) first. Check for broken bones and other injuries. **If you think you have an emergency medical condition and you cannot safely go to a Plan hospital, call 911 or go to the nearest hospital.**

Emergency services are available at Kaiser Permanente hospital emergency departments 24 hours a day, 7 days a week.

Legal Protection

If you are needed in an emergency, give what help you can. Most states have a Good Samaritan law to protect people who help in an emergency. You cannot be sued for giving first aid unless it can be shown that you are guilty of gross negligence.

Accidental Tooth Loss

If a permanent tooth is knocked out, a dentist may be able to reimplant it. Baby teeth need to come out anyway, so they are not usually reimplanted.

A chipped tooth can be repaired. A blow that was hard enough to chip a tooth may have moved several teeth out of alignment or broken the portion of bone that holds the tooth in place.

Home Treatment

- Call your dentist immediately for an emergency visit. Reimplanting a tooth works best when it is done within 30 minutes. After 2 hours, it is unlikely the procedure will be successful.
- Clean the tooth gently and place it back in the socket, between the gum and cheek (use care not to swallow the tooth), or in a small container of milk. Do not transport the tooth in tap water.

When to Call a Dentist

- If a permanent tooth is knocked out or chipped.
- If a baby tooth is knocked out, schedule an appointment within 2 weeks to determine if a spacer is needed until a permanent tooth comes in.

Animal and Human Bites

When bitten by an animal, most people want to know if they need a rabies shot. The main wild animal carriers of rabies are bats, raccoons, skunks, and foxes. Pet dogs, cats, and ferrets that have been vaccinated rarely have rabies. However, many stray animals have not been vaccinated. Rabies is quite rare, but it is fatal if not treated. The treatment is no more painful than a typical injection. Report all wild animal bites to your physician and the health department.

Bites that break the skin can cause bacterial infections. Cat and human bites are particularly prone to infection. You can get tetanus from a bite if your tetanus shots are not up to date. See page 16.

Prevention

- Vaccinate all pets against rabies. Do not keep wild animals as pets.
- Do not disturb animals—not even your pets—while they are eating.
- Teach children not to approach or play with stray animals.
- Do not touch wild animals or provoke them to attack. Do not handle sick or injured animals.

Home Treatment

- Scrub the bite immediately with soap and water. Treat it as a puncture wound. See page 65.
- If you are bitten by a pet dog, cat, or ferret, find out whether the animal has been vaccinated for rabies.
- A healthy pet that has bitten someone should be confined and observed for 10 days by a veterinarian to see if the pet develops symptoms of rabies. If the pet's owner cannot be located, contact the health department.
- If you are bitten by a wild animal, contact your physician and the health department. The health department can tell you whether that animal is a rabies carrier in your area, and whether treatment is needed.

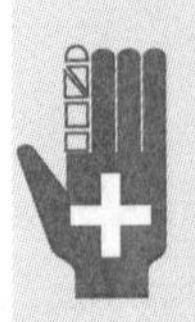

When to Call Kaiser Permanente

- If the bite is from a wild animal.
- If the bite is from a human or a cat.
- If the bite is from a dog, cat, or ferret that is acting strangely and/or foaming at the mouth, or if the animal attacked for no apparent reason.
- If the bite is from a pet whose owner cannot be found or cannot confirm that the animal has been vaccinated for rabies.
- If the bite is severe and may need stitches or if it is on your face, hand, or foot. If stitches are needed, they usually should be done within 8 hours.
- If signs of infection develop:
  - Increased pain, swelling, redness, or tenderness.
  - Heat or red streaks extending from the bite.
  - Discharge of pus.
  - Fever of 100° or higher with no other cause.

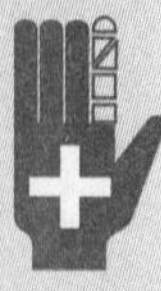

Blood Under a Nail

Fingernails and toenails often get crunched, bashed, or smashed. These injuries usually aren't too serious, but if there is bleeding under the nail, the pressure can be very painful. The only way to relieve the throbbing and pain is by making a hole in the nail to drain the blood.

Draining is helpful only if you have severe, throbbing pain (you can feel the pulse beating under the nail) that is bad enough to keep you from sleeping. If you aren't having a lot of pain, draining the nail is not recommended.

Home Treatment

- Apply ice and elevate the injured area as soon as possible to minimize swelling and relieve pain. Acetaminophen will also ease discomfort.
- If you have severe, throbbing pain, make a hole in the nail to relieve the pressure. (Do not do this unless you are confident you can do it without burning yourself. Do not do this if you have diabetes or circulation problems.) Follow these steps:
  - Straighten a paper clip and heat the tip in a flame until it is red-hot.
  - Place the tip of the paper clip on the nail and let it melt through. You do not need to push. This will not be painful, because the nail has no nerves. Go slowly and reheat the clip as necessary. A thick nail may take several tries.
  - As soon as the hole is complete, blood will escape and the pain will be relieved. If your pain is not relieved by this procedure, you may have a more serious injury, such as a broken finger or toe or a deep cut. In this case, you should see your physician.

- Soak the finger 3 times a day in a half-and-half mixture of hydrogen peroxide and warm water.
- If the pressure builds up again in a few days, repeat the procedure, using the same hole.

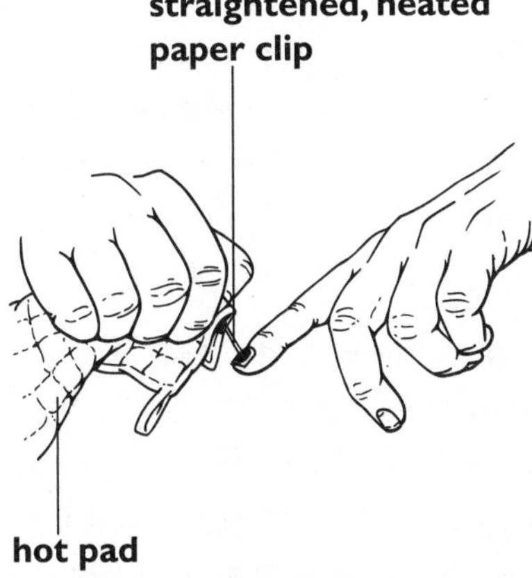

Use a red-hot paper clip to relieve the pain caused by blood under a fingernail or toenail.

When to Call Kaiser Permanente

- If blood under a nail is causing severe pain and you are not willing to drain the blood from the nail yourself.
- If you drained the blood from under the nail, but your fingertip or the tip of your toe still hurts a lot.
- If you smashed your toenail and you have a condition such as diabetes or peripheral vascular disease, which decreases blood flow to the feet.
- If signs of infection develop:
  - Increased pain, swelling, redness, or tenderness.
  - Heat or red streaks extending from the injured area.
  - Discharge of pus.
  - Fever of 100° or higher with no other cause.
- If your nail has torn or separated from the nail bed and you need help removing it.

Blunt Abdominal Wounds

Blunt abdominal wounds caused by a blow to the stomach can cause severe bruising of the abdominal wall and bleeding from the internal organs. Such injuries are often caused by automobile, bicycle, sledding, or skiing accidents, when the victim is thrown into an object or to the ground.

An abdominal injury may cause the abdomen to become tender or rigid. The injured person may become confused and may not be able to remember what caused the injury. Signs of shock (faintness, weakness, drowsiness, or confusion; sweating and cool, clammy skin) may also develop.

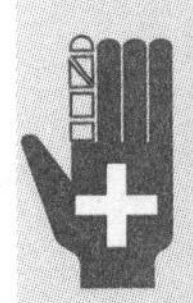

Home Treatment

- Monitor the injured person's pulse and respiration rate. See pages 57 and 68. If possible, monitor the person's blood pressure as well. A rapid, weak pulse, very rapid or very slow breathing, or falling blood pressure may indicate internal bleeding. If these signs develop, **call 911 or take the person to the emergency room immediately**.
- Have the injured person lie down with the feet elevated above the heart. Loosen the person's clothing and cover him or her with a blanket for warmth. Do not give the person anything to eat or drink, even though he or she may be thirsty.
- Watch for signs of shock (see page 67).

When to Call Kaiser Permanente

- If signs of shock or internal bleeding (see page 67) develop up to 48 hours after an abdominal injury.
- If there is bleeding from the rectum, blood in the urine, or unexpected vaginal bleeding following a blow to the abdomen.
- If the injury causes nausea, vomiting, heartburn, or loss of appetite.
- If the person's abdomen is swollen and hard, or if pressing on the abdomen causes severe pain.
- If you have any concerns about the symptoms you observe.

Breathing Emergencies

Who needs to be trained to help a person who is having a breathing emergency? You do. If you have children, drive a car, shop at the mall, or go anyplace where a person may be in a life-threatening situation, you need to know how to respond. An added benefit is the confidence you will have when you know you can help a person when it matters most.

The guidelines presented in this book are not meant to replace formal training from a certified instructor. They are here for you to use to refresh your memory between trainings or to read aloud to a person who is performing a rescue procedure. (Note, however, that your first responsibility as a helper is to call 911 or seek emergency services and to make the area safe for the victim and the rescuer.)

Rescue Breathing and CPR

WARNING: CPR (cardiopulmonary resuscitation) that is done improperly or on a person whose heart is still beating can cause serious injury. Do not perform CPR unless:

1. The person has stopped breathing.

2. The person does not have signs of circulation, such as normal breathing, coughing, or movement in response to rescue breathing.

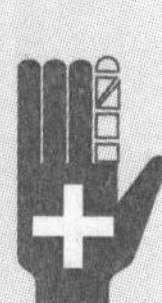

3. No one with more training in CPR is present.

For basic life support, think **ABC: A**irway, **B**reathing, and **C**irculation, in that order. You must give rescue breaths before you can begin the chest compressions, which will help circulate blood for a person whose heart has stopped beating.

Step 1: Check for consciousness. Tap or gently shake the person and shout, "Are you okay?" If you suspect a neck or spinal injury, do not shake the person.

If the person does not respond:

- **Adult (age 9 and older): Call 911 or other emergency services immediately** (have someone else make the call if possible). Then proceed to Step 2.
- **Infant or child through 8 years:** Check to see if the infant or child is breathing (Step 2). If the infant or child is not breathing, give rescue breaths for 1 full minute (Step 3).

Then **call 911 or other emergency services.** If the child is small enough, carry him or her to the telephone with you so you can continue to give rescue breaths. Keep the child's head and neck steady.

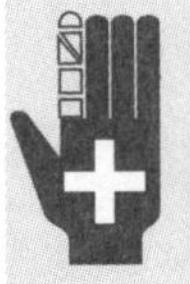

CPR Ready Reference

	Adults	Children Age 1 through 8	Infants Under 1 Year
If the person is not breathing, begin rescue breathing:	Give 2 full breaths.	Give rescue breaths for 1 full minute.	Give rescue breaths for 1 full minute.
If the person does not breathe or show signs of circulation in response to rescue breaths, locate the compression landmark:	Trace the ribs into the sternal notch; place 2 fingers on the sternum. See illustration on p. 39.	Same as for an adult.	1 finger-width below nipple line.
Do chest compressions with:	2 hands stacked; heel of 1 hand on sternum	Heel of 1 hand on sternum	2 or 3 fingers on sternum
Rate of compressions per minute:	100	100	100
Compression depth:	1½ to 2 inches	1 to 1½ inches	½ to 1 inch
Ratio of compressions to breaths:	15:2	5:1	5:1
Guidelines from the American Heart Association			

Step 2: Check for breathing. Look, listen, and feel for breathing for 5 seconds. Kneel next to the person with your head close to his or her head.

- Look to see if the person's chest rises and falls.
- Listen for breathing sounds, wheezing, gurgling, or snoring.
- Put your cheek near the person's mouth and nose to feel whether air is moving out.

If the person is not breathing (or if you can't tell), roll the person onto his or her back. If he or she may have a spinal injury, gently roll the person's head, neck, and shoulders together as a unit until the person is on his or her back.

Step 3: Begin rescue breathing.

- Place your hand on the person's forehead and pinch the person's nostrils shut with your thumb and forefinger. With your other hand, continue tilting the chin forward to keep the airway open.

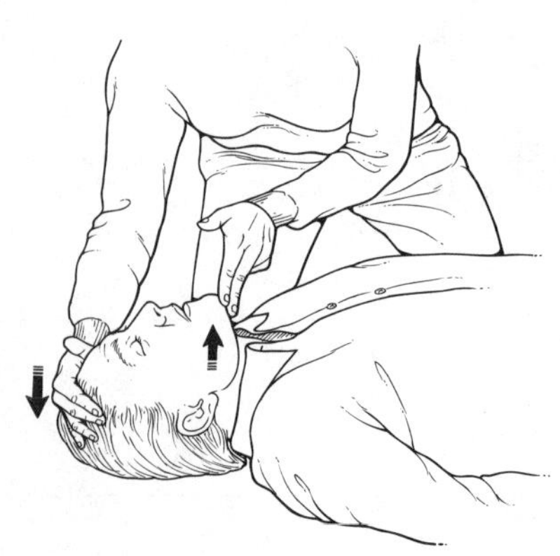

Airway: Position the head to open the airway.

- Take a deep breath and place your mouth over the person's mouth, making a tight seal. For an infant, place your mouth over the baby's mouth and nose. As you slowly blow air into the person, watch to see if his or her chest rises.

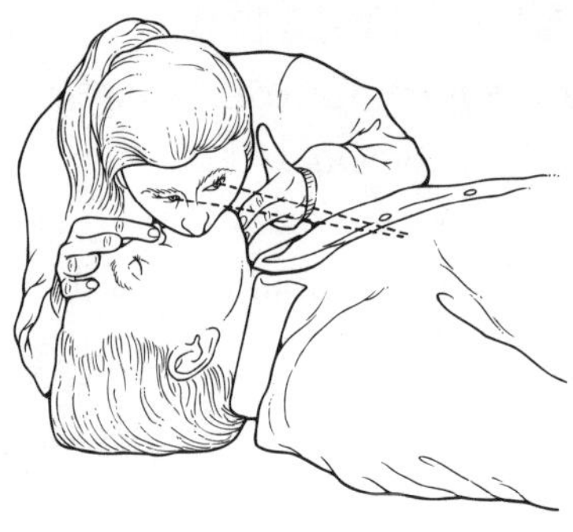

Breathing: Blow air in slowly; look to see if chest rises.

- If the first breath does not go in, try tilting the person's head again and give another breath.
- Slowly blow air in until the person's chest rises. Take 1½ to 2 seconds to give each breath. Between rescue breaths, remove your mouth from the person's mouth and take a deep breath. Allow his or her chest to fall and feel the air escape.
- Give the person 2 full breaths. Then check for circulation.

Step 4: Check for circulation. Look for signs of circulation, such as breathing, coughing, or movement in response to rescue breathing.

If there are **no signs of circulation**, begin chest compressions. See Step 5.

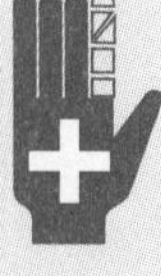

If there are signs of circulation, continue to give rescue breaths until help arrives or until the person starts breathing on his or her own. If the person starts breathing again, he or she still needs to be seen by a health professional.

Give rescue breaths:

- Adult (age 9 and older): 2 breaths every 15 seconds
- Infant or child through 8 years: 1 breath every 3 seconds

Step 5: Begin chest compressions. Adult (age 9 and older):

- Kneel next to the person. Use your fingers to locate the end of the person's breastbone (sternum), where the ribs come together. Place 2 fingers at the tip of the sternum. Place the heel of the other hand directly above your fingers (on the side closest to the person's face).

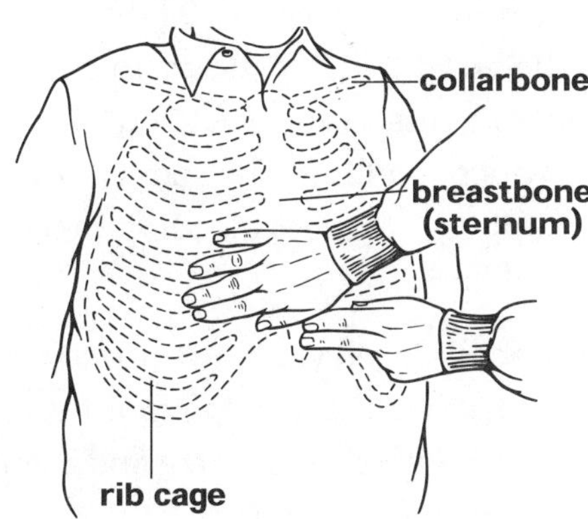

Put your hand 2 fingers'-width above the bottom of the breastbone.

- Place your other hand on top of the one that you just put in position. Lock the fingers of both hands together, and raise the fingers so they don't touch the person's chest.
- Straighten your arms, lock your elbows, and center your shoulders directly over your hands.
- Press down in a steady rhythm, using your body weight and keeping your elbows locked. The force from each thrust should go straight down onto the sternum, compressing it 1½ to 2 inches. It may help to count "one and two and three and four...," giving 1 downward thrust each time you say a number. Lift your weight, but not your hands, from the chest each time you say "and." Give 15 compressions.

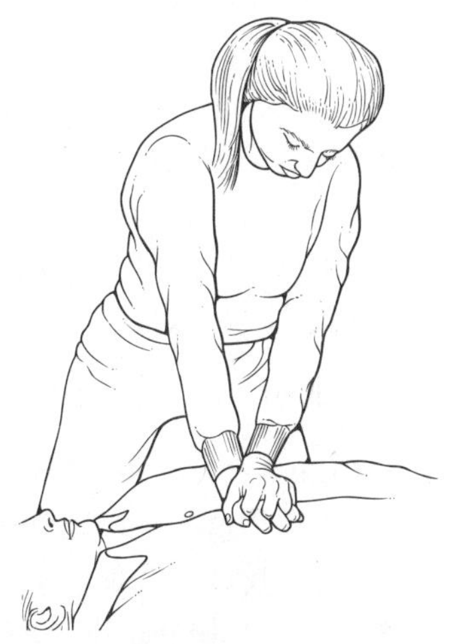

Chest Compressions: Keep your shoulders directly over your hands with your elbows straight as you give chest compressions.

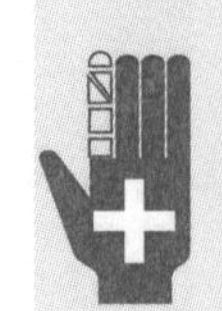

- After 15 compressions, give 2 full, slow breaths.
- Repeat the 15 compressions/2 breaths cycle 4 times (1 minute); then check again for signs of circulation. If there are still no signs of circulation, continue to give chest compressions and rescue breaths

until help arrives or until signs of circulation are present and breathing is restored.

Child (age 1 through 8 years):

- Position the heel of one hand 2 fingers'-width above the tip of the sternum. Press with less force than you would for an adult, compressing the sternum 1 to 1½ inches.
- Give 5 chest compressions. Then give 1 rescue breath. Repeat the 5 compressions/1 breath cycle 12 times (1 minute); then check again for signs of circulation, such as normal breathing, coughing, or movement in response to rescue breaths. If there are still no signs of circulation, continue to give chest compressions and rescue breaths until help arrives or until signs of circulation are present and breathing is restored.

Infant (younger than 1 year):

- Place 2 fingers on the baby's sternum, about 1 finger-width below an imaginary line connecting the nipples. Press with gentle force, compressing the sternum about ½ to 1 inch.
- Give 5 chest compressions. Then give 1 rescue breath. Repeat the cycle of 5 compressions and 1 breath 12 times (1 minute); then check again for signs of circulation. If there are still no signs of circulation, continue to give chest compressions and rescue breaths until help arrives or until signs of circulation are present and breathing is restored.

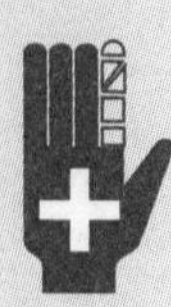

Bruises

Bruises (contusions) are caused by ruptured blood vessels under the skin. Blood seeps into the surrounding tissues, causing the black-and-blue color of a bruise.

Bruises usually develop after a bump or fall. People who take aspirin or blood thinners (anticoagulants) may bruise easily. A bruise may also develop after blood is drawn.

A black eye is a type of bruise. If you have a black eye, apply home treatment for a bruise and inspect the eye for blood. If there is any loss of or change in your vision or if you cannot move your eye in all directions, see a physician.

Home Treatment

- Apply ice or cold packs for up to 10 minutes every 1 to 2 hours. Do this for the first 48 hours to help blood vessels constrict and to reduce swelling. The sooner you apply ice, the less bleeding there will be.
- If possible, elevate the bruised area above the level of your heart. Blood will leave the area and there will be less swelling.
- Rest the injured limb so you don't injure it further.
- If the area is still painful after 48 hours, use ice or apply heat with warm towels, a hot water bottle, or a heating pad.

When to Call Kaiser Permanente

- If signs of infection develop:
  - Increased pain, swelling, redness, or tenderness (after the initial bruise).
  - Heat or red streaks extending away from the area.
  - Discharge of pus.
  - Fever of 100° or higher with no other cause.
- If pain increases or if your ability to use or move the bruised part decreases.
- If a blow to the eye causes:
  - Blood in the colored part of the eye or blood in the white part of the eye (see page 173).
  - Loss of or change in vision.
  - Inability to move the eye normally in all directions.
  - Severe pain in the eyeball rather than in the eye socket.
- If you suddenly begin to bruise easily, or if you have unexplained recurrent or multiple bruises.

Burns

Burns are classified as first-, second-, or third-degree depending on their depth, not on the amount of pain or the extent of the burn. A first-degree burn involves only the outer layer of skin. The skin is dry, painful, and sensitive to touch. A mild sunburn is an example.

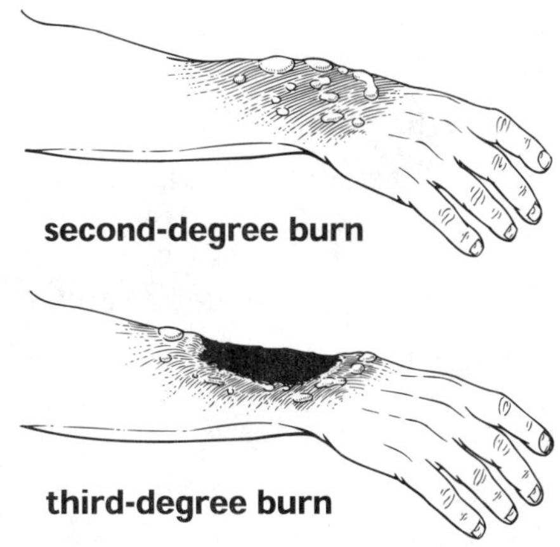

A second-degree burn will cause skin to swell and blister, and it may also weep fluid. A third-degree burn may cause skin to look pale white or charred black.

A second-degree burn involves several layers of skin. The skin becomes swollen, puffy, weepy, or blistered.

A third-degree burn involves all layers of skin and may include any underlying tissue or organs. The skin is dry, pale white or charred black, swollen, and sometimes breaks open. Nerves are destroyed or damaged, so there may be little pain except on the edges, where there may be second-degree burns.

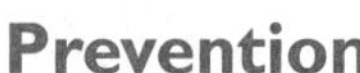

Prevention

- Install smoke detectors on each story of your home. Check and replace the batteries regularly.
- Keep a fire extinguisher near the kitchen. Have it inspected yearly.
- Set your water heater at 120° or lower to avoid burns.
- Don't smoke in bed.

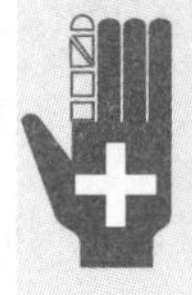

If your clothing catches fire:

- Do not run, because running will fan the flames. Stop, drop, and roll on the ground to smother the flames. Or smother the flames with a blanket, rug, or coat.
- Use water to douse the fire and cool the skin.

To avoid kitchen burns:

- Use caution when handling hot foods.
- Turn pot handles toward the back of the stove.
- Smother burning food or grease with a pot or pot lid.
- Supervise children closely.

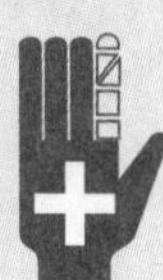

Home Treatment

Third-degree burns require immediate medical treatment. Call Kaiser Permanente and apply home treatment:

- Make sure the source of the burn has been extinguished.
- Have the person lie down to prevent shock.
- Cover the burned area with a clean sheet.
- Do not apply any salve or medication to the burn.

First- and second-degree burns can be treated at home as follows:

- Run cool tap water over the burn until the pain stops (10 to 30 minutes). Cool water is the best immediate treatment for minor burns. The cold lowers skin temperature and lessens the severity of the burn. Do not use ice or ice water, because it may further damage the injured skin.
- Remove rings, bracelets, watches, or shoes from the burned limb. Swelling may make these items difficult to remove later.
- Clean the burn area with mild soap and water. If the burned skin or blisters have broken open, a bandage is needed. Otherwise, don't cover the burn unless clothing rubs on it. If clothing rubs the burned area, cover the burn with a nonstick gauze pad taped well away from the burn. Do not encircle a hand, arm, or leg with tape. Keep the bandage clean and dry.
- Do not put salve, butter, grease, oil, or ointment on a burn. They increase the risk of infection and don't help the burn heal.
- After 2 to 3 days of healing, apply the juice from an aloe leaf to soothe minor burns.

If the burn causes blisters to form:

- Do not break blisters. If blisters break, clean the area by running tap water over it and applying a mild soap. Apply an antibiotic ointment, such as Polysporin or Bacitracin, and cover the burn with a sterile dressing. Don't touch the burned area with your hands or any unsterile objects. Remove the dressing every day, clean the burned area with mild soap, and cover it again.

- Take aspirin or ibuprofen to help relieve pain. Don't give aspirin to anyone younger than 20.

When to Call Kaiser Permanente

- For all third-degree burns.
- If you are in doubt about the extent of a burn, or in doubt whether it is a second- or third-degree burn.
- If a second-degree burn involves the face, hands, feet, genitals, or a joint and is more than 1 inch in diameter.
- If the burn encircles an arm or leg, or if it covers more than ¼ of the body part involved.
- If the pain lasts longer than 48 hours.
- If signs of infection develop:
    - Increased pain, swelling, redness, or tenderness.
    - Heat or red streaks extending from the area.
    - Discharge of pus.
    - Fever of 100° or higher with no other cause.
- If a child younger than 5, an older adult, or a person with a weakened immune system or a chronic health problem (such as cancer, heart disease, or diabetes) is burned.

Chemical Burns

Chemical burns occur when something caustic, such as a cleaning product, gasoline, or turpentine, is splashed into an eye or onto the skin.

The vapors or fumes of strong chemicals can also burn or irritate the eyes, the respiratory passages, and the lungs.

A chemically burned eye becomes red and watery and may be sensitive to light. If the damage is severe, the eye will look whitish. Chemically burned skin may become red, blistered, or blackened, depending on how strong the caustic material is.

Home Treatment

- Immediately flush your eye or skin with water. Use a cold shower for skin burns. For eye burns, fill a sink or dishpan with water, immerse your face in the water, and open and close your eyelids with your fingers to force the water to all parts of the eye. Or flush your eye under a running faucet or shower.
- Continue flushing for 15 to 20 minutes or until the pain stops, whichever takes longer.

When to Call Kaiser Permanente

Call 911 or seek other emergency services immediately if a strong chemical such as acid or lye is splashed into your eye.

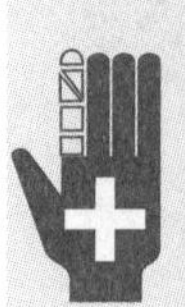

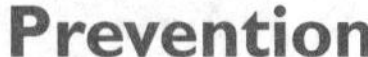

Call Kaiser Permanente or the local poison control center if any one of the following occurs:

- Major skin exposure (more than ¼ of any part of the body or on the face) to a strong acid, such as battery acid, or to a caustic substance, such as lye or Drano.
- A chemically burned eye still hurts after 20 minutes of home treatment.
- A chemically burned eye appears to be damaged. Symptoms include:
    - Persistent redness.
    - Discharge or watering.
    - Any visual impairment, such as double vision, blurring, or sensitivity to light.
    - Colored part of the eye (iris) appears white.
- Your skin shows signs of a chemical burn (see page 43).

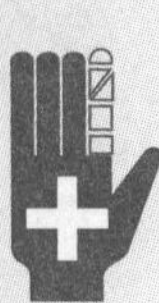

Choking

Choking is usually caused by food or an object stuck in the windpipe. A person who is choking cannot cough, talk, or breathe, and may turn blue or dusky. The **Heimlich maneuver**, described on page 45, can help dislodge the food or object.

Prevention

- Don't drink too much alcohol before eating. It may dull your senses, and you might not chew food properly or might try to swallow too large a portion of food.
- Take small bites. Cut meat into small pieces. Chew your food thoroughly.
- Do not give popcorn, peanuts, or hard candy to children younger than 3, and supervise older children when they eat these foods.
- Do not allow children younger than 3 to play with toys that have very small parts (smaller than a 50-cent piece) that could be swallowed.
- Keep balloons away from any child who may put them in his or her mouth.

When to Call Kaiser Permanente

Call 911 or seek other emergency services immediately if you are unable to dislodge the object using the Heimlich maneuver (see page 45) or if the person loses consciousness. Attempt rescue breathing while waiting for help to arrive. See page 36.

Call Kaiser Permanente even if the object has been dislodged. The person's throat could be damaged by the object, or there could be abdominal damage from doing the Heimlich maneuver.

Choking Rescue Procedure (Heimlich Maneuver)

WARNING: Do *not* begin the choking rescue procedure unless the person *cannot breathe* or is turning blue and cannot speak, and you are *certain* that the person is choking.

If an object is not easily dislodged by the Heimlich maneuver or if the victim loses consciousness, have someone **call 911 or emergency services** while you continue trying.

Adult or child older than 1 year:

If the victim is standing or sitting

- Stand behind the victim and wrap your arms around his or her waist. If the victim is standing, place one of your feet between the victim's legs so you can support the victim's body if he or she loses consciousness.

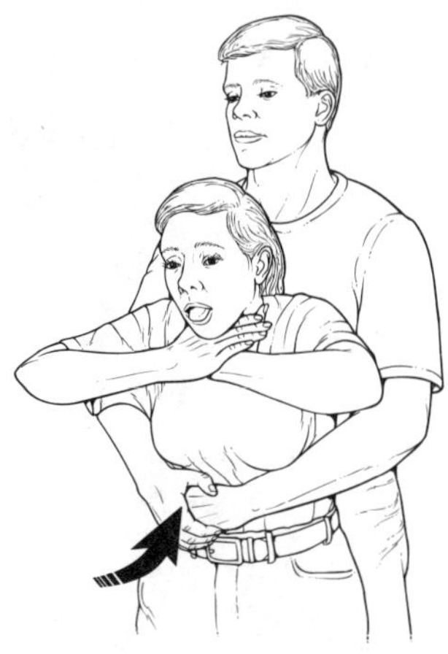

A. Heimlich maneuver: Give quick upward thrusts to dislodge the object.

- Make a fist with one hand. Place the thumb side of your fist against the victim's abdomen, just above the navel but well below the sternum. See illustration A on page 45.
- Grasp your fist with the other hand. Give a quick upward thrust into the victim's abdomen. This may cause the object to pop out. Use less force for a child. See illustration A on page 45.
- Repeat thrusts until the object pops out or the victim loses consciousness.
- **If you choke while you are alone**, do abdominal thrusts on yourself, or lean over the back of a chair and press forcefully to pop out the object.

If the victim loses consciousness, gently lower the victim to the ground. Call 911 or seek other emergency services immediately.

- Begin standard CPR, including chest compressions.
- Each time the airway is opened during CPR, look for an obstructing object in the back of the mouth or throat.
  - If you see an object, remove it.
  - Do not perform blind finger sweeps of the mouth.
- Do not perform abdominal thrusts (such as the Heimlich maneuver).
- Continue doing CPR until the object is dislodged and the victim is breathing on his or her own or until an ambulance arrives.

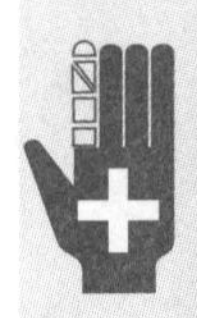

Infant (younger than 1 year):

- Hold infant as in illustration B on page 46.
- Use the heel of one hand to jar the child between the shoulder blades in an attempt to dislodge the object. Repeat 4 times.

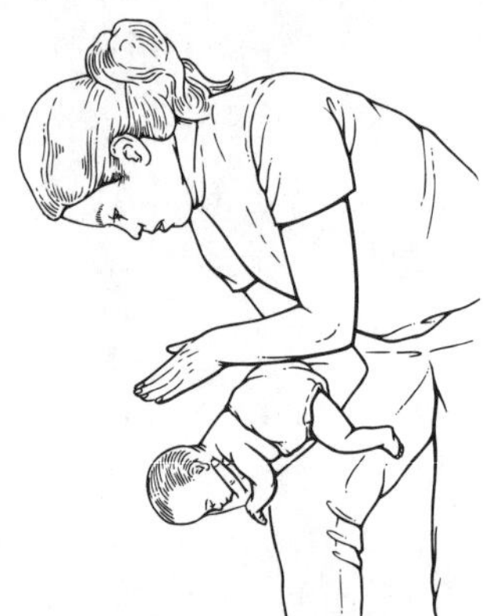

B. To help a baby who is choking, put him face down on your forearm so his head is lower than his chest. Support the baby's head in your palm against your thigh (don't cover the baby's mouth or twist his neck). Use the heel of your other hand to give back blows between the baby's shoulders.

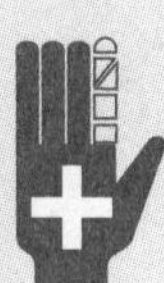

- If the airway remains blocked, support the infant's head and turn the infant face up on your thigh with his or her head down.
- Place 2 or 3 fingers just below a line between the nipples, and give up to 5 upward thrusts until the object pops out.
- Look for the object in the infant's mouth. If you can see it, remove it with your finger. Then give 2 rescue breaths (see page 38).

When to Call Kaiser Permanente

- **Call 911 or seek other emergency services immediately** if back blows and chest thrusts do not dislodge the object or if the person loses consciousness. Attempt rescue breathing while waiting for help to arrive. See page 36.
- Call even if the object has been dislodged. The throat could be damaged by the object, or there could be abdominal damage from doing the Heimlich maneuver.

Cuts

When you see a cut (laceration), the first steps are to stop the bleeding and determine whether stitches are needed.

If the cut is bleeding heavily or spurting blood, see "Stopping Severe Bleeding" on page 47.

Bleeding from minor cuts will usually stop on its own or after you apply a little direct pressure.

To decide whether stitches are needed, see "Are Sutures Necessary?" on page 49.

If stitches are needed, apply home treatment and seek medical care as soon as possible, certainly within 8 hours. If stitches are not needed, you can clean and bandage the cut at home.

Stopping Severe Bleeding

- Wash your hands well with soap and water. Put on medical gloves or place several layers of fabric or plastic bags between your hands and the wound.
- Elevate the site that is bleeding.
- Remove any visible objects from the surface of the wound. Do not attempt to clean out the wound.
- Press firmly on the wound with a clean cloth or the cleanest material available. If there is an object deep in the wound, apply pressure around the object, not directly over it.
- Apply steady pressure for a full 15 minutes. Don't peek after a few minutes to see if bleeding has stopped. If the bleeding does not seem to be slowing down during this time, **call 911 or seek other emergency services immediately**. Continue to apply pressure to the wound. If blood soaks through the cloth, apply another cloth without lifting the first one.
- If severe bleeding decreases after you apply pressure for 15 minutes, but minimal bleeding starts again once you release the pressure, apply direct pressure to the wound for another 15 minutes. Direct pressure may be applied up to 3 times (total of 45 minutes) for minimal bleeding. If bleeding (more than just oozing small amounts of blood) continues after 45 minutes of direct pressure, call a health professional.
- Watch for signs of shock. See page 67.

Home Treatment

- Wash the cut well with soap and water. Treat an animal bite like a puncture wound. See page 65.
- Stop any bleeding by applying direct, continuous pressure over the wound for 15 minutes.
- If you think the cut may need stitches, see a health professional (see "Are Sutures Necessary?" on page 49). If the cut does not need stitches, proceed with home treatment.
- Consider bandaging the cut, especially if it is in an area that may get dirty or irritated.
- If a cut needs bandaging, but not stitches, apply antibiotic ointment (such as Polysporin or Bacitracin). The ointment will keep the cut from sticking to the bandage. Do not use rubbing alcohol, hydrogen peroxide, iodine, or mercurochrome, which can harm tissue and slow healing.
- Use an adhesive strip (such as Band-Aid) to provide continuous pressure. Always put an adhesive strip across a cut rather than lengthwise. A butterfly bandage (made at home or purchased) can help hold cut skin edges together:
  - Using a clean scissors, cut a strip from a roll of 1-inch adhesive tape and fold it sticky side out. Cut notches into the tape as shown in illustration A on page 48.

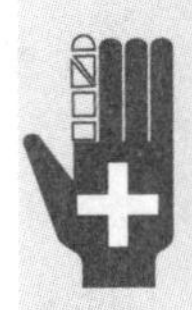

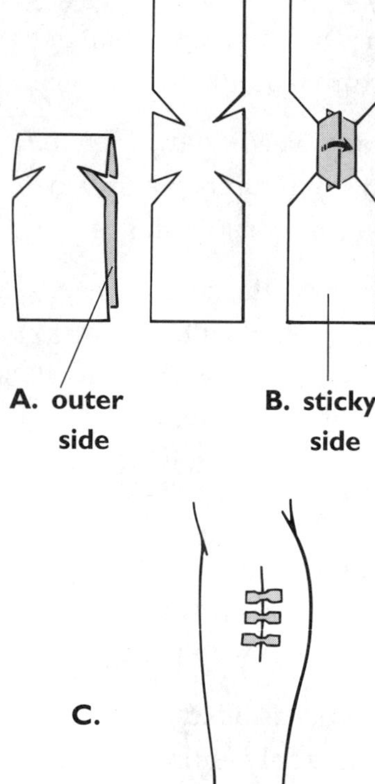

Butterfly bandages are best for closing a long cut.

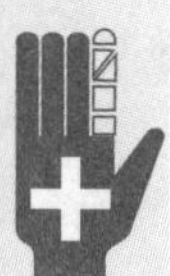

- Unfold the tape; then fold the notched pieces together, sticky side in as in illustration B on page 48. The center of the tape will not be sticky. Keep the part that will be over the cut clean.
- Place one end of the tape on the skin. Then pull the other end to close the wound tightly as in illustration C on page 48.
- If the cut is long, use more than one bandage.

- Apply a clean bandage at least once a day, or when the old bandage gets wet or dirty.

When to Call Kaiser Permanente

- If a person who has been cut goes into shock, even if bleeding has stopped. See Shock on page 67.
- If a cut continues to bleed through bandages after you apply direct pressure for 15 minutes.
- If the skin near the wound is blue, white, or cold; if you have numbness, tingling, loss of feeling; or if you are unable to move a limb below the wound.
- If the cut contains, or might contain, foreign objects such as wood or gravel.
- If the cut needs stitches. Stitches usually need to be done within 8 hours.
- If you have been cut and your tetanus shots are not up to date. See page 16. If you need a tetanus booster, you should have it within 2 days of being injured.
- If signs of infection develop:
  - Increased pain, swelling, redness, or tenderness.
  - Heat or red streaks extending away from the cut.
  - Discharge of pus.
  - Fever of 100° or higher with no other cause.

Are Sutures Necessary?

For best results, cuts that need stitches should be sutured within 8 hours. Wash the cut well with soap and water and stop the bleeding; then pinch the sides of the cut together. If it looks better, you may want to consider stitches. If stitches are needed, avoid using an antibiotic ointment until after a health professional has examined the cut.

Sutures may be needed for:

- Deep cuts (more than ¼ inch deep) that have jagged edges or gape open.
- Deep cuts on a joint: elbow, knuckle, knee.
- Deep cuts on the palm side of the hand or fingers.
- Cuts on the face, eyelids, or lips.
- Cuts in an area where you are worried about scarring, especially the face.
- Cuts that go down to the muscle or bone.
- Cuts that continue to bleed after you apply direct pressure for 15 minutes.

Cuts like these that are sutured usually heal with less scarring than similar cuts that are not sutured.

Sutures may not be needed for:

- Cuts with smooth edges that tend to stay together during normal movement of the affected body part.
- Shallow cuts that are less than ¼ inch deep and less than 1 inch long.

Electrical Burns

Electrical burns are a medical emergency. An electrical burn may look minor on the outside, but electricity can cause serious internal damage, including burns and heart rhythm disturbances.

Prevention

- Keep electrical cords out of the reach of small children and pets. Plug bare electrical sockets with plastic inserts.
- Have frayed power cords on electric appliances replaced.
- Unplug lamps before replacing light bulbs. Turn off the power at the circuit breaker when replacing bulbs in ceiling or wall lights.
- Unplug all appliances (including your computer) when making minor repairs.
- During a lightning storm, take cover inside a car, large building, or house, or seek low ground. Do not stand under a tree during a lightning storm.

Home Treatment

- Do not approach a victim who has been electrocuted until you are sure the area surrounding the victim is safe. Disconnect the power source if possible. If you feel tingling in your lower body, turn around and hop to a safe place.
- Do not attempt to move wires off of a victim unless you are sure the power has been disconnected.

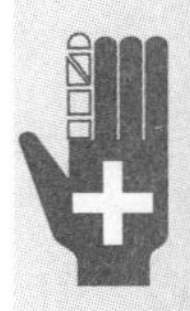

- If it is safe to approach the victim, check ABCs (Airway, Breathing, Circulation). If necessary, begin rescue breathing and CPR. See page 36.
- To prevent shock, raise the victim's legs 8 to 12 inches and keep the victim warm.
- Cover burns with dry, sterile dressing.

When to Call Kaiser Permanente

- **Call 911 or seek other emergency services immediately:**
    - If a person who has been electrocuted stops breathing or has no pulse.
    - If a person who has been electrocuted fell and may have a spinal injury.
- Call Kaiser Permanente for any electrical burn. Even an electrical burn that looks minor can be serious and needs to be evaluated.

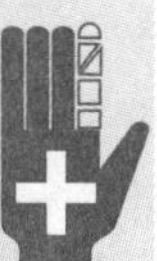

Fishhook Removal

In the excitement of fishing, sometimes fingers are hooked instead of fish. It is useful to know how to remove a fishhook, especially if you are far from medical help.

Home Treatment

Remove the hook as follows:

- Use ice, cold water, or hard pressure to provide temporary numbing.

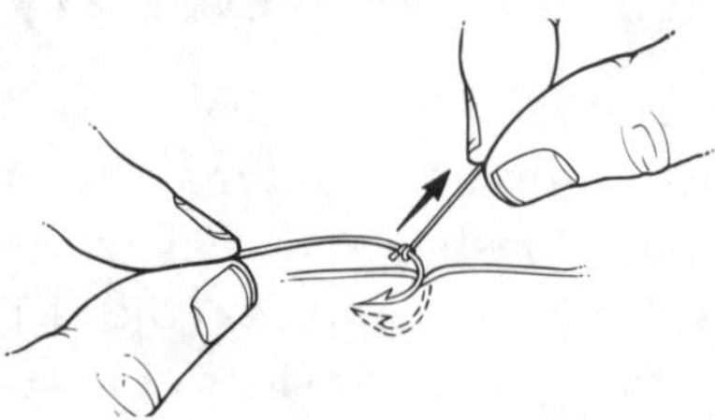

Removing a fishhook

- **Step A:** Tie a piece of fishing line to the hook near the skin's surface.
- **Step B:** Grasp the eye of the hook with one hand and press down about 1/8 of an inch to disengage the barb.
- **Step C:** While still pressing the hook down (barb disengaged), jerk the line near the skin's surface so that the hook shaft leads the barb out of the skin.
- If the fishhook is deeply embedded, another option is to push the hook the rest of the way through the skin, snip off the barb, and then pull the hook out the same way it entered the skin.
- Wash the wound thoroughly with soap if possible. Treat it as a puncture wound. See page 65.
- Do not try to remove a fishhook from an eyeball. Seek medical care immediately.

When to Call Kaiser Permanente

- If the hook is in the eyeball.
- If you cannot remove the hook.
- If your skin was punctured by a fishhook and your tetanus shots are not up to date. See page 16. If

you need a tetanus booster, you should have it within 2 days of being injured.

- If signs of infection develop:
  - Increased pain, swelling, redness, or tenderness.
  - Heat or red streaks extending from the area.
  - Discharge of pus.
  - Fever of 100° or higher with no other cause.

Freeing Trapped Limbs

Fingers, arms, or legs sometimes get caught in objects such as bottles, jars, or pipes. Stay calm; panic will only make the situation worse.

Home Treatment

- Don't try to force the limb from where it is stuck, because doing so will make it swell and become more difficult to remove.
- Try to relax the limb. Relaxation alone will sometimes enable you to free the limb.
- If possible, elevate the limb.
- Apply ice around the exposed part of the limb. This may reduce any swelling and allow the limb to be released.
- If ice doesn't work, dribble soapy water or cooking oil on the limb. Turn the limb or the object so you "unscrew" it rather than pulling it out directly.

When to Call Kaiser Permanente

Call if you are unable to free the trapped limb.

Frostbite

Frostbite is freezing of the skin or underlying tissues that occurs as a result of prolonged exposure to cold.

Frostbitten skin is pale or blue, stiff or rubbery to touch, and feels cold and numb. The severity is divided into 3 degrees:

First degree: Frostnip. Skin is whitish and numb, but there is little likelihood of blistering if it is rewarmed promptly.

Second degree: Superficial frostbite. Outer skin feels hard and frozen, but tissue underneath has normal resilience. Blistering is likely.

Third degree: Deep frostbite. Skin is white or blotchy and blue. Skin and tissue underneath are hard and very cold.

Prevention

Stay dry and out of the wind in extreme cold, and cover areas of exposed skin. Keep your body's core temperature up:

- Wear layers of clothing. Wool and polypropylene are good insulators. Wear windproof, waterproof outer layers. Wear wool socks and well-fitting, waterproof boots.
- Wear a hat to prevent heat loss from your head. Wear mittens rather than gloves.

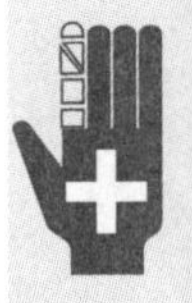

- Keep protective clothing and blankets in your car in case of a breakdown in an isolated area.
- Don't drink alcohol or smoke when you are out in extreme cold.

Home Treatment

- Get inside or take shelter from the wind.
- Check for signs of hypothermia (see page 57) and treat it before treating frostbite.
- Protect the frozen body part from further exposure. Don't rewarm the area if refreezing is possible. Wait until you reach shelter.
- Warm small areas (ears, face, nose, fingers, toes) with warm breath or by tucking hands or feet inside warm clothing next to bare skin.
- Don't rub or massage the frozen area, because doing so will further damage tissues. Avoid walking on frostbitten feet if possible.
- Keep the frostbitten body part warm and elevated. Wrap it with blankets or soft material to prevent bruising. If possible, immerse it in warm water (104° to 108°) for 15 to 30 minutes.
- Blisters may appear as the skin warms. Do not break them. The skin may turn red, burn, tingle, or be very painful. Aspirin or acetaminophen may help.

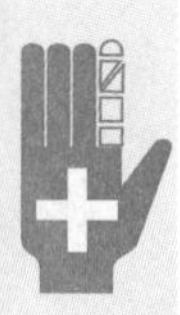

When to Call Kaiser Permanente

- If the skin is white or blue, hard, and cold (third-degree frostbite). Careful rewarming and antibiotic treatment are needed to prevent permanent tissue damage and infection.
- If blisters develop during rewarming (second- or third-degree frostbite). Do not break blisters. The risk of infection is very high.
- If signs of infection develop:
  - Increased pain, swelling, redness, or tenderness.
  - Heat or red streaks extending from the area.
  - Discharge of pus.
  - Fever of 100° or higher with no other cause.

Head Injuries

Most bumps on the head are minor and heal as easily as bumps anywhere else. Head injuries that cause cuts often bleed heavily because the blood vessels of the scalp are close to the skin's surface. In children, blood loss from a scalp injury may be enough to cause symptoms of shock.

Head injuries that do not cause visible external bleeding may have caused life-threatening bleeding and swelling inside the skull. Anyone who has experienced a head injury should be watched carefully for 24 hours for signs of a severe head injury.

Prevention

- Wear a seat belt when in a motor vehicle. Use child safety seats.
- Wear a helmet while biking, motorcycling, and skating.
- Don't dive into shallow or unfamiliar water.

Home Treatment

- If the victim is unconscious, assume he or she has a spinal injury. Do not move the victim without first protecting the neck from movement (see page 69). Check for other injuries.
- If there is bleeding, apply firm pressure directly over the wound with a clean cloth or bandage for 15 minutes. If the blood soaks through, apply additional cloths over the first one. See "Stopping Severe Bleeding" on page 47.
- Apply ice or cold packs to reduce the swelling. A "goose egg" may appear anyway, but ice will help ease the pain.
- For the first 24 hours after a head injury, watch the victim for signs of a severe head injury. Check for the following every 2 hours:
    - Confusion. Ask the person his or her name, address, age, the date, etc.
    - Inability to move the arms and legs on one side of the body, or slower movement of the limbs on one side than on the other.
    - Lethargy, abnormally deep sleep, or difficulty waking up.
    - Vomiting that continues after the first 2 hours, or violent vomiting that persists after the first 15 minutes.
    - Seizures or convulsions.
- Continue observing the person every 2 hours during the night. Wake the person up and check for any unusual symptoms. **Call 911 or go to an emergency room immediately** if you cannot wake the person or if he or she has any of the above symptoms.
- Check for injuries to other parts of the body, especially if the person has fallen. The alarm from seeing a head injury may cause you to overlook other injuries that need attention.

When to Call Kaiser Permanente

- If the person loses consciousness at any time after being injured.
- If double vision or speech difficulty persists after the first minute.
- If weakness or numbness occurs on one side of the body.
- If blood or clear fluid drains from the ears or nose following a blow to the head (not due to a cut or direct blow to the nose).
- If the person is confused or does not remember being injured.
- If the person develops a severe headache.
- If vomiting occurs after the first 2 hours or violent vomiting persists after the first 15 minutes.

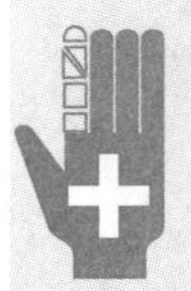

- If the person has seizures or convulsions.
- If bleeding cannot be stopped (see page 47) or the wound needs stitches (see page 49).

Heart Attack

Call 911 or seek other emergency services immediately if you think you may be having a heart attack. A heart attack (myocardial infarction) is caused by a complete blockage of the blood flow to a part of the heart muscle. This usually occurs when a small blood clot forms in one of the blood vessels that supply the heart muscle.

Many people mistake heart attack symptoms for other problems, such as indigestion, heartburn, or a pulled muscle. It is important to recognize the signals your body sends during the early stages of a heart attack and

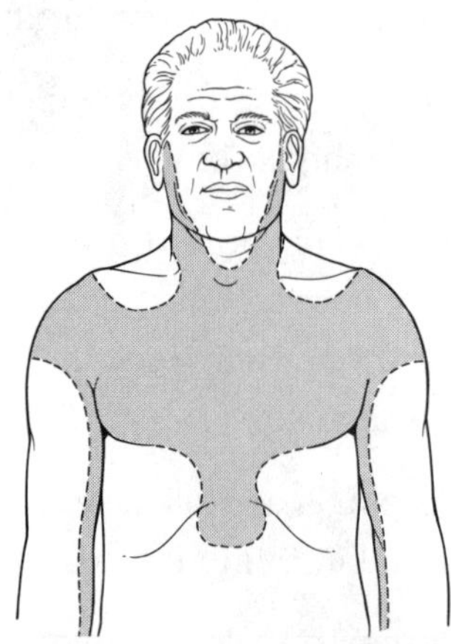

Discomfort caused by a heart attack can occur in any of the shaded areas, as well as the upper back.

Am I Having a Heart Attack?

You may be having a heart attack if you feel **any** of these symptoms:

Chest discomfort or pain that:

❑ Lasts longer than 20 minutes AND is not relieved by rest or nitroglycerin AND feels like:
- Pressure
- Tightness
- Squeezing
- Crushing
- Intense burning
- Aching

In addition to the symptoms above, you may also have:

❑ Pain radiating to your:
- Back
- Shoulder
- Neck
- Jaw/teeth
- Arm
- Wrist

❑ Sweating

❑ Shortness of breath

❑ Dizziness

❑ Fainting

❑ Nausea (feeling sick to your stomach)

❑ Vomiting (throwing up)

❑ Unusual weakness

❑ Rapid and/or irregular heartbeat

❑ Sense of doom

The more boxes you check, the more likely it is that you are having a heart attack. There may be other explanations for chest pain, but it is important to get medical help **immediately**.

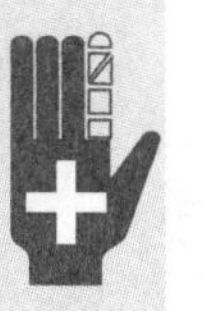

seek emergency care. Medical treatment is needed **immediately** to prevent muscle damage or death. Sometimes, medications can be given to avoid the heart muscle damage caused by a heart attack.

Heat Exhaustion and Heat Stroke

Heat exhaustion occurs when your body cannot sweat enough to cool you off. It generally develops when you are working or exercising in hot weather. Symptoms include:

- Fatigue, weakness, headache, dizziness, or nausea.
- Skin that is cool, moist, pale, or flushed.

Heat exhaustion can sometimes lead to **heat stroke**, which requires emergency treatment. Heat stroke happens when you stop sweating and your body temperature continues to rise, often to 105° or higher. Symptoms of heat stroke include:

- Confusion, delirium, or unconsciousness.
- Skin that is red, hot, and dry, even under the armpits.

Prevention

- Avoid strenuous physical activity outdoors during the hottest part of the day.
- Wear light-colored, loose-fitting clothing to reflect the sun.
- Avoid sudden changes of temperature. Air out a hot car before getting into it.
- If you take diuretics, ask your physician about taking a lower dose during hot weather.
- Drink 8 to 10 glasses of water per day. Drink even more if you are working or exercising in hot weather.
- If you exercise strenuously in hot weather, drink more liquid than your thirst seems to require. For example, runners should drink about 1 cup of water 10 to 15 minutes before running and another cup of water every 2 miles or so.

Home Treatment

- Get out of the sun to a cool spot, and drink lots of cool water, a little at a time. If you are nauseated or dizzy, lie down.
- If a person's temperature exceeds 102°, call for immediate help and try to lower the temperature as quickly as possible:
    - Apply cool (not cold) water to the person's whole body; then fan the person. Or apply ice packs to the groin, neck, and armpits. Do not immerse the person in ice water.
    - If you can get the person's temperature down to 102°, take care to avoid overcooling. Stop cooling the person once his or her temperature is lowered to 98.6°.

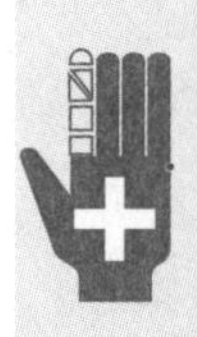

- Do not give aspirin or acetaminophen to reduce the temperature.
- Watch for signs of heat stroke (confusion or unconsciousness; red, hot, dry skin).
- If the person stops breathing, call for immediate help and start rescue breathing (see page 36).

When to Call Kaiser Permanente

Call 911 or seek other emergency services immediately if the person's body temperature reaches 102° and keeps rising, or if signs of heat stroke develop:

- Confusion, disorientation, unconsciousness.
- Skin that is red, hot, and dry, even under the armpits.

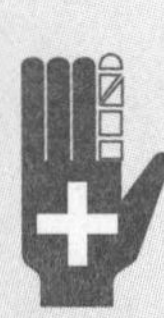

Hyperventilation

When you breathe very fast and deep (hyperventilate), the carbon dioxide (CO_2) level in your blood can drop too low. Symptoms that may occur with hyperventilation include:

- Numbness or tingling in your hands, feet, or around your mouth or tongue.
- Pounding, racing heartbeat and anxiety.
- Feeling like you can't get enough air.
- Lightheadedness (feeling like you might pass out).
- Chest pain.
- Loss of consciousness (if hyperventilation is severe).

Prevention

If you have hyperventilated before:

- Ask people to tell you if you start to breathe too fast.
- As soon as you notice fast breathing or other symptoms, slow your breathing to 1 breath every 5 seconds, or slow enough that symptoms gradually go away.

Home Treatment

- Sit down and concentrate on slowing your breathing. Try breathing through pursed lips or through your nose.
- Practice a relaxation technique. See page 328.
- Hold a paper bag over your nose and mouth and take 6 to 12 easy, natural breaths. This will help bring the amount of CO_2 in your blood back to normal. Continue doing this off and on for 5 to 15 minutes. Do not breathe continuously into the bag. Do not use this technique at all if you have heart or lung problems or if you are at an altitude above 6,000 feet.

When to Call Kaiser Permanente

- If hyperventilation occurs in a person who doesn't appear tense or anxious. See page 312 to help determine if a person is anxious.

- If anxiety and hyperventilation are frequent and interfere with your daily activities.

Hypothermia

Hypothermia occurs when your body temperature drops below normal. It develops when your body loses heat faster than heat can be produced by metabolism, muscle contractions, and shivering.

Early symptoms indicating mild to moderate hypothermia include:

- Shivering
- Cold, pale skin
- Apathy (listlessness)
- Impaired judgment

Later symptoms of severe hypothermia include:

- Cold abdomen
- Slow pulse and breathing
- Weakness or drowsiness
- Confusion

Shivering may stop if your body temperature drops below 90°.

Hypothermia is an emergency. It can quickly lead to unconsciousness and death if the heat loss continues. Hypothermia can happen at temperatures of 45° or even higher in wet and windy weather. Frail and inactive people can develop hypothermia indoors if they are not dressed warmly.

Taking a Pulse

The pulse is the rate at which a person's heart beats. As the heart pumps blood through the body, you can feel a throbbing in the arteries wherever they come close to the skin's surface. Most of the time, the pulse is taken at the wrist, neck, or upper arm.

- Count the pulse after a person has been sitting or resting quietly for 5 to 10 minutes.
- Place 2 fingers gently against the wrist as shown (don't use your thumb).
- If it is hard to feel the pulse in the wrist, locate the carotid artery in the neck, just to either side of the windpipe. Press gently.
- Count the beats for 30 seconds; then double the result to calculate beats per minute.

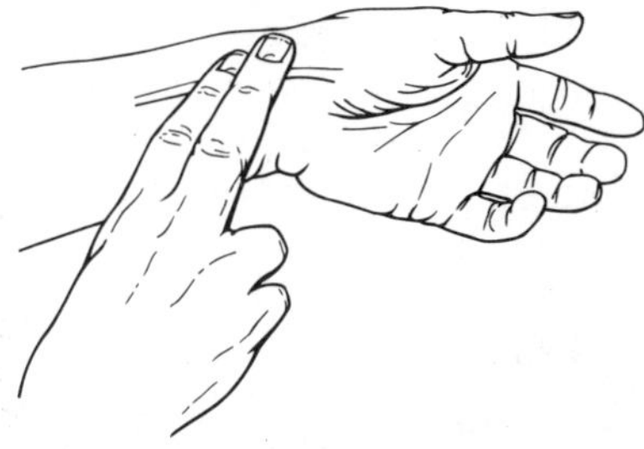

Normal resting pulse:

- Newborn to 12 months: 100–160 beats/minute
- 1 through 6 years: 65–140 beats/minute
- 7 through 10 years: 60–110 beats/minute
- 11 years through adult: 50–100 beats/minute

Certain illnesses can cause the pulse to increase, so it is helpful to know what your resting pulse rate is when you are well. The pulse rate rises about 10 beats per minute for every degree of fever.

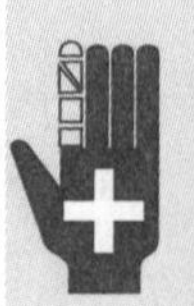

Early recognition is very important in the treatment of hypothermia. Often a hiker or skier will lose heat to a critical degree before others notice anything is wrong. If someone starts to shiver violently, stumble, or respond incoherently to questions, suspect hypothermia and warm the person quickly.

Prevention

Whenever you plan to be outdoors for several hours in cold weather, take the following precautions:

- Dress warmly and wear windproof, waterproof clothing. Wear fabrics that remain warm even when wet, such as wool or polypropylene.
- Wear a warm hat. An unprotected head loses a great deal of the body's total heat.
- Head for shelter if you get wet or cold.
- Eat well before going out and carry extra food.
- Don't drink alcohol while in the cold. Alcohol makes your body lose heat faster.
- Older or less active people can prevent indoor hypothermia by dressing warmly and keeping room temperatures above 65°.

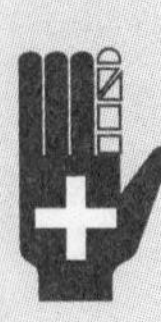

Home Treatment

The goal of home or "in-the-field" treatment is to stop additional heat loss and slowly rewarm the person. Warming 1° per hour is best.

- For mild cases, get the person out of the cold and wind. Give the person dry or wool clothing to wear.
- For moderate cases, remove cold, wet clothes first. Then warm the person with your own body heat by wrapping a blanket or sleeping bag around both of you.
- Give warm liquids to drink and high-energy foods, such as candy, to eat. Do not give food or drink if the person is disoriented or unconscious. Do not give alcoholic beverages.
- Rewarming the person in warm water can cause shock or heart attack. However, in emergency situations when help is not available and other home treatments are not working, you can use a warm water bath (100° to 105°) as a last resort.

When to Call Kaiser Permanente

Call 911 or seek other emergency services immediately if the person seems confused or loses consciousness and remains unconscious.

Call Kaiser Permanente:

- If the victim is a child or an older adult. It's a good idea to call regardless of the severity of the symptoms.
- If the person's body temperature does not return to normal after 4 hours of warming.

Insect and Spider Bites and Stings

Insect and spider bites and bee, yellow jacket, and wasp stings usually cause a localized reaction with pain, swelling, redness, and itching. In some people, especially children, the redness and swelling may be worse, and the local reaction may last up to a few days. In most cases, bites and stings do not cause reactions all over the body. (In a few areas, mosquitoes may spread illnesses, including encephalitis and malaria.)

Some people have severe skin reactions to insect or spider bites or stings, and a few have allergic (anaphylactic) reactions that affect the whole body. Symptoms may include hives all over the body; shortness of breath and tightness in the chest; dizziness; wheezing; or swelling of the tongue and face. If these symptoms develop, immediate medical attention is needed.

Spider bites are rarely serious, although any bite may be serious if it causes a person to have an allergic reaction.

Black widow spiders can be up to 2 inches across (although they are generally much smaller) and are shiny black with a red hourglass mark on their undersides. Their bites may cause chills, fever, nausea, and abdominal muscle pain. A person having a severe reaction may have difficulty breathing. People with high blood pressure, elderly people, and children have the greatest risk of having a severe reaction.

Brown recluse (fiddler) spiders are smaller than black widows and have long legs. They are brown with a violin-shaped mark on their heads. Their bites result in intense pain (although the bite itself may be painless) and a blister may develop that turns into a large, open sore. Their bites also may cause nausea, vomiting, headaches, and chills.

Also see Tick Bites on page 71.

Prevention

- To avoid bee stings, wear white or light-colored, solid fabrics. Bees are attracted to dark colors and flowered prints.
- Avoid wearing perfumes and colognes when you are outside.
- Apply an insect repellent containing DEET every few hours when in insect- and spider-infested areas. Use a lower-concentration DEET product for small children and pregnant women. Wash DEET off when you come inside. Alpha Keri and Skin-So-Soft bath oils also seem to repel insects.
- Wear gloves and tuck pants into socks when working in woodpiles, sheds, and basements where spiders are found.

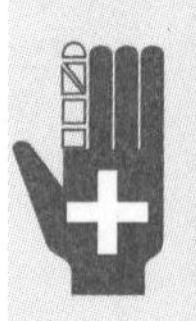

Home Treatment

- Remove a bee stinger by scraping or flicking it out (if the stinger isn't visible, assume there isn't one). Don't squeeze the stinger; you may release more venom into the skin.
- If the bite is from a black widow or brown recluse spider, apply ice to the bite and call your physician.
- Apply a cold pack or ice cube to the bite or sting. Some people also find that applying a paste of baking soda, meat tenderizer, or activated charcoal mixed with a little water helps relieve pain and decrease the reaction.
- Take an oral antihistamine (such as Benadryl or Chlor-Trimeton) to relieve pain, swelling, and itching if there are many bites. Calamine lotion or hydrocortisone cream may also help.
- Carry an emergency kit containing a syringe and adrenaline (epinephrine) if you have had a severe allergic reaction to insect venom in the past. Ask your physician or pharmacist how to use the kit.
- Trim your fingernails to prevent scratching, because scratching can lead to infection.

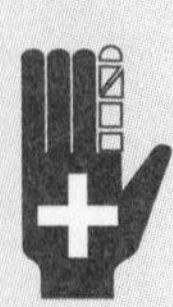

When to Call Kaiser Permanente

Call 911 or seek other emergency services immediately if signs of a severe allergic reaction develop soon after you have been bitten or stung by an insect or spider:

- Wheezing or difficulty breathing.
- Swelling around the lips, tongue, or face, or significant swelling around the site of the bite or sting (e.g., entire arm or leg is swollen).
- Spreading skin rash, itching, feeling of warmth, or hives.

Call Kaiser Permanente:

- If you have been bitten by the same type of spider or insect that previously caused a serious reaction.
- If a blister appears at the site of a spider bite, or if the surrounding skin becomes discolored.
- If symptoms are not improving in 2 to 3 days or if signs of infection develop:
  - Increased pain, swelling, redness, or tenderness.
  - Heat or red streaks extending from the area.
  - Discharge of pus.
  - Fever of 100° or higher with no other cause.
- To talk about adrenaline kits or allergy shots (immunotherapy) for insect venom if you have had a serious allergic reaction.

Nosebleeds

Nosebleeds are inconvenient and messy, but they can usually be stopped with home treatment. Some common causes of nosebleeds are low humidity, colds and allergies, blows to the nose, medications (especially aspirin), high altitude, and blowing or picking your nose.

Prevention

- Low humidity is a common cause of nosebleeds. Humidify your home, especially the bedrooms, and keep the heat low (60° to 64°) in sleeping areas.
- If your nose becomes very dry, breathe moist air for a while (e.g., in the shower) and then put a little petroleum jelly on the inside of your nose to help prevent bleeding. A saline nasal spray may also help. See page 346.
- Limit your use of aspirin, which can contribute to nosebleeds.

Home Treatment

- Sit up straight and tip your head slightly forward. Tilting your head back may cause blood to run down your throat.
- Blow all the clots out of your nose. Pinch your nostrils shut between your thumb and forefinger or apply firm pressure against the bleeding nostril for 10 full minutes. Resist the urge to peek after a few minutes to see if your nose has stopped bleeding.

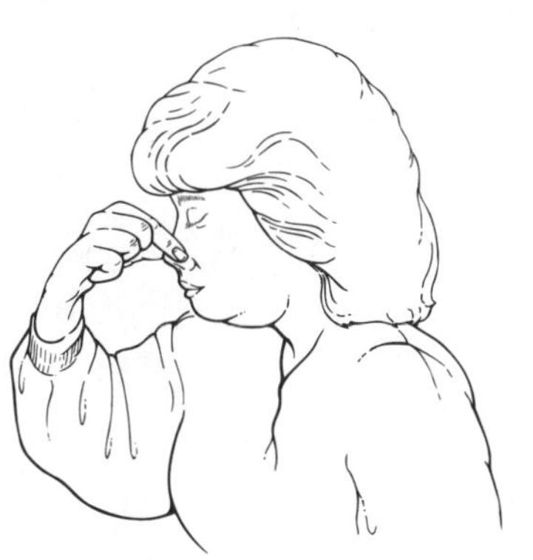

Stopping a nosebleed

- After 10 minutes, check to see if your nose is still bleeding. If it is, hold it for 10 more minutes. Most nosebleeds will stop after you apply direct pressure for 10 to 30 minutes.
- Stay quiet for a few hours and do not blow your nose for at least 12 hours after the bleeding has stopped.

When to Call Kaiser Permanente

- If the bleeding hasn't stopped after you have applied direct pressure for 30 minutes.
- If blood runs down the back of your throat even when you pinch your nose.
- If your nose is deformed after an injury and may be broken.
- If nosebleeds recur often.

Objects in the Ear

Children sometimes put small objects in their ears, or an insect may crawl into the ear. It may be hard to know if an insect is in the ear. Your child may say, "My ear is bumping around."

Home Treatment

- Don't try to kill an insect inside a person's ear. Pull the ear up and back and point it toward the sun or a bright light. Insects are attracted to light, so the insect may crawl out.

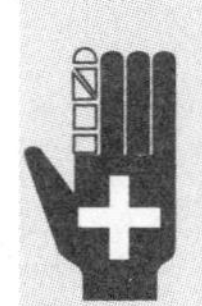

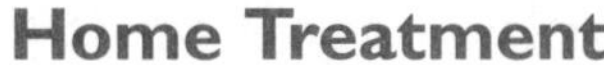

- If the insect doesn't crawl out, fill the ear canal with mineral, olive, or baby oil. The insect may float out.
- To remove other objects from the ear, tilt the person's head to the side and shake it gently. Gently pulling the ear up and back may straighten the ear canal and help dislodge the object.
- If the object is soft and can be easily seen, try carefully to remove it with tweezers. Do not try this if the person will not hold very still or if the object is in the ear so far that you can't see the tips of the tweezers. Use care not to push the object in farther.

When to Call Kaiser Permanente

Call if you cannot remove the insect or object.

Objects in the Eye

A speck of dirt or small object in the eye will often wash out with your tears. If the object is not removed, it may scratch the eye (corneal abrasion). Most corneal abrasions are minor and will heal on their own in 1 to 2 days.

When an object is thrown forcefully into the eye (e.g., from a machine), it is likely that the eyeball will be punctured and emergency care will be needed.

Home Treatment

- Wash your hands before touching the eye.
- Don't rub the eye; you could scratch the cornea. You may have to restrain a small child to keep the child from rubbing his or her eye.
- Do not try to remove an object that is on the colored part of the eye or stuck in the white of the eye. Call a health professional.
- If the object is at the side of the eye or on the lower lid, moisten a cotton swab or the tip of a twisted piece of tissue and touch the end to the object. The object should cling to the swab or tissue. Some minor irritation is common after you have removed the object.
- Gently wash the eye with cool water. An eyedropper helps.
- Never use tweezers, toothpicks, or other hard items to remove an object from the eye. Eye damage may result.

When to Call Kaiser Permanente

Call 911 or seek other emergency services immediately if the eyeball seems to be punctured.

Call Kaiser Permanente:

- If the object is on the colored part of the eye or is embedded in the eye. Do not pull out an object that is stuck in the eye.
- If you cannot remove the object.

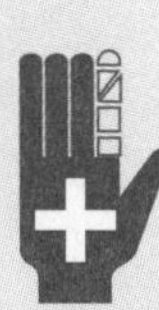

- If pain is severe or persists; if it feels like there is still something in your eye; if your eye is sensitive to light; or if your vision is blurred after the object has been removed. Your cornea may be scratched. Keep your eye closed.

Objects in the Nose

Children sometimes put small objects, like beads or popcorn, up their noses. If the child doesn't tell you about it, your first clue may be a foul-smelling, green or yellow discharge from just one nostril. The nose may also be tender and swollen.

Home Treatment

- Have the child pinch the other nostril closed and try to blow the object out.
- If you can see the object, try to remove it with blunt-nosed tweezers. Hold the child's head still and use care not to push the object in farther. If the child resists, do not try tweezers. Minor bleeding from the nostril is not serious.
- Spray a nasal decongestant (see page 346) in the affected nostril to reduce the swelling, unless you suspect the object is a disc battery.

When to Call Kaiser Permanente

- If a disc battery is stuck in the nose. The moist tissue in the nose can cause the battery to release harmful chemicals, often in less than an hour.
- If you are unable to remove the object after several tries.
- If removing the object causes a severe nosebleed. See page 60.

Poisoning

FOR ANY POISONING: Call 911 or your local poison control center immediately.

Children will swallow just about anything, including poisons. When in doubt, assume the worst.

Always believe a child who indicates that he or she has swallowed poison, no matter how unappetizing the substance is.

If you suspect food poisoning, see page 93.

Prevention

About 80 percent of poisonings occur in children between the ages of 1 and 4. Develop poison prevention habits before your child is born or certainly before he or she is crawling. Infants grow so fast that sometimes they are crawling and walking before you have time to protect them.

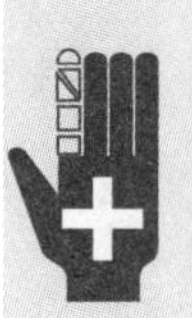

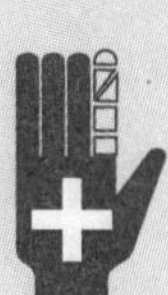

Carbon Monoxide Poisoning

Carbon monoxide is a colorless, odorless, tasteless gas produced from burning fuels such as natural gas, gasoline, fuel oil, or wood. If fuel-burning appliances are not used properly, dangerous levels of carbon monoxide can build up in enclosed areas.

When a person inhales carbon monoxide, the carbon monoxide begins to replace the oxygen in the blood. This condition is called carbon monoxide poisoning. Symptoms include headache, dizziness, and nausea. If the exposure to carbon monoxide continues, the person may lose consciousness and even die. Infants, small children, older adults, and people with chronic health problems are more easily affected by high amounts of carbon monoxide in the blood, and their symptoms may be more severe.

A good way to protect yourself and your family from carbon monoxide poisoning is to install a carbon monoxide detector in your home. Also, have your heating appliances, chimneys, and vents inspected each year. Do not leave your car's engine running when the car is in an enclosed area such as a garage, even if the garage door is open.

If you know or suspect that someone has carbon monoxide poisoning, seek medical care immediately.

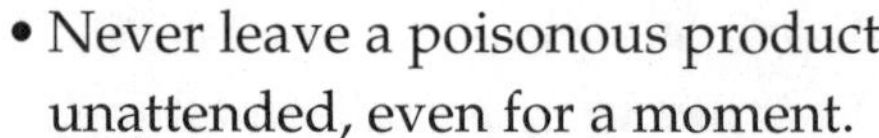

- Never leave a poisonous product unattended, even for a moment.
- Lock all drugs and vitamins away from children. Aspirin is the most common source of childhood poisoning, especially flavored baby aspirin. Lock up drugs between doses.
- Do not keep poisons, such as drain opener, dishwasher detergent, oven cleaner, or plant food, under your kitchen sink. Keep them completely out of the reach of children. Dishwasher detergent is especially dangerous.
- Keep products in their original containers. Never store poisonous products in food containers.
- Use childproof latches on your cupboards.
- Use "Mr. Yuk" stickers and teach your children to recognize them.
- Purchase syrup of ipecac (see page 350), and keep the poison control center number near your phone.

Home Treatment

- Call a poison control center or Kaiser Permanente immediately. Have the poison container with you so you can describe the poison. You will be told whether it is safe to make the person vomit.
- Do not have the person vomit if he or she:
  - Is having convulsions.
  - Is unconscious.

  - Has a burning sensation in the mouth or throat.
  - Has swallowed a corrosive agent or petroleum product (dishwasher detergent, lye, bleach, disinfectant, drain opener, floor wax, kerosene, grease remover).
- If suggested by the poison control center, induce vomiting by:
  - Giving syrup of ipecac, if available. See page 350.
  - Placing a spoon or finger at the back of the person's throat.
- When vomiting begins, place the person's head lower than his or her chest to keep vomited material from entering the lungs.

Puncture Wounds

Puncture wounds are caused by sharp, pointed objects that penetrate the skin. Nails, tacks, ice picks, knives, needles, and animal bites can all cause puncture wounds. Puncture wounds become infected easily because they are difficult to clean and provide a warm, moist place for bacteria to grow.

Home Treatment

- Make sure nothing is left in the wound, such as the tip of a needle. Check to see if the object is intact.
- Allow the wound to bleed freely to clean itself out, unless there has been a large loss of blood or the blood is squirting out. If bleeding is heavy, see "Stopping Severe Bleeding" on page 47.

Lead Poisoning

Infants and young children who eat or drink things that contain lead are at risk for developing learning disabilities and growth problems.

Lead is present in old paint, water pipes, and other substances. Lead-based paint may be a hazard in older homes, especially if the paint is flaking or peeling and a child eats the paint flakes.

To reduce the risk of lead poisoning:

- Keep painted surfaces in good repair. Clean paint flakes and chips from older painted surfaces (such as floors and windowsills) carefully.
- Keep young children away from home remodeling and refinishing projects.
- If your home has lead or lead-soldered water pipes, use cold water and let the water run for a few minutes before using it for cooking or formula.
- Have your child's blood tested for lead at about 1 year of age.
- Call your local health department for more information about preventing lead poisoning.

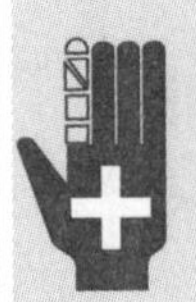

- Clean the wound thoroughly with soap and water.
- Watch for signs of infection (see When to Call Kaiser Permanente on page 66). If the wound closes, an infection under the skin may not be detected for several days.

When to Call Kaiser Permanente

- If the wound is in your head, neck, chest, or abdomen, unless it is minor.
- If the skin near the wound is blue, white, or cold; if there is numbness, tingling, loss of feeling; or if you are unable to move a limb below the wound.
- If an animal bite is severe and may need stitches, or if it is on your face, hand, or foot. Stitches usually need to be done in 8 hours.
- If you are unable to remove an object from the wound or if you think part of the object may still be in the wound.
- If the wound was caused by a cat or human bite.
- If you have a puncture wound and your tetanus shots are not up to date (see page 16).
- If a deep wound to the foot occurred through a shoe.
- If signs of infection develop:
  - Increased pain, swelling, redness, or tenderness.
  - Heat or red streaks extending from the wound.
  - Discharge of pus.
  - Fever of 100° or higher with no other cause.

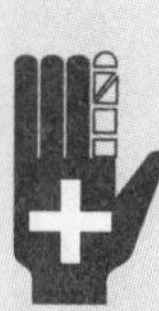

Scrapes

Scrapes or abrasions happen so often that they seem unimportant. Good home treatment will reduce scarring and prevent infection.

Home Treatment

- Scrapes are usually very dirty. Remove large pieces of debris with tweezers. Then scrub vigorously with soap and water and a washcloth. The injured person will probably complain loudly, but cleaning is necessary to prevent infection and scarring. Using a water sprayer from the kitchen sink is a good way to wash a scrape.
- Apply steady pressure with a clean bandage or cloth to stop bleeding.
- Applying ice may help reduce swelling and bruising.
- If the scrape is large or in an area that may be rubbed by clothing, apply an antibiotic ointment to the scrape and cover it with a non-stick (such as Telfa) bandage.

When to Call Kaiser Permanente

- If your tetanus shots are not up to date. See page 16.
- If the scrape is very large and dirty.

- If you cannot remove dirt and debris that are embedded under the skin. They may cause permanent skin discoloration or infection if they are not removed.
- If signs of infection develop:
  - Increased pain, swelling, redness, or tenderness.
  - Heat or red streaks extending from the scrape.
  - Discharge of pus.
  - Fever of 100° or higher with no other cause.

Removing Splinters

If you can grasp the end of the splinter with tweezers, gently pull it out. If the splinter is embedded in the skin, clean a needle with alcohol and make a small hole in the skin over the end of the splinter. Then lift the splinter with the tip of the needle until it can be grasped with the tweezers and pulled out.

After the splinter has been removed, wash the area with soap and water. Apply a bandage if needed to keep the wound clean; otherwise, leave it open to the air. Watch for signs of infection.

Call a health professional if the splinter is very large or deeply embedded and cannot be easily removed, or if the splinter is in the eye.

Shock

Shock may develop as a result of sudden illness or injury. When the circulatory system is unable to get enough blood to the vital organs, the body goes into shock. Sometimes even a mild injury will lead to shock.

The signs of shock include:

- Cool, pale, clammy skin.
- Weak, rapid pulse.
- Shallow, rapid breathing.
- Low blood pressure.
- Thirst, nausea, or vomiting.
- Confusion or anxiety.
- Faintness, weakness, dizziness, or loss of consciousness.

Shock is a life-threatening condition. Prompt home treatment can save the person's life.

Home Treatment

- Have the person lie down and elevate his or her legs 12 inches or more. If the injury is to the head, neck, or chest, keep the legs flat. If the person vomits, roll the person to one side to let fluids drain from the mouth. Use care if there could be a spinal injury (see page 69).
- Control any bleeding (see Cuts on page 46) and splint any fractures (see page 134).
- Keep the person warm, but not hot. Place a blanket underneath the person, and cover the person with

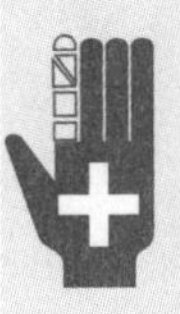

a sheet or blanket, depending on the weather. If the person is in a hot place, try to keep the person cool.

- Take and record the person's pulse every 5 minutes. See page 57.
- Comfort and reassure the person to relieve anxiety.

When to Call Kaiser Permanente

Call 911 or seek other emergency services immediately if the person develops signs of shock.

Counting Respiration Rates

The respiration rate is the number of breaths a person takes in 1 minute. It increases with fever and some illnesses. The best time to count the respiration rate is when a person is resting, perhaps after taking the person's pulse while your fingers are still on the person's wrist. The person's breathing is likely to change if he or she knows you are counting it.

- Count the number of times the chest rises in 1 full minute.
- Notice whether there is any sucking in beneath the ribs or any apparent wheezing or difficulty breathing.

Normal resting respiration rate:

- Newborn to 1 year: 40–60 breaths/minute
- 1 through 6 years: 18–26 breaths/minute
- 7 years through adult: 12–24 breaths/minute

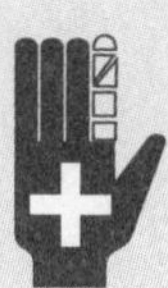

Snake Bites

While thousands of people are bitten by snakes every year in the United States, only about 10 people die as a result. Rattlesnakes inflict most poisonous snake bites. Other poisonous snakes in North America are copperheads, cottonmouths (also called water moccasins), and coral snakes. Even if a poisonous snake bites you, it may not inject poison. However, if your skin is broken by the bite, assume that poison has been injected.

If you are bitten by a snake and it is safe for someone who is with you to kill the snake, have the person do so, and take the dead snake with you when you get medical care. Be very careful when handling the dead snake. The snake's biting reflex remains for up to 60 minutes after it has died. By knowing what kind of snake has bitten you, a health professional can quickly select the correct treatment.

Get medical care as quickly as possible. Medication for snake bites is most effective when given within 4 hours and is less effective after more than 12 hours have passed.

Prevention

- Be aware if the area you are in is inhabited by poisonous snakes.
- Wear high leather boots and long pants when you are in areas that snakes inhabit.

- Do not put your hands or feet anywhere until you can see that it is safe to do so. Do not step over logs or rocks if you cannot see the other side.
- Avoid walking in snake-infested areas at night.
- Do not handle snakes, even if they are dead, unless you know how to identify snakes and know their habits.

Home Treatment

If you think you have been bitten by a poisonous snake:

- Keep calm. Frantic activity will cause the poison to spread faster.
- If possible, lie down and keep the area of the bite lower than your heart.
- Tie a band or strip of cloth around the limb between the bite and the heart. This band should be tight enough to indent the skin like a rubber band, but not tight enough to stop blood flow.
- Do not eat or drink anything, especially alcoholic beverages.
- Get medical attention as soon as possible.
- Snake bite kits are of minimal benefit. Use them only if you have been instructed how to do so by an expert.

When to Call Kaiser Permanente

Call 911 or seek other emergency services immediately if you think that you or someone you are with has just been bitten by a poisonous snake.

Spinal Injuries

Injury to the spine must be considered any time there has been an accident involving the neck or back. Permanent paralysis may be avoided if the injured person is immobilized and transported correctly.

Signs of a spinal injury include:

- Severe pain in the neck or back.
- Bruises on the head, neck, shoulders, or back.
- Weakness, tingling, or numbness in the arms or legs.
- Loss of bowel or bladder control.
- Bleeding or clear fluid discharge from the ears or nose (not due to a cut or direct blow to the nose).
- Loss of consciousness.

Home Treatment

- If you suspect a spinal injury, do not move the person unless there is an immediate threat to life, such as fire. Don't drag victims from automobile accidents.

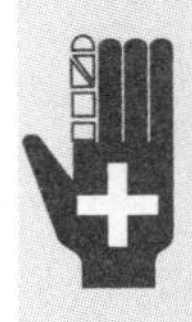

Removing a Ring

If you did not remove a ring before an injured finger started to swell, try the following method to remove the ring:

- Stick the end of a slick piece of string, such as dental floss, under the ring toward your hand.
- Starting at the side of the ring closest to the middle knuckle, wrap the string snugly around your finger, wrapping beyond the middle knuckle. Each wrap should be right next to the one before it.
- Grasp the end of the string that is stretched under the ring and start unwrapping it. Push the ring ahead of the unwrapped string as you go, until the ring passes the middle knuckle.

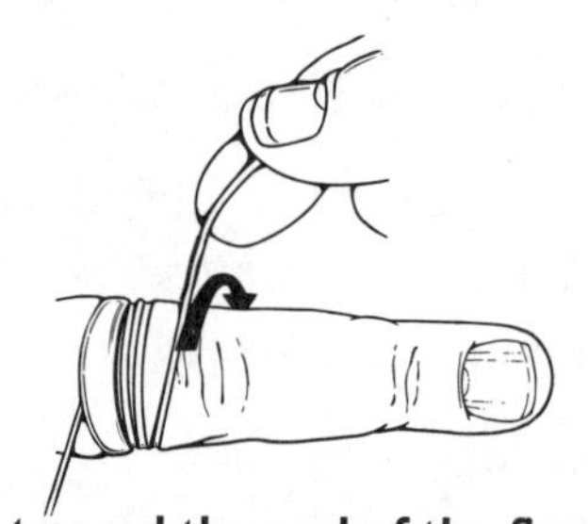

Wrap toward the end of the finger.

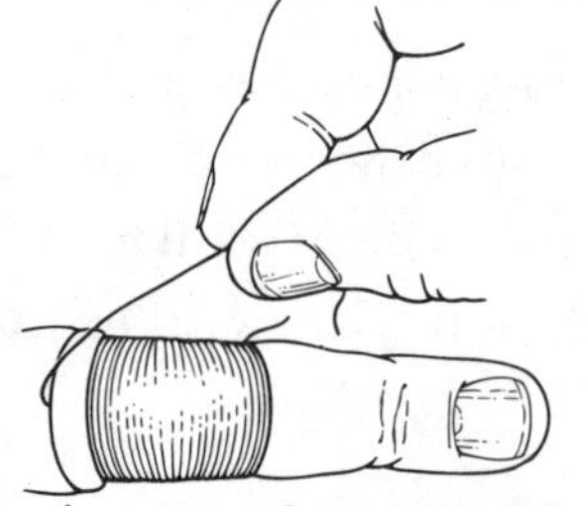

Pull the ring over the wrapped joint.

- If the person is in immediate danger, and must be moved, do whatever you can to move the person's head, neck, and shoulders together as a unit while you move him or her to safety.
- If the person was injured in a diving accident, don't pull the injured person from the water, because you may cause permanent damage. Float the person face up in the water until help arrives. The water will act as a splint and keep the person's spine immobile.

When to Call Kaiser Permanente

Call 911 or seek other emergency services immediately to transport the injured person if you suspect a spinal injury.

Stroke

A stroke occurs when a blood vessel (artery) supplying blood to the brain bursts or becomes blocked by a blood clot. Within minutes, the nerve cells in that area of the brain are damaged and die. As a result, the part of the body controlled by those cells cannot function properly.

A person having symptoms of a stroke needs to seek care immediately. If medical treatment is sought as soon as stroke symptoms are noticed, fewer brain cells may be permanently damaged by the stroke.

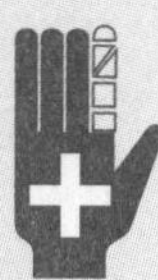

The effects of a stroke may range from mild to severe and may be temporary or permanent. A stroke can affect vision, speech, behavior, thought processes, and the ability to move parts of the body. Sometimes it can cause a coma or death. The effects of a stroke depend on:

- Which brain cells are damaged.
- How much of the brain is affected.
- How quickly blood supply is restored to the affected area.

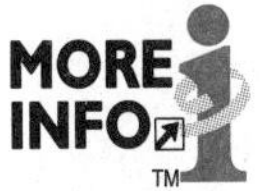

One or more transient ischemic attacks (TIAs) often occur before a person has a stroke. TIAs are often called mini strokes because their symptoms are similar to those of a stroke. However, unlike stroke symptoms, TIA symptoms disappear within minutes (usually within 10 to 20 minutes) to 24 hours. A TIA can occur months before a stroke occurs. The first TIA needs to be treated as an emergency because it is a warning signal that a stroke may soon occur.

When to Call Kaiser Permanente

Call 911 or seek other emergency services immediately if you have any of the following symptoms of stroke:

- Any new weakness, numbness, or paralysis in your face, arm, or leg, especially on only one side of your body.
- Blurred or decreased vision in one or both eyes that does not clear with blinking.
- Newly developed difficulty speaking or understanding simple statements.
- Sudden, unexplainable, and intense headache that is different from any headache you have had before.
- Severe dizziness, loss of balance, or loss of coordination, especially if another warning sign is present at the same time.

If a symptom was definitely there and then went away after a few minutes, call your physician immediately. Symptoms that go away in a few minutes may be caused by a TIA. A TIA is a strong sign that a major stroke may soon occur.

Tick Bites

Ticks are small, spider-like insects that bite into the skin and feed on blood. Ticks live in the fur and feathers of many birds and other animals. Tick bites occur more often from early spring to late summer.

Most ticks do not carry diseases, and most tick bites do not cause serious health problems. However, it is important to remove a tick as soon as you find one.

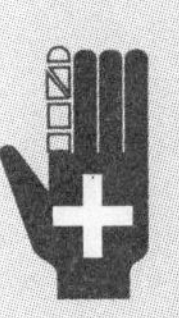

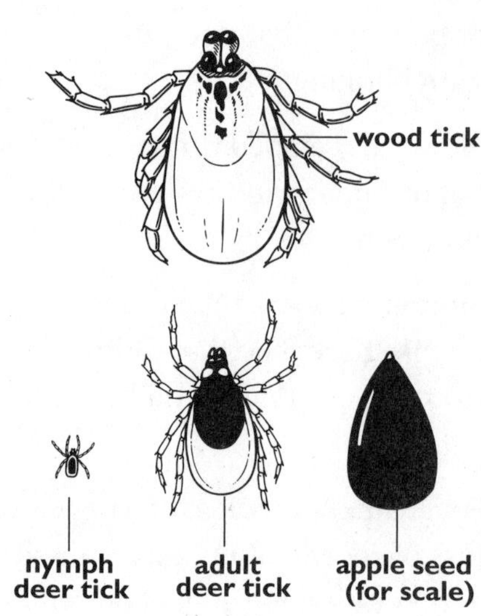

Lyme disease is usually spread by nymph deer ticks, which are difficult to see. Adult deer ticks are about the size of an apple seed. All ticks grow larger as they fill up with blood.

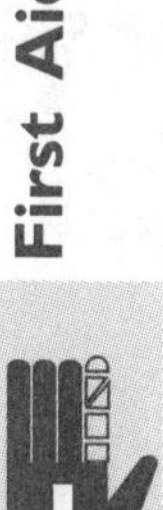

Many of the diseases ticks may pass to humans (including Rocky Mountain spotted fever, relapsing fever, Colorado tick fever, and Lyme disease) have the same flu-like symptoms: fever, headache, muscle aches, and a general feeling of illness. Sometimes a rash or crater-like sore (ulcer) may accompany the flu-like symptoms. An expanding rash that looks like a bull's-eye is an early symptom of Lyme disease. It may appear 1 day to 1 month after you have been bitten by a deer tick. If you develop any of the symptoms described here after being bitten by a tick, be sure to tell your health professional.

Prevention

Before going outdoors in a tick-infested area:

- Put on light-colored clothing and tuck pant legs into socks.
- Apply an insect repellent containing DEET to exposed areas of skin or to clothing. Apply carefully around eyes and mouth.
  - Children and pregnant women should use a lower-concentration DEET product.
  - Don't put repellent on small children's hands, because they often put their hands in their mouths.
  - After returning indoors, wash the repellent off with soap and water.

Home Treatment

- Check regularly for ticks when you are out in the woods, and thoroughly examine your skin and scalp when you return home. Check your pets too. The sooner ticks are removed, the less likely they are to spread infection.
- Remove a tick by gently pulling on it with tweezers, as close to the skin as possible. Pull straight out and try not to crush the body. Save the tick in a jar for tests in case you develop flu-like symptoms after you have been bitten.
- Wash the area and apply an antiseptic.

When to Call Kaiser Permanente

- If you are unable to remove the entire tick.
- If a tick has been attached for more than 24 hours and you live in an area where Lyme disease is common.
- If you develop a red rash that expands over several days, especially if you know you were recently exposed to ticks. The rash may be accompanied by flu-like symptoms, such as fatigue, headache, stiff neck, fever, chills, or body aches.

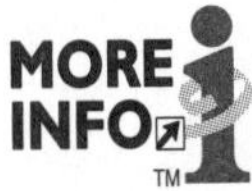
Your physician will probably be able to tell if you have Lyme disease based on your symptoms and whether you may have been exposed to deer ticks. In most cases, blood tests to diagnose Lyme disease are not useful.

Unconsciousness

An unconscious person is completely unaware of what is going on and is unable to make purposeful movements. Fainting is a brief form of unconsciousness; a coma is a deep, prolonged state of unconsciousness.

Causes of unconsciousness include stroke, epilepsy, heat stroke, diabetic coma, insulin shock, head injury, suffocation, alcohol or drug overdose, shock, bleeding, irregular heartbeat, and heart attack.

Fainting is a short-term loss of consciousness, usually lasting only a few seconds. It is most often caused by a momentary drop in blood flow to the brain. When you fall or lie down, blood flow is improved and you regain consciousness. Fainting is a mild form of shock and is usually not serious. If it happens often, there may be a more serious problem. Dizziness and fainting can also be brought on by sudden emotional stress or injury. See page 178.

Home Treatment

- Make sure the unconscious person can breathe. Check for breathing, and if necessary, begin rescue breathing. See page 36.
- Check for signs of circulation, such as coughing, normal breathing, or movement in response to rescue breaths. If there are none, call for help and start cardiopulmonary resuscitation (CPR). See page 36.
- Keep the person lying down.
- Look for a medical identification bracelet, necklace, or card that identifies a medical problem such as epilepsy, diabetes, or drug allergy.
- Treat any injuries.
- Do not give the person anything to eat or drink.

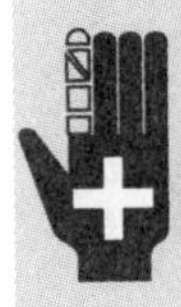

When to Call Kaiser Permanente

Call 911 or seek other emergency services immediately if a person remains unconscious.

Call Kaiser Permanente:

- If a person has completely lost consciousness, even if the person is now awake.
- If unconsciousness follows a head injury and the victim is now awake. A person with a head injury needs to be carefully observed. See page 52.
- Whenever a person with diabetes loses consciousness, even if he or she is now awake. He or she may have insulin shock (low blood sugar) or be in a diabetic coma (too much sugar in the blood).

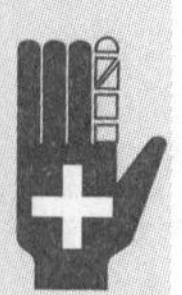

One laughs when joyous, sulks when angry, (is) at peace with all when the stomach is satisfied with food.
Hawaiian proverb

4

Abdominal Problems

The cause of abdominal problems can be hard to pinpoint. Sometimes serious and minor abdominal problems start with the same symptoms. Fortunately, most abdominal problems are minor and home treatment is all that is needed.

Use the chart on page 76 to find the symptoms that most closely match the ones you are having. Some illnesses that can cause abdominal problems are covered more thoroughly in other chapters. Use the chart or the index to find those topics.

Abdominal Pain

You can get clues about the cause of abdominal pain and how serious the problem may be by noting the following:

- The severity of the pain. A visit to a health professional is usually needed when severe abdominal pain comes on suddenly and continues, or when new or different pain becomes more severe over several hours or days.
- The location of the pain. See illustration on page 77.

Generalized pain is pain that occurs in more than half of the abdomen. Generalized pain can occur with many different illnesses, most of which will go away without medical treatment. Heartburn (indigestion) and stomach flu are common problems that can cause generalized abdominal pain. **Cramping**, which can be very painful, is rarely serious if passing gas or a stool relieves it. Many women have cramping pain with their periods. Unless it is significantly different than usual, or it localizes, generalized pain is usually not a cause for concern.

Localized pain is pain that is most intense in one part of the abdomen. Localized pain that comes on suddenly and persists, that gradually becomes more severe, or that gets

Abdominal Problems	
Symptoms	**Possible Causes**
Nausea or vomiting	Nausea and Vomiting, p. 90; Hepatitis, p. 97; Medication reaction—call your physician or pharmacist; Adverse Drug Reactions, p. 353.
Bowel Movements	
Frequent, watery stools	Diarrhea, p. 82; Stomach Flu and Food Poisoning, p. 93; Antibiotics, p. 351.
Stools are dry and difficult to pass	Constipation, p. 78.
Bloody or black, tarry stools	Ulcers, p. 95; Diarrhea, p. 82.
Pain during bowel movements; bright red blood on surface of stool or on toilet paper	Rectal Problems, p. 91.
Abdominal Pain	
Pain and tenderness localized to one place with possible nausea, vomiting, and fever	Appendicitis, p. 77; Urinary Tract Infections, p. 100; Ovarian cyst, p. 77; Gallstones, p. 88; Kidney Stones, p. 85; also see p. 75.
Bloating and gas with diarrhea, constipation, or both	Irritable Bowel Syndrome, p. 87.
Burning or discomfort behind or below breastbone	Heartburn, p. 83; Ulcers, p. 95; Chest Pain, p. 151.
Pain in lower abdomen and lower back just before menstrual period	Menstrual Cramps, p. 262; Ovarian cyst, p. 77.
Pain on one side of lower abdomen with possible pregnancy	Ectopic pregnancy, p. 259.
Urination	
Pain or burning while urinating	Urinary Tract Infections, p. 100; Kidney Stones, p. 85; Prostate problems, pp. 273 to 276; Sexually Transmitted Diseases, p. 283.
Difficulty urinating or weak urine stream (men)	Prostate problems, pp. 273 to 276.
Blood in urine	Urinary Tract Infections, p. 100; Kidney Stones, p. 85; also see p. 102.
Abdominal Lumps or Swelling	
Painless lump or swelling in groin that comes and goes	Hernia, p. 85.
Very rigid or distended abdomen	Blunt Abdominal Wounds, p. 35; Watch for shock, p. 67.

worse when you move or cough may indicate a problem in an abdominal organ, such as appendicitis, pancreatitis, diverticulitis, ovarian cyst, or gallbladder disease.

Any abdominal pain that lasts more than a few days needs to be evaluated by a health professional.

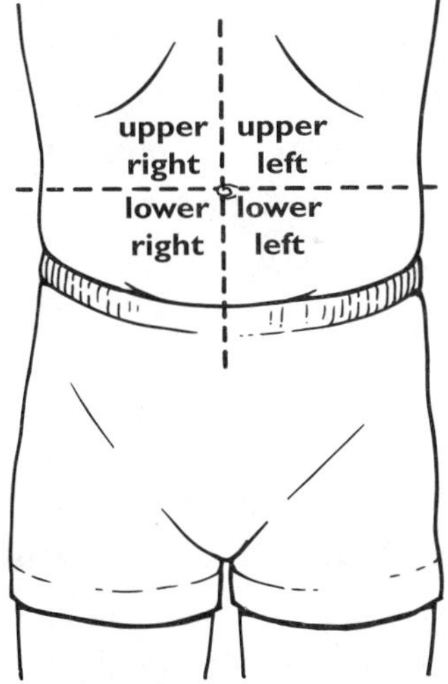

If you have abdominal pain, it helps to tell your physician exactly where the pain is.

Home Treatment

Most of the time, abdominal pain improves with home treatment and does not require a visit to a health professional.

Specific home treatment for abdominal pain often depends on the symptoms that accompany the pain, such as diarrhea or nausea and vomiting. Be sure to review the home treatment guidelines for any other symptoms you have that are covered in this or other chapters.

Appendicitis

Sometimes the appendix becomes inflamed or infected (appendicitis). If not treated, appendicitis can cause the appendix to burst and spread infection throughout the abdomen (peritonitis).

Typical symptoms of appendicitis include:

- Pain in the abdomen that begins around the navel or a little higher. The pain becomes more intense and then moves (localizes) below the navel or to the lower right part of the abdomen. The pain is steady and gets worse when you walk or cough.
- Loss of appetite, nausea, vomiting, and constipation.
- Fever and chills.

Call your health professional:

- If you think you have appendicitis.
- If continuous pain in the lower right abdomen lasts longer than 4 hours.

Also see When to Call Kaiser Permanente on page 78.

If you have mild abdominal pain without other symptoms, try the following:

- Rest until you are feeling better.
- Drink plenty of fluids to avoid dehydration. You may find that taking small, frequent sips of a

beverage is easier on your stomach than trying to drink a whole glass at once.

- Try eating several small meals instead of 2 or 3 large ones. Eat mild foods, such as rice, dry toast or crackers, bananas, and applesauce. Avoid spicy foods, other fruits, alcohol, and drinks that contain caffeine until 48 hours after all symptoms have gone away.

When to Call Kaiser Permanente

Call 911 or seek other emergency services immediately if you have any of the following:

- Signs of shock (see page 67).
- Pain in the upper abdomen with chest pain that is crushing or squeezing, feels like a heavy weight on your chest, or occurs with any other symptoms of a heart attack (see page 54).
- Signs of severe dehydration (see page 80).
- Severe abdominal pain following an injury to the abdomen.

Call Kaiser Permanente if you have:

- Ongoing severe abdominal pain.
- Localized pain that lasts longer than 4 hours.
- Generalized abdominal pain or cramping pain that has lasted longer than 24 hours and is not improving.
- Inability to keep down fluids.
- Pain that gets worse when you move or cough and does not feel like a pulled muscle.
- Any abdominal pain that has lasted longer than 3 days.

Constipation

Constipation occurs when stools are difficult to pass. Some people are overly concerned with frequency because they have been taught that a healthy person has a bowel movement every day. This is not true. Most people pass stools anywhere from 3 times a day to 3 times a week. If your stools are soft and pass easily, you are not constipated.

Constipation may occur with cramping and pain in the rectum caused by straining to pass hard, dry stools. There may be some bloating and nausea. There may also be small amounts of bright red blood on the stools caused by slight tearing as the stools are pushed through the anus. The bleeding should stop when the constipation is relieved.

If a stool becomes lodged in the rectum (impacted), mucus and fluid may leak out around the stool, which sometimes leads to leakage of fecal material (fecal incontinence). You may experience this as constipation alternating with diarrhea.

Lack of fiber and inadequate water in the diet are common causes of constipation. Other causes include inactivity, delaying bowel movements, medications, pain caused by a tear (fissure) in the lining of the rectum, and laxative overuse. Irritable bowel syndrome (see page 87) may also cause constipation.

Toilet training may contribute to constipation in young children. Children who are involved in play or other activities and ignore the urge to pass stools may become constipated. Children and adults who are reluctant to use toilets away from home may become constipated.

Prevention

- Eat plenty of high-fiber foods such as fruits, vegetables, and whole grains. You can also add fiber to your diet in the following ways (also see page 299):
    - Eat a bowl of bran cereal with 10 grams of bran per serving.
    - Add 2 tablespoons of wheat bran to cereal or soup.
    - Try a product, such as Citrucel, FiberCon, or Metamucil, that contains a bulk-forming agent. Start with 1 tablespoon or less and drink extra water to avoid bloating.
- Avoid foods that are high in fat and sugar.
- Drink 1½ to 2 quarts of water and other fluids every day. Drink extra fluids in the morning.
- Be more physically active. A walking program is a good start. See Chapter 16.
- Set aside relaxed times for having bowel movements. Urges usually occur sometime after meals. Establishing a daily routine (after breakfast, for example) may help.
- Go when you feel the urge. Your bowels send signals when a stool needs to pass. If you ignore the signal, the urge will go away and the stool will eventually become dry and difficult to pass.

Home Treatment

- Follow the diet outlined in Prevention to help relieve and prevent constipation.
- If necessary, use a stool softener or a very mild laxative such as milk of magnesia. Do not use mineral oil or any other laxative for more than 2 weeks without consulting your physician.
- If an infant or child up to age 10 is having rectal pain because he or she is unable to have a bowel movement, put the child in a warm bath with 2 ounces of baking soda in the tub. This may help relax the muscles that normally keep stool inside the rectum, allowing the child to pass the stool.
- If your child is 6 months old or older and the warm bath does not work, use 1 or 2 glycerin suppositories to make the stool easier to pass. Use glycerin suppositories only once or twice. If constipation is not relieved or develops again, discuss the problem with your physician.

- Do not give laxatives or enemas to a child without talking to your child's physician first.

When to Call Kaiser Permanente

- If constipation persists after home treatment has been followed for several days for an adult or according to a pediatrician's recommendation for an infant.
- If rectal bleeding is heavy (more than a few bright red streaks) or if the blood is reddish brown or black.
- If rectal bleeding lasts longer than 2 to 3 days after constipation has improved, or if bleeding occurs more than once.
- If you have sharp or severe abdominal pain.
- If you have rectal pain that either continues after you pass a stool or keeps you from passing stools at all.
- If constipation and major changes in bowel movements continue after 1 week of home treatment, and there is no clear reason for such changes.
- If you experience stool leakage (fecal incontinence).
- If your stools have become consistently more narrow (may be no wider than a pencil).
- If you are unable to have bowel movements without using laxatives.

Dehydration

Dehydration occurs when your body loses too much water. When you stop drinking water or lose large amounts of fluids because of diarrhea, vomiting, or sweating, your body's cells reabsorb fluid from the blood and other tissues. Severe dehydration can lead to shock, which can be life-threatening.

Dehydration is very dangerous for infants, small children, and older adults. Watch closely for its early signs anytime there is an illness that causes high fever, vomiting, or diarrhea. The early symptoms are:

- Dry mouth and sticky saliva.
- Urinating smaller amounts than usual; dark yellow urine.

Prevention

- Prompt home treatment for illnesses that cause diarrhea, vomiting, or fever will help prevent dehydration. See the chart on page 76.
- To prevent dehydration during hot weather or exercise, drink 8 to 10 glasses of fluid (water and/or sport drinks) each day. Drink extra water before, during, and after exercise.

Home Treatment

Treatment of mild dehydration involves stopping the fluid loss and gradually replacing lost fluids.

- To stop vomiting or diarrhea, do not eat any solid foods for several hours or until you are feeling better. In the first 24 hours, take frequent, small sips of water or a rehydration drink.
- Once the vomiting or diarrhea is controlled, drink water, diluted broth, or sport drinks a sip at a time until your stomach can handle larger amounts. Drinking too much fluid too soon can cause vomiting to recur.
- If vomiting or diarrhea lasts longer than 24 hours, sip a rehydration drink to replace lost minerals.
- Watch for signs of more severe dehydration (see below).

For infants and children age 3 and younger:

- Give small sips of an oral electrolyte solution (such as Pedialyte or Lytren) as soon as vomiting or diarrhea starts. See page 228 for home treatment of vomiting or diarrhea in children.

When to Call Kaiser Permanente

- If the following signs of severe dehydration develop:
  - Sunken eyes, no tears, dry mouth and tongue.
  - Sunken soft spot on an infant's head.
  - Little or no urine for 8 hours.
  - Skin that is doughy or doesn't bounce back when pinched.

Rehydration Drinks

Diarrhea and vomiting can cause your body to lose large amounts of water and essential minerals called electrolytes. If you are unable to eat for a few days, you are also losing nutrients. This happens faster and is more serious in infants, young children, and older adults.

A rehydration drink (Pedialyte, Lytren, Rehydralyte) will replace fluids and electrolytes in amounts that are best used by your body. Sports drinks and other sugared drinks will replace fluid, but most contain too much sugar (which can make the diarrhea worse) and not enough of the other essential ingredients. Plain water won't provide any necessary nutrients or electrolytes.

Rehydration drinks won't make diarrhea or vomiting go away faster, but they will prevent serious dehydration from developing.

You can make an inexpensive rehydration drink. However, do not give this homemade drink to children under age 12.

Measure all ingredients precisely. Small variations can make the drink less effective or even harmful.

- 1 quart water
- ½ teaspoon baking soda
- ½ teaspoon table salt
- 3 to 4 tablespoons sugar
- ¼ teaspoon salt substitute ("lite" salt), if available

  - Extreme dizziness or lightheadedness when moving from lying down to sitting upright.
  - Rapid breathing and heartbeat.
  - Sleepiness, difficulty awakening, listlessness, and extreme irritability.
- If vomiting lasts longer than 24 hours in an adult.
- If a person is unable to hold down even small sips of fluid, and therefore cannot drink enough to replace lost fluids.
- If severe diarrhea (large, loose stools every 1 to 2 hours) lasts longer than 2 days in an adult.

Diarrhea

Diarrhea occurs when the intestines push stools through before the water in the stools can be reabsorbed by the body. This causes bowel movements to occur more frequently and stools to become watery and loose. A person with diarrhea may also have abdominal cramps and nausea. Diarrhea can help your body clear out viruses, bacteria, and toxins.

Viral stomach flu (gastroenteritis) or food poisoning often causes diarrhea. Many medications, especially antibiotics, can cause diarrhea; so can laxatives, if they are overused. Sorbitol (a sugar substitute) and olestra (a fat substitute used in some processed foods) may cause diarrhea. For some people, emotional stress, anxiety, or food intolerance may bring on this problem. Irritable bowel syndrome (see page 87) may also cause diarrhea.

Drinking untreated water that contains parasites, viruses, or bacteria is another cause of diarrhea. Symptoms usually develop 1 to 4 weeks after you drink the contaminated water.

Home Treatment

To treat diarrhea in infants and children under age 4, see Home Treatment on page 228.

- Don't eat any food for several hours or until you are feeling better. Take frequent, small sips of water or a rehydration drink.
- Avoid antidiarrheal drugs for the first 24 hours. After that, use them only if there are no other signs of illness, such as fever, and if cramping or discomfort continues. See antidiarrheal preparations on page 345.
- After the first 24 hours (or sooner, depending on how you feel), begin eating mild foods, such as rice, dry toast or crackers, bananas, and applesauce. Avoid spicy foods, other fruits, alcohol, and drinks that contain caffeine until 48 hours after all symptoms have disappeared. Avoid dairy products for 3 days after symptoms disappear.
- Take care to avoid dehydration. See page 80.

When to Call Kaiser Permanente

- If you develop signs of dehydration (see page 80).
- If you develop severe diarrhea (large, loose bowel movements every 1 to 2 hours).
- If diarrhea lasts longer than 2 weeks.
- If stools are bloody or black.
- If abdominal pain increases or localizes, especially to the lower right or lower left part of the abdomen.
- If your symptoms become more severe or frequent.
- If diarrhea occurs after drinking untreated water.

Heartburn

Heartburn occurs when there is an abnormal backflow of stomach acid into the tube (esophagus) that leads from the mouth to the stomach. The acid backflow (reflux) causes a feeling of burning, warmth, or heat beneath the breastbone. The discomfort may spread in waves upward into the neck, and you may get a sour taste in your mouth. Heartburn can last up to 2 hours or longer. Symptoms often start after you eat. They grow worse when you lie down or bend over and improve when you sit or stand up.

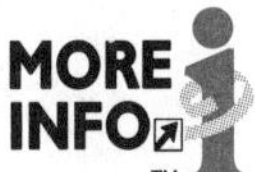

Don't be concerned if you have heartburn now and then; nearly everyone does. Following the home treatment tips can prevent most cases of heartburn. However, if backflow of stomach acid into your esophagus happens regularly, you may have gastroesophageal reflux disease (GERD). GERD can cause continuous irritation of the lining of the esophagus, which can lead to other health problems. It is important to visit a health professional if you have frequent heartburn and home treatment does not relieve the discomfort.

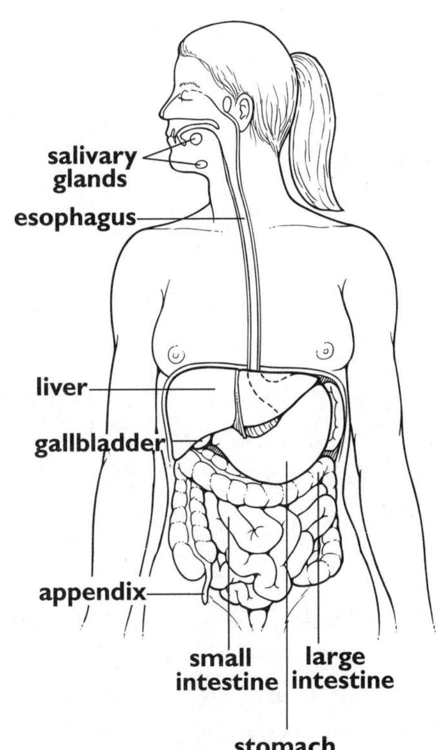

Organs of the digestive tract

Home Treatment

Try other home treatment measures before taking antacids or stomach acid blockers to relieve heartburn. If you take medications to relieve your heartburn without doing other home treatment, your heartburn is likely to keep coming back. If symptoms are not relieved by home treatment, or if symptoms last longer than 2 weeks, call your physician.

- Eat smaller meals, and avoid late-night snacks. Don't lie down for 2 to 3 hours after eating.
- Avoid foods that bring on heartburn. These include chocolate, fatty or fried foods, peppermint- or spearmint-flavored foods, coffee, alcohol, and carbonated drinks.
- Limit acidic foods that can irritate your esophagus. This includes citrus fruits and juices such as orange juice and tomato juice. Limit spicy foods.
- Avoid clothes with tight belts or waistbands.
- If you smoke or use other tobacco products, consider getting help to quit. See page 26 for tips on quitting. Smoking promotes heartburn.
- Lose weight if you are overweight. Being overweight can worsen heartburn, and the loss of even a few pounds can help prevent heartburn.
- Raise the head of your bed 6 to 8 inches by putting blocks underneath your bed frame or placing a foam wedge under the head of your mattress. (Adding extra pillows does not work well.)
- Aspirin, ibuprofen, naproxen sodium, and other anti-inflammatory drugs can cause heartburn. Try acetaminophen instead.
- Take a nonprescription product for heartburn. Antacids, such as Maalox, Mylanta, Tums, and Gelusil, neutralize stomach acid. Stomach acid blockers, such as Pepcid AC, Tagamet HB, and Zantac, reduce the production of stomach acid. Ask your pharmacist to help you choose one of these medications, and follow the package instructions and your physician's advice for its use.

When to Call Kaiser Permanente

Call 911 or seek other emergency services immediately if you have any of the following:

- Pain in the upper abdomen with chest pain that is crushing or squeezing, feels like a heavy weight on your chest, or occurs with any other symptoms of a heart attack (see page 54).
- Signs of shock (see page 67).

Call Kaiser Permanente:

- If there is blood in your vomit or stools.

- If you suspect that a medication is causing heartburn. Antihistamines, central nervous system depressants, birth control pills, and anti-inflammatory drugs including aspirin, ibuprofen, and naproxen sodium can sometimes cause heartburn.
- If you are routinely having pain or difficulty when swallowing solid foods.
- If you are losing weight and you don't know why.
- If heartburn persists for more than 2 weeks despite home treatment. Call sooner if symptoms are severe or are not relieved at all by antacids or acid blockers. See Ulcers on page 95.

Hernia

A hiatal hernia is a common problem that occurs when a portion of the stomach bulges into the chest cavity. Hiatal hernias often do not cause symptoms. However, sometimes a hiatal hernia will cause a backflow of stomach acid into the esophagus (the tube leading from the mouth to the stomach), which can cause heartburn and a sour taste in the mouth.

An inguinal hernia occurs when abdominal tissue bulges through a weak spot in the abdominal wall in the groin area. Inguinal hernias are more common in men than in women. In a man, an inguinal hernia may bulge into the scrotum.

Kidney Stones

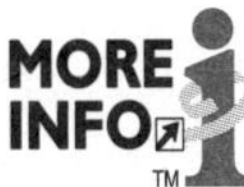

Kidney stones can form from the minerals in urine. The most common cause of kidney stones is not drinking enough water.

As long as they stay in the kidneys, kidney stones usually cause no problems. A stone may move out of the kidney into the tube that leads to the bladder (ureter). If the stone blocks the flow of urine, there may be severe pain.

Symptoms that may develop when a kidney stone moves through a ureter include:

- Pain in the side, groin, or genital area that begins suddenly and gets worse over 15 to 60 minutes until it is steady and nearly unbearable. The pain may stop for a while when the stone is not moving, and pain often vanishes suddenly when the stone moves into the bladder.
- Nausea and vomiting.
- Blood in the urine.
- Feeling like you need to urinate often or pain when urinating.
- Loss of appetite, diarrhea, or constipation.
- Inability to find a comfortable body position.

Call your physician immediately if you suspect that you are passing a kidney stone. Most small kidney stones pass without the need for any medical treatment other than pain medication. In rare cases, surgery may be needed.

A person with an inguinal hernia may sense that something has "given way." Other symptoms may include:

- A tender bulge in the groin or scrotum. The bulge may appear gradually, or it may form suddenly after heavy lifting, coughing, or straining. The bulge may disappear when the person lies down.
- Groin discomfort or pain that may extend into the scrotum. Discomfort may increase with bending or lifting.
- Nausea and abdominal swelling.

Inguinal hernias can be caused by increased abdominal pressure resulting from lifting heavy weights, coughing, or straining to pass stools. Sometimes a weak spot in the abdominal wall is present at birth. An inguinal hernia is called reducible if the protruding tissue can be pushed back into place in the abdomen. If the tissue cannot be pushed back into place, the hernia is called irreducible.

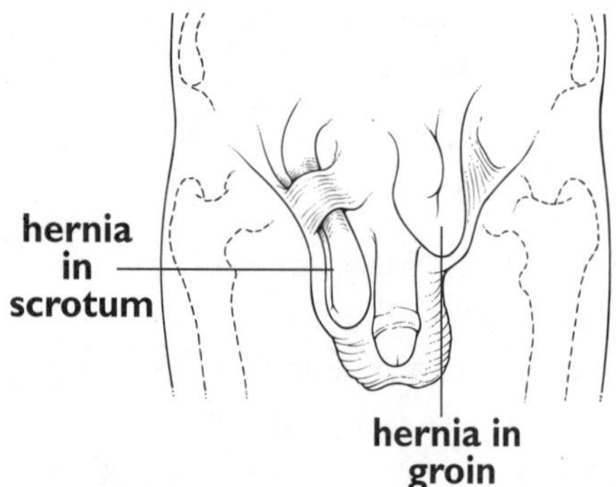

A hernia can cause a bulge or lump in the groin or scrotum.

If an inguinal hernia is irreducible, the tissue may become trapped outside the abdominal wall. If the blood supply to the tissue is cut off (strangulated hernia), the tissue will swell and die. The dead tissue will quickly become infected, requiring immediate medical attention. Rapidly increasing pain in the groin or scrotum is a sign that a hernia has become strangulated.

A hernia can develop anywhere there is a weakness in the abdominal wall. Common places for hernias to develop are the bellybutton (umbilical hernia) and at the site of an incision from abdominal surgery (incisional hernia).

Prevention

- Use proper lifting techniques (see page 107), and avoid lifting weights that are too heavy for you.
- Lose weight if you are overweight.
- Avoid constipation and do not strain during bowel movements and urination.
- If you smoke or use other tobacco products, consider getting help to quit (especially if you have a chronic cough). See page 26 for tips on quitting.

When to Call Kaiser Permanente

- If mild groin pain or an unexplained bump or swelling in the groin continues for more than 1 week.

- If the skin over a hernia or bulge in the groin or abdomen becomes red.
- If heartburn persists for more than 2 weeks despite home treatment. Call sooner if symptoms are severe or are not relieved at all by antacids or acid blockers. See Heartburn on page 83.

If you have been diagnosed with a hernia, call a health professional:

- If you have sudden, severe pain in the groin area, along with nausea, vomiting, and fever.
- If the hernia cannot be pushed back into place with gentle pressure when you are lying down.

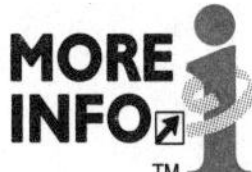

If you suspect that you have a hernia, see your physician to confirm the diagnosis and discuss your treatment options.

Irritable Bowel Syndrome

Irritable bowel syndrome (IBS) is one of the most common disorders of the digestive tract. Symptoms of IBS often increase with stress or after eating and include:

- Abdominal bloating, pain, and gas.
- Mucus in the stool.
- Feeling as if a bowel movement hasn't been completed.
- Irregular bowel habits, with constipation, diarrhea, or both.

The cause of IBS is unknown. Symptoms are thought to be related to abnormal muscle contractions in the intestines. However, when tests are done, they find no changes (such as inflammation or tumors) in the physical structure of the intestines.

IBS can persist for many years. An episode may be more severe than the one before it, but the disorder itself does not worsen over time or lead to more serious diseases such as cancer. Symptoms tend to get better over time.

If you have not yet been diagnosed with IBS, try to rule out other causes of stomach problems, such as eating a new food, nervousness, or stomach flu. Try home treatment for 1 to 2 weeks. If there is no improvement, or if your symptoms worsen, call your physician for an appointment.

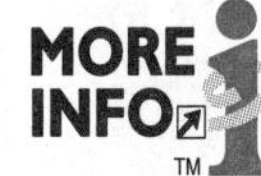

Your physician may prescribe medication for you to take in addition to doing home treatment. There are no tests that can diagnose irritable bowel syndrome, but your physician may recommend testing to rule out other possible causes of your symptoms. The amount of testing your physician will do to determine the cause of your symptoms depends on your age; how your symptoms come on and how severe they are; and how you respond to initial treatment.

Gallstones

Gallstones are tiny stones (usually made of cholesterol) that form in the gallbladder.

Sometimes gallstones cause the gallbladder to become inflamed. The main symptom is a dull aching or cramping pain that starts in the upper right abdomen and may radiate to the center of the upper abdomen or to the right upper back or shoulder blade. The pain may be severe and usually lasts several hours. Fever and vomiting also may be present.

Symptoms often occur at night, usually at about the same time every night. Symptoms may be worse after you eat a high-fat meal.

Risk factors for gallstones include a high-fat, high-sugar diet, obesity, lack of exercise, rapid weight loss, estrogen therapy, diabetes, high cholesterol, and high blood pressure.

Gallstones that don't cause symptoms don't require treatment. If gallstones cause pain or infection, surgery to remove the gallbladder is the most common treatment.

If you have mild symptoms, it is safe to wait until symptoms recur several times before seeking treatment. See When to Call Kaiser Permanente on page 78 to decide what to do if your symptoms become more severe.

Prevention

There is no way to prevent IBS. However, symptoms often worsen or improve because of changes in your diet, your stress level, medications, the amount of exercise you are getting, and for other reasons that may or may not be known. Identifying the things that trigger your symptoms may help you avoid or minimize attacks.

Home Treatment

If constipation is your main symptom:

- Eat more fruits, vegetables, legumes, and whole grains. Add these fiber-rich foods to your diet slowly so they do not worsen gas or cramps. See page 299.
- Add unprocessed wheat bran to your diet. Start by using 1 tablespoon per day, and gradually increase to 4 tablespoons per day. Sprinkle bran on cereal, soup, and casseroles. Drink extra water to avoid becoming bloated.
- Try a product (such as Citrucel, FiberCon, or Metamucil) that contains a bulk-forming agent. Start with 1 tablespoon or less and gradually increase. Drink extra water to avoid bloating.
- Use laxatives only if your physician recommends them.

If diarrhea is your main symptom:

- Using the fiber-rich food and wheat bran suggestions for relieving constipation can sometimes help relieve diarrhea by absorbing liquid in the large intestine.
- Avoid foods that make diarrhea worse. Try eliminating one food at a time; then add it back gradually. If a food doesn't seem to be related to symptoms, there is no need to avoid it. Many people find that the following foods or drinks make their symptoms worse:
  - Alcohol, caffeine, nicotine
  - Beans, broccoli, cabbage, apples
  - Spicy foods
  - Foods high in acid, such as citrus fruit
  - Fatty foods, including bacon, sausage, butter, oils, and anything deep-fried
- Avoid dairy products that contain lactose (milk sugar) if they seem to worsen symptoms. However, get enough calcium in your diet from other sources. See "Lactose Intolerance" on page 304.
- Avoid sorbitol (an artificial sweetener found in some sugarless candies and gum) and olestra (a fat substitute used in some processed foods, such as potato chips).
- Avoid foods that don't digest well, such as corn, carrots, peas, etc.
- Add more starchy food (bread, rice, potatoes, pasta) to your diet.
- If diarrhea persists, a nonprescription medication such as loperamide (the active ingredient in products such as Imodium) may help. Check with your physician if you are using loperamide twice a month or more.

To reduce stress:

- Keep a record of the life events that occur with your symptoms. This may help you see any connection between your symptoms and stressful occasions.
- Get regular, vigorous exercise such as swimming, jogging, or brisk walking to help reduce tension.
- See page 328 for more tips on managing stress.

When to Call Kaiser Permanente

- If you have been diagnosed with irritable bowel syndrome and your symptoms get worse, begin to disrupt your usual activities, or do not respond as usual to home treatment.
- If you are becoming increasingly fatigued.
- If your symptoms frequently wake you.
- If your pain gets worse with movement.
- If you have abdominal pain and a fever.
- If you are losing weight and you don't know why.

- If your appetite has decreased.
- If you have abdominal pain that does not get better when you pass gas or stools.
- If there is blood in your stools that is not obviously related to previously diagnosed hemorrhoids.

Nausea and Vomiting

Nausea is a very unpleasant feeling in the pit of the stomach. A person who is nauseated may feel weak and sweaty and produce lots of saliva. Intense nausea often leads to vomiting, which forces stomach contents up the esophagus and out of the mouth. Home treatment will help ease the discomfort.

Nausea and vomiting may be caused by:

- Viral stomach flu or food poisoning (see page 93).
- Stress or nervousness.
- Medications, especially antibiotics and anti-inflammatory drugs (aspirin, ibuprofen, naproxen sodium, etc.).
- Pregnancy (see "Morning Sickness" on page 255).
- Diabetes.
- Migraine headache (see page 192).
- Head injury (see page 52).

Nausea and vomiting can also be signs of other serious illnesses involving abdominal organs such as the liver (hepatitis, see page 97), pancreas, gallbladder (see page 88), stomach (ulcers, see page 95), or appendix (appendicitis, see page 77).

Home Treatment

For home treatment of vomiting in children under age 4, see pages 229 and 230. For older children and adults:

- If vomiting lasts longer than 24 hours, sip a rehydration drink to restore lost fluids and nutrients. See page 81.
- Rest in bed until you are feeling better.
- Watch for and treat early signs of dehydration. See page 80. Older adults and young children can quickly become dehydrated from vomiting.
- After vomiting has stopped for 1 hour, drink 1 ounce of a clear liquid every 20 minutes for 1 hour. Clear liquids include apple or grape juice mixed to half strength with water, rehydration drinks, weak tea with sugar, clear broth, and gelatin dessert. Avoid citrus juices.
- When you are feeling better, begin eating clear soups, mild foods, and liquids until all symptoms have been gone for 12 to 48 hours. Gelatin dessert, dry toast, crackers, and cooked cereal are good choices.

When to Call Kaiser Permanente

- If signs of severe dehydration develop (see page 80).
- If vomiting occurs with:
  - Severe headache, sleepiness, lethargy, or stiff neck. See "Encephalitis and Meningitis" on page 160.
  - Chest pain and fever.
  - Fever and increasing pain in the lower right abdomen.
  - Fever and shaking chills.
  - Abdominal swelling.
  - Pain in the upper right or upper left abdomen.
- If vomit contains blood or material that looks like coffee grounds. See Shock on page 67.
- If vomiting and fever last longer than 48 hours.
- If you suspect that a medication is causing the problem. Antibiotics and anti-inflammatory medications (aspirin, ibuprofen, naproxen sodium, etc.) may cause nausea or vomiting. Learn which of your medications can cause these symptoms.
- If vomiting occurs after a head injury, see page 52.
- If vomiting comes and goes and lasts longer than 1 week.

Rectal Problems

The rectum is the lower part of the large intestine. At the end of the rectum is the anus, where stools pass out of the body.

Rectal problems are common. Most everyone experiences itching, pain, or bleeding in the rectal or anal area at some time. These problems are often minor and will go away on their own or with home treatment.

Anal itching can have many causes. Skin around the anus may become irritated because of stool leakage. Caffeine and spicy foods can irritate the lining of the rectum, causing anal itching and discomfort. If the anus is not kept clean, itching may result. However, trying to keep the area too clean by rubbing it with dry toilet paper or using harsh soap may injure the skin.

Hemorrhoids are enlarged and inflamed veins that may develop inside or outside of the anus. Straining to pass hard stools, being overweight or pregnant, and prolonged sitting or standing can all cause hemorrhoids.

The symptoms of hemorrhoids include bright red streaks of blood on stools or spurting from the anus; leakage of mucus from the anus; and irritation or itching around the anus. Sometimes an internal hemorrhoid will actually stick out of the anus, and it may have to be pushed back into place with a finger. Pain is not usually a symptom, unless a blood clot forms in a hemorrhoid. A clotted hemorrhoid may be extremely painful but is not dangerous. Hemorrhoids generally last several days and often come back (recur).

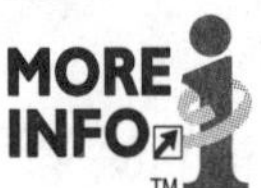

You may want to consider surgery if you have hemorrhoids that bleed persistently, are very uncomfortable, or make it difficult to keep your anal area clean. Talk to your physician about your options for surgery.

An **anal fissure** may cause pain during bowel movements and streaks of blood on stools. Anal fissures are long, narrow sores that usually develop when the tissue in the anal area is torn during a bowel movement.

Prevention

- Keep your stools soft. Include plenty of water, fresh fruits and vegetables, and whole grains in your diet. Include up to 2 tablespoons of bran or a commercial stool softener, such as Citrucel or Metamucil, in your diet each day. Regular exercise promotes smooth bowel movements. Also see Constipation on page 78.
- Try not to strain during bowel movements, and never hold your breath. Take your time, but don't sit on the toilet too long.
- Avoid sitting or standing too much. Take short walks to increase blood flow in your pelvic region.
- Keep the anal area clean, but be gentle when cleansing it. Use water and a fragrance-free soap, such as Ivory, or use baby wipes or Tucks pads.

Flexible Sigmoidoscopy

Flexible sigmoidoscopy is a screening test for precancerous growths and cancers of the colon and rectum. The sigmoidoscope is a flexible viewing instrument that is inserted into the rectum to examine the lower bowel. The exam takes about 10 to 15 minutes, is only mildly uncomfortable, and is very safe.

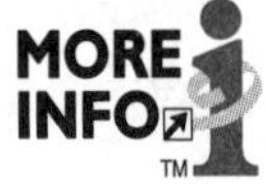

Having flexible sigmoidoscopy exams reduces your risk of dying from colorectal cancer. Most experts recommend that you have a flexible sigmoidoscopy exam around age 50. However, experts disagree about how often you should have repeat exams. Recommendations usually range from every 3 years to every 10 years. In addition to screening for cancer, physicians sometimes wish to examine the colon to check for the cause of rectal bleeding, diarrhea, or constipation.

Home Treatment

- Take warm baths. They are soothing and cleansing, especially after you have a bowel movement. Sitz baths (warm baths with just enough water to cover the anal area) are also helpful for hemorrhoids but may worsen anal itching.
- Wear cotton underwear and loose clothing to decrease moisture in the anal area.
- Apply a cold compress on the anus for 10 minutes, 4 times a day.
- Ease itching and irritation with zinc oxide, petroleum jelly, or hydrocortisone (1 percent) cream. Use medicated suppositories to relieve pain and lubricate the anal canal during bowel movements. Ask your physician before using any product that contains a local anesthetic (these products have the suffix "-caine" in the name or ingredients). Such products cause allergic reactions in some people.

When to Call Kaiser Permanente

- If rectal bleeding occurs for no apparent reason and is not associated with trying to pass stools.
- If rectal bleeding continues for more than 1 week or occurs more than once.
- If stools become more narrow than usual (may be no wider than a pencil).
- If pain caused by hemorrhoids is severe, or if moderate anal pain lasts longer than 1 week after home treatment.
- If any unusual material or tissue seeps or sticks out of the anus.
- If a lump near the anus gets bigger or becomes more painful and you develop a fever.
- If fever accompanies bloody stools.

Stomach Flu and Food Poisoning

Stomach flu and food poisoning are different ailments with different causes. However, many people confuse the two because the symptoms are so similar. Most people who get food poisoning attribute their symptoms of nausea, vomiting, diarrhea, and stomach pain to a sudden case of stomach flu, and vice versa.

Stomach flu is usually caused by a viral infection in the digestive system. To prevent stomach flu, you must avoid contact with the virus, which is not always easy to do.

Food poisoning is usually caused by a toxin produced by bacteria in food that is not handled or stored properly. Bacteria can grow rapidly when certain foods, especially meats, dairy products, and sauces, are not handled properly during preparation or are kept at temperatures between 40° and 140°.

Suspect food poisoning when symptoms are shared by others who ate the same food, or after eating unrefrigerated foods. Symptoms of food poisoning may begin as soon as 1 or 2 hours or as long as 48 hours after eating. Nausea, vomiting, and diarrhea may last from 12 to 48 hours for common food poisoning.

Botulism is a rare but often fatal type of food poisoning. It is generally caused by improper home canning methods for low-acid foods like beans and corn. Bacteria that survive the canning process may grow and produce toxin in the jar. Symptoms include blurred or double vision and difficulty swallowing or breathing.

Prevention

To prevent food poisoning:

- Keep hot foods hot and cold foods cold.
- Follow the 2-40-140 rule. Don't eat meat, dressings, salads, or other foods that have been kept for more than 2 hours between 40° and 140°.
- Use a thermometer to check your refrigerator. It should be between 34° and 40°.
- Defrost meats in the refrigerator or microwave, not on the kitchen counter.
- Keep your kitchen clean. Wash your hands, cutting boards, and countertops frequently. After handling raw meats, especially chicken, wash your hands and utensils before preparing other foods.
- Cook hamburger until it is well done. Cook chicken until the juices run clear.
- Do not eat raw eggs or uncooked sauces made with raw eggs.
- Discard any cans or jars with bulging lids or leaks.
- Follow home canning and freezing instructions carefully. Contact your county agricultural extension office for advice.

Home Treatment

- Viral stomach flu and food poisoning will usually go away within 24 to 48 hours. Good home care can speed recovery. For adults and children age 4 and older, see Nausea and Vomiting on page 90 and Diarrhea on page 82. For children younger than 4, see page 228.
- Watch for and treat early signs of dehydration (see page 80). Older adults and young children can quickly become dehydrated from diarrhea and vomiting.

When to Call Kaiser Permanente

- If vomiting lasts longer than 1 day in an adult.
- If severe diarrhea (large, loose stools every 1 to 2 hours) lasts longer than 2 days in an adult.
- If signs of severe dehydration develop. See page 80.
- If you suspect food poisoning from a canned food or have symptoms of botulism (blurred or double

vision, difficulty swallowing or breathing). If you still have a sample of the food you suspect caused your symptoms, take it to the physician for testing.

Ulcers

An ulcer (peptic ulcer) is a sore or crater in the lining of the digestive tract. Most ulcers develop in the stomach (gastric ulcers) or in the upper part of the small intestine (duodenal ulcers).

Until recently, the cause of ulcers was not well understood. It is now believed that most people who develop ulcers are infected with *Helicobacter pylori (H. pylori)* bacteria. Many people who are infected with *H. pylori* do not develop ulcers unless other factors are also present. Such factors may include:

- Use of certain medications.
- Excessive alcohol use.
- Smoking.
- Stress.
- Other illnesses.

Most ulcers that are not caused by *H. pylori* infection are caused by frequent use of aspirin or other non-steroidal anti-inflammatory drugs (ibuprofen, indomethacin, naproxen sodium, clinoril, etc.), which can damage the digestive tract's lining.

The symptoms of an ulcer are often similar to symptoms of other stomach problems like heartburn (indigestion) or inflammation of the stomach lining (gastritis). Symptoms may include a burning or gnawing pain between the navel and the breastbone. The pain often occurs between meals and may wake you during the night. Eating something or taking an antacid usually relieves the pain. Ulcers may also cause bloating, nausea, or vomiting after meals.

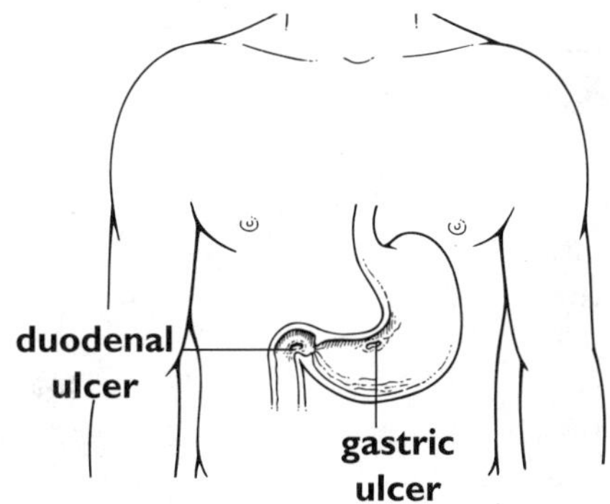

Most ulcers occur in the stomach (gastric ulcer) or in the opening to the small intestine (duodenal ulcer).

Ulcers can cause bleeding in the stomach, which may cause stools to turn dark red, black, or tarry. Without treatment, ulcers may occasionally cause a blockage between the stomach and the small intestine. An ulcer may break through (perforate) the stomach wall, causing severe abdominal pain. Ulcers that bleed or perforate the stomach wall require immediate medical treatment.

If you think you have an ulcer and your symptoms do not improve after 10 to 14 days of home treatment, make an appointment with your physician. He or she can evaluate your symptoms and prescribe a treatment plan that may include antacids or other medications.

Home Treatment

- Avoid foods, especially alcohol, caffeine, and spicy foods, that seem to bring on symptoms. It isn't necessary to eliminate any particular food from your diet if it doesn't cause you problems.
- Try eating smaller, more frequent meals. If it doesn't help, return to a regular diet.
- If you smoke or use other tobacco products, consider getting help to quit. See page 26 for tips on quitting. Smoking slows healing of ulcers and increases the likelihood that they will come back.
- Do not take aspirin, ibuprofen, or naproxen sodium. Try acetaminophen instead.
- Antacids (such as Tums, Maalox, and Mylanta) reduce the amount of acid in your stomach. Acid blockers (such as Pepcid AC, Tagamet HB, Zantac 75, and Axid AR) reduce the amount of acid your stomach produces. Reducing the amount of acid in your stomach helps your ulcer heal. If you are taking antacids, you may need frequent, large doses to do the job. Talk with your physician about the best dose. Also see page 344.
- Too much stress may slow ulcer healing. Practice the relaxation techniques on page 328.

When to Call Kaiser Permanente

- If you have pain in the upper abdomen with chest pain that is crushing or squeezing, feels like a heavy weight on your chest, or occurs with any other symptoms of a heart attack (see page 54).
- If you have been diagnosed with an ulcer and you have severe, continuous abdominal pain, severe vomiting, blood in vomit or stools, dizziness or lightheadedness, or signs of shock (see page 67).
- If your symptoms continue or get worse after 10 to 14 days of treatment with antacids or acid blockers.
- If you are losing weight and you don't know why.
- If nausea or vomiting often occurs right after meals.
- If abdominal pain awakens you from sleep.
- If you have pain or difficulty when swallowing.

Hepatitis

Hepatitis means "liver inflammation." Viruses cause hepatitis A, B, and C, the most common types of hepatitis.

Most people in the U.S. get hepatitis A after having intimate contact with someone who is infected with the hepatitis A virus (HAV). Large groups of people can become infected with HAV if someone who has hepatitis A prepares food for them. HAV infection usually goes away without medical treatment, causing no long-term problems.

The hepatitis B virus (HBV) lives in blood and other body fluids. It is commonly spread during sexual contact and when people share needles to inject drugs. A pregnant woman who is infected with HBV can pass the virus to her baby. Young people who become infected with HBV are more likely to develop chronic HBV infection and long-term liver problems than are people who become infected later in life.

The hepatitis C virus (HCV) is spread when HCV-infected blood enters a person's body. Blood transfusions were once a common means of spreading HCV. The virus is also spread among people who share needles to inject drugs. Many people develop chronic HCV infection, which can lead to severe liver damage after many years.

Hepatitis symptoms are similar to flu symptoms. They include nausea, headache, sore muscles, and fatigue. Some people have pain in the upper right side of the abdomen. Jaundice may develop, causing the skin and whites of the eyes to turn yellow and making the urine dark. Call a health professional if you develop hepatitis symptoms or if you have had intimate contact or shared needles or other "drug works" with someone who has hepatitis. Because all 3 types of viral hepatitis have similar symptoms, blood tests are needed to determine which hepatitis virus is causing the infection.

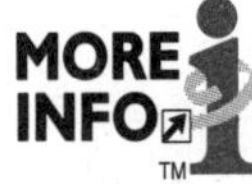

Vaccines can prevent hepatitis A and B, but there is no vaccine for hepatitis C. If you are exposed to HAV or HBV before you have been vaccinated, getting a shot of immune globulin is likely to keep you from becoming infected. Drug treatment is available for people with chronic hepatitis infection (HBV or HCV) who are likely to develop liver problems.

Urinary Incontinence

If you suffer from loss of bladder control (urinary incontinence), you are not alone. Many people are coping with this problem.

Many cases of incontinence can be controlled or cured if the underlying problem is corrected. Water pills (diuretics) and many other common medications can cause temporary incontinence. Constipation, urinary tract infections, stones in the urinary tract, multiple pregnancies, and being overweight are other causes of incontinence.

The 2 most common types of persistent or chronic loss of bladder control are described here.

Stress incontinence occurs when small amounts of urine leak out during exercise or when you cough, laugh, or sneeze. It is more common in women than in men, but it may affect some men after prostate surgery. For women, Kegel exercises often help relieve stress incontinence. See page 98. Ask your physician about devices that can be used to prevent urine from leaking.

Urge incontinence happens when the need to urinate comes on so quickly that there is not enough time to get to the toilet. Causes include bladder infection, prostate enlargement, tumors that press on the bladder, Parkinson's disease, and nerve-related disorders such as multiple sclerosis or stroke.

Kegel Exercises

Kegel exercises can help cure or improve stress incontinence by strengthening the muscles that control the flow of urine. No one will know you are doing them except you.

- Locate the muscles by repeatedly stopping your urine in midstream and starting again.
- Practice squeezing these muscles while you are not urinating. If your stomach or buttocks move, you are not using the right muscles.
- Hold the squeeze for 3 seconds, then relax for 3 seconds.
- Repeat the exercise 10 to 15 times per session. Do at least 3 Kegel exercise sessions per day.

Home Treatment

- Don't let incontinence keep you from doing the things you like to do. Absorbent pads or briefs, such as Attends and Depend, are available in pharmacies and supermarkets. No one will know you are wearing an absorbent pad.
- Avoid beverages that contain caffeine, which overstimulates the bladder. Do not cut down on fluids overall; you need fluids to keep the rest of your body healthy.

- If you smoke or use other tobacco products, consider getting help to quit. See page 26 for tips on quitting. This may reduce your coughing, which may in turn reduce your problem with incontinence.
- Lose weight if you are overweight.
- Practice "double-voiding." Empty your bladder as much as possible, relax for a minute, and then try to empty it again.
- If you have stress incontinence, practice Kegel exercises daily (women only). See "Kegel Exercises" on page 98.
- Urinate on a schedule, perhaps every 3 to 4 hours during the day, whether the urge is there or not. This may help you restore control.
- Wear clothing that can be removed quickly, such as pants with elastic waistbands.
- Clear a path from your bed to the bathroom, or consider placing a portable commode by your bed.
- Keep skin in the genital area dry to prevent rashes. Vaseline or Desitin ointment will help protect the skin from irritation caused by urine.
- Incontinence is sometimes caused by a urinary tract infection. If you feel pain or burning when you urinate, see Urinary Tract Infections on page 100.
- Pay special attention to any medications you are taking, including nonprescription drugs, since some affect bladder control.

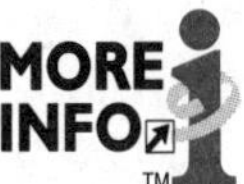

Don't let incontinence embarrass you. Take charge and work with your physician to treat any underlying condition that may be causing the problem.

For more information about urinary incontinence, contact the National Association for Incontinence, P.O. Box 8310, Spartanburg, SC 29305, 1-800-252-3337.

When to Call Kaiser Permanente

- If you suddenly become incontinent.
- If you are urinating frequently, but only passing small amounts of urine.
- If your bladder feels full even after you urinate.
- If you have difficulty urinating when your bladder feels full.
- If you feel burning or pain while urinating.
- If your urine looks bloody. See "Blood in the Urine" on page 102.
- If your urine has an unusual odor.

Urinary Tract Infections

The urinary tract is composed of the kidneys, ureters, bladder, and urethra. The kidneys filter the blood, and the waste products from the blood become urine. The ureters carry urine from the kidneys to the bladder. The bladder holds the urine until the urine is expelled through the urethra (the tube that carries urine from the bladder to the outside of the body).

Urinary tract infections (UTIs), including bladder infections (cystitis) and kidney infections (pyelonephritis), are generally caused by bacteria that are normally present in the digestive system. Females get UTIs more often than males do.

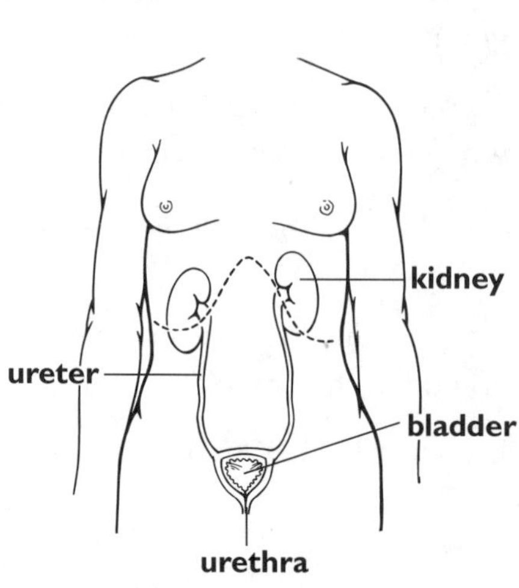

Infections can occur in any of the structures of the urinary tract.

Early symptoms of a UTI may include burning or pain during urination and itching or pain in the urethra. There may also be discomfort in the lower abdomen or back and a frequent urge to urinate without being able to pass much urine. The urine may be cloudy or reddish in color and may have an unusual odor.

Chills and fever may also be present if the infection is severe, especially if it has spread to the kidneys. Men with symptoms similar to those caused by a UTI may have an infection of the prostate gland or the epididymis (the tube that transports sperm from the testicle). See Prostatitis on page 273 and Testicular Problems on page 276.

Men who have enlarged prostates, women who have had multiple pregnancies, people with kidney stones or diabetes, and those who are paralyzed from the waist down may be at higher risk for chronic urinary tract infections.

Other causes of irritation to the genital area that may be associated with UTIs include having sexual intercourse, using a diaphragm for birth control, wearing tight pants, riding a bike, using perfumed soaps and powders, or even eating spicy foods.

If urinary pain or vaginal burning and redness occur in a young girl, consider the possibility of an allergy to bubble bath or soap. Urinary pain or vaginal burning may also be a symptom of a sexually transmitted disease (STD) or sexual abuse. If you are concerned about sexual abuse of a child, call your physician.

Prevention

- Drink plenty of fluids; water is best. Aim for at least 2 quarts per day.
- Urinate frequently.
- Females should wipe from front to back after going to the toilet. This will reduce the spread of bacteria from the anus to the urethra. Teach young girls this habit during toilet training.
- Avoid douching, and don't use vaginal deodorants or perfumed feminine hygiene products.
- Wash the genital area once a day with plain water or mild soap and water. Rinse well and dry the area thoroughly.
- Drink extra water before sexual intercourse and urinate promptly afterwards. This is especially important if you tend to get UTIs.
- Wear cotton underwear, cotton-lined panty hose, and loose clothing.
- Avoid alcohol, caffeine, and carbonated beverages, which can irritate the bladder.
- Drinking cranberry and blueberry juice may protect against UTIs, especially in females.

Home Treatment

Start home treatment at the first sign of genital irritation or painful urination. A day or so of self-care may eliminate minor symptoms. However, if your symptoms last longer than 1 day or worsen despite home treatment, call your physician. Because the organs of the urinary tract are connected, untreated UTIs can spread, which may lead to kidney infections and other serious problems.

- Drink extra fluids (think in terms of gallons) as soon as you notice symptoms and for the next 24 hours. This will help dilute the urine, flush bacteria out of the bladder, and decrease irritation.
- Urinate frequently and follow the other tips outlined in Prevention.
- Check your temperature twice daily. Fever may indicate a more serious infection.
- A hot bath may help relieve pain. Avoid using bubble bath and harsh soaps. Apply a heating pad over your genital area to help relieve the pain. Never go to sleep with a heating pad in place.
- Avoid sexual intercourse until symptoms improve. Do not use a diaphragm. It may put pressure on your urethra and slow down or prevent complete emptying of the bladder.
- Drink cranberry juice and/or blueberry juice.

When to Call Kaiser Permanente

- If painful urination occurs with any of the following symptoms:
  - Fever of 101° or higher and chills.
  - Inability to urinate when you feel the urge.
  - Pain in the back, side, groin, or genital area.
  - Blood or pus in the urine.
  - Unusual vaginal discharge.
  - Nausea and vomiting.
- If symptoms get worse despite home treatment.
- If symptoms do not improve after 24 hours of home treatment.
- If you are pregnant or have diabetes and you have symptoms of a urinary tract infection.
- If you suspect that your child has a urinary tract infection or has been sexually abused.

Blood in the Urine

A blow to the kidneys, kidney stones, excessive running, or a urinary tract infection can cause blood in the urine. Blood in the urine can be a sign of a serious illness and should always be discussed with a health professional.

Eating foods such as beets, blackberries, and foods containing red artificial food colorings can temporarily color the urine pink or red.

Stand up straight!
Mom

5

Back and Neck Problems

Although back and neck problems are usually preventable, most of us will suffer from one or both at some time in our lives. Fortunately, 9 out of 10 acute back problems will improve on their own within 4 to 6 weeks.

By following the prevention and home treatment guidelines in this chapter, you can recover from most back and neck problems and prevent them from recurring.

Quick Reference Guide

- First aid for back problems, page 104.
- Back problems due to arthritis, page 117.
- Neck problems, page 113.

Back Problems

Your back includes the bones of the spine (vertebrae that support body weight), their joints (facets that guide the direction of the movement of the spine), the discs that separate the vertebrae and absorb shock as you move, and the muscles and ligaments that hold it all together. One or more of these structures can be injured.

- You can strain or sprain the ligaments or muscles by a sudden or improper movement or by overuse.
- You can damage your discs the same way so that they bulge or tear. If the tear is large enough, the disc may press against a nerve. The nerve may also become irritated due to swelling or inflammation of the other parts of the back.

First Aid for Back Problems

When you first feel a catch or strain in your back, try these steps to avoid or reduce expected problems. These are the most important home treatments for the first few days of a back problem. Also see Home Treatment on page 110.

First Aid #1: Activity

Stick to your usual routine as much as you can. Take a short walk for a few minutes every hour or 2 on a flat surface. Try to work up to 20-minute walks. If you have pain down your leg, start with shorter walks less often. Walk only distances you can manage without making your back or leg worse. Swimming is also a good activity for a back problem.

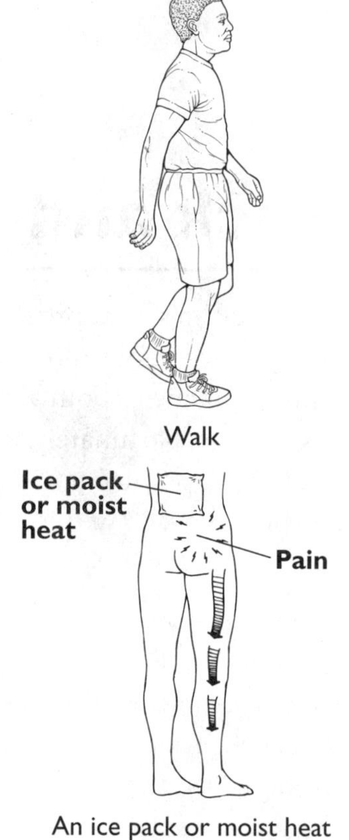

Walk

An ice pack or moist heat in middle of low back

First Aid #2: Ice and/or Heat

If your problem is in your neck, upper back, or shoulders, place the ice or moist heat on the back and sides of your neck. Otherwise, put it in the middle of your low back. Go for a walk afterward, when you feel more comfortable.

First Aid #3: Medicine

Medication can relieve pain and help you move around more easily. See page 111 for specific suggestions.

First Aid #4: Good Posture

Keep the small curves in your spine all the time. See pages 106, 107, and 114. Avoid sitting for very long.

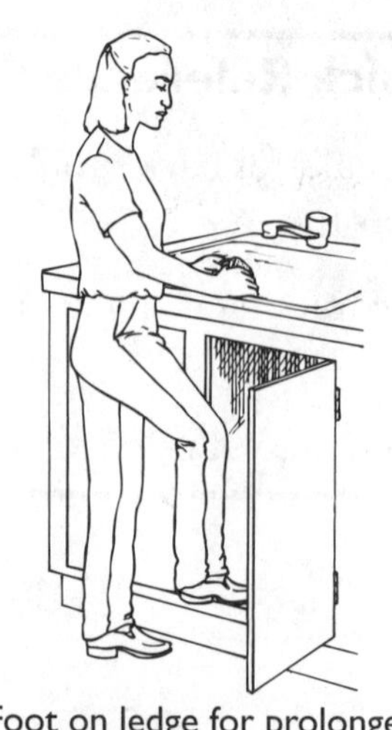

Foot on ledge for prolonged standing activities

Any of these injuries can result in 2 or 3 days of acute pain and swelling in the injured tissue, followed by slow healing and a gradual reduction in pain. The problem may be felt in the low back, in the buttock, or down the leg. The goals of self-care are to relieve the inflammation, promote healing, and avoid reinjury.

Back problems can also be caused by conditions that affect the bones and joints of the spine. Arthritis pain may be a steady ache, unlike the sharp, acute pain of strains, sprains, or disc injuries. If you think your back problem may be caused by arthritis, combine the self-care guidelines for back problems with those for arthritis on page 117.

Osteoporosis weakens the bones of the spine, which can cause the bones to compress and lead to varying degrees of pain. See page 129.

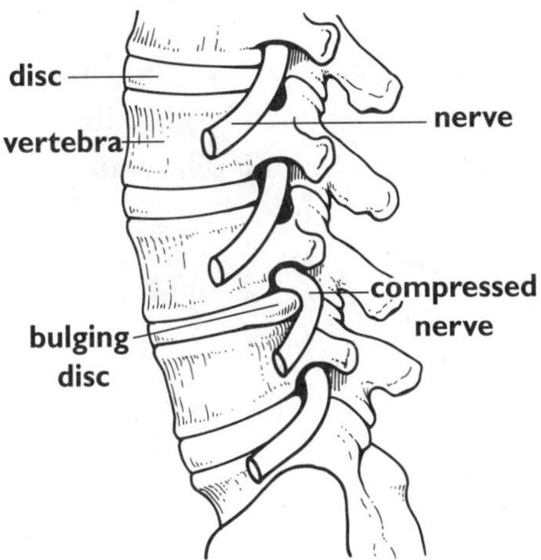

A spinal disc that bulges or ruptures can put pressure on a nerve, causing pain.

Sciatica

Sciatica is an irritation of the sciatic nerve, which runs from the low back down through the buttocks to the feet. It can occur when an injured disc presses against the nerve. Its main symptom is radiating pain, numbness, tingling, or weakness that is usually worse in the leg than in the back. In addition to the Home Treatment for back problems on page 110, the following may help:

- Avoid sitting, if possible, unless it is more comfortable than standing.
- Alternate standing or lying down with short walks. Increase the distance as you are able to tolerate without increasing your pain.
- Ice or moist heat will probably do the most good placed in the middle of your low back. See pages 104 and 133.

The Upper Back

Tension, tightness, or aches in the upper back usually connect to a neck problem.

Prevention

The more time we spend sitting at desks, in cars, or in front of the TV, the more we must do to prevent back problems. Good posture and body mechanics will reduce the stress on your back.

For both men and women, extra weight in the abdomen area can make it harder to keep the natural curves in your back. For this reason, it is especially important to watch your posture and, if necessary, to reduce your weight. Also, smokers tend to have more back problems and take longer to recover from them.

Exercise (stretching, strengthening, and aerobic exercise) will help maintain your flexibility, strengthen the muscles that support your spine, and maintain your overall fitness.

Back Posture

Improper posture puts too much stress on your back and can lead to discomfort and damage. The key to good back posture is to keep the right amount of curve in your low back. Too much curve ("swayback") or too little curve ("flat back") can result in problems.

Standing and Walking

When you stand and walk with good posture, your ear, shoulder, hip, and ankle should be in a line. Do not lock your knees. Keep the small curve in your low back.

Sitting

When you sit, keep your shoulders back and down, chin back, abdomen in, and your low back supported in its natural curve. Slouching can stress the ligaments and muscles in your low back.

- Avoid sitting in one position for more than 1 hour at a time. Get up or change positions often.
- If you must sit a lot, the exercises on page 109 are particularly important.
- If your chair doesn't give enough support, use a small pillow or rolled towel to support your low back.
- See the illustration of proper sitting posture on page 114.
- To rise from a chair, keep the curves in your back and scoot forward to the edge of the chair. Use your leg muscles to stand up without leaning forward at the waist.
- For driving, pull your seat forward so that the pedals and steering wheel are within comfortable reach. Stop often to stretch and walk around. Consider using a small pillow for your low back.

Sleeping

A firm bed is better than a soft mattress or waterbed. Sleep so that your back keeps its natural curves.

- If you sleep on your back, you may want to use a towel roll to support your low back or a pillow under your knees.

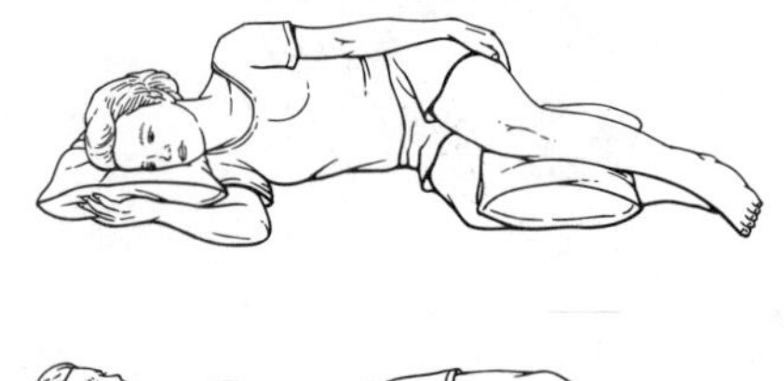

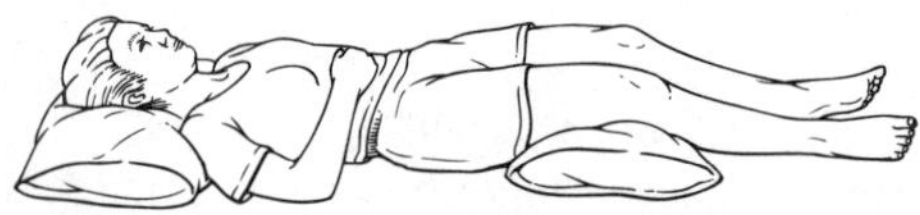

Use pillows while sleeping to prevent back or neck problems.

- If you sleep on your side, try placing a pillow between your knees.
- To rise from bed, lie on your side, bend both knees, and drop your feet over the side of the bed as you push with both arms to sit up. Scoot to the edge of the bed and position your feet under your buttocks. Stand up, keeping a small curve in your low back.

Body Mechanics

Good body mechanics means practicing good posture during daily activities. Use good body mechanics all the time, not just when you have a back problem.

- Keep the small curve in your low back.
- When you must stay in one position for long periods, take regular breaks to walk and stretch.
- When standing for long periods, stand with one foot on a small stool, ledge, or box.

Lifting

- Bend your knees and let your arms and legs do the work. Tighten your buttocks and abdomen to further support your back.
- Keep your upper back straight and keep the curve in your low back. Do not bend forward from the waist to lift.
- Keep the load as close to your body as possible, even if it is light.
- While holding a heavy object, turn your feet, not your back. Do not turn or twist your body.

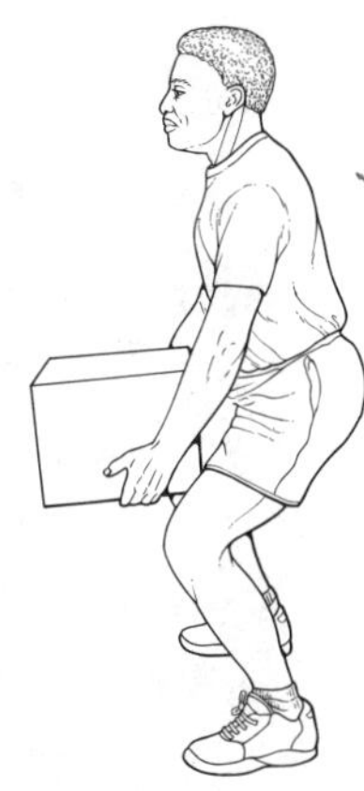

Avoid back strain when lifting heavy objects by keeping your upper back straight, bending your knees, and keeping the load close to your body.

- Never lift a heavy object above shoulder level.
- Get close to objects you need to reach. Use a stool or ladder for items that are above your head, and place it close to what you are doing.
- Use a hand truck or ask someone to help with heavy or awkward objects.

Exercises to Prevent Back Problems

Strengthening your entire body prevents future back problems and also improves your general health. Many exercises and sports strengthen your arms and legs. Doing special exercises to strengthen your abdominal muscles is also encouraged. See curl-ups and pelvic tilts on page 108.

Keeping your body flexible helps you to use proper body mechanics that protect your back.

These exercises are *not recommended* for use during an acute back problem or spasm. Instead, see First Aid for Back Problems on page 104.

- If any exercise causes increased or continuing back pain, stop the exercise and try something else. Stop any exercise that causes the pain to radiate away from your spine into your buttocks or legs, either during or after the exercises.
- You do not need to do every exercise. Stick with the ones that help you most.
- Start with 5 repetitions 3 to 4 times a day, and gradually increase to 10 repetitions. Do all exercises slowly.

The basic types of exercises that can help your back include: flexion, extension, and stretching and strengthening.

Flexion Exercises

Flexion exercises stretch the low back muscles and strengthen the stomach muscles.

1. Pelvic Tilts

This exercise gently moves the spine and stretches the low back.

- Lie on your back with knees bent and feet flat on the floor.
- Slowly tighten your stomach muscles and press your low back against the floor. Hold for 10 seconds (do not hold your breath). Slowly relax.

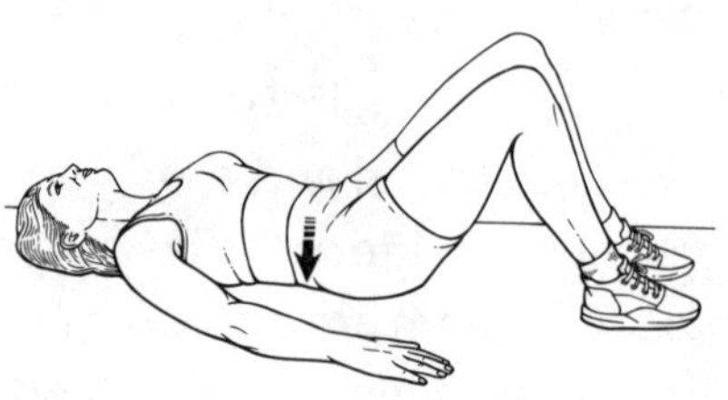

1. Pelvic tilt

2. Curl-Ups

Curl-ups strengthen your abdominal muscles, which work with your back muscles to support your spine.

- Lie on your back with knees bent (60° angle) and feet flat on the floor, arms crossed on your chest. Do not hook your feet under anything.
- Slowly curl your head and shoulders a few inches up until your shoulder blades barely rise from the floor. Keep your low back pressed to the floor. To avoid neck problems, remember to lift your shoulders and do not force your head up or forward. Hold for 5 to 10 seconds (do not hold your breath), then curl down very slowly. Do not do full sit-ups.

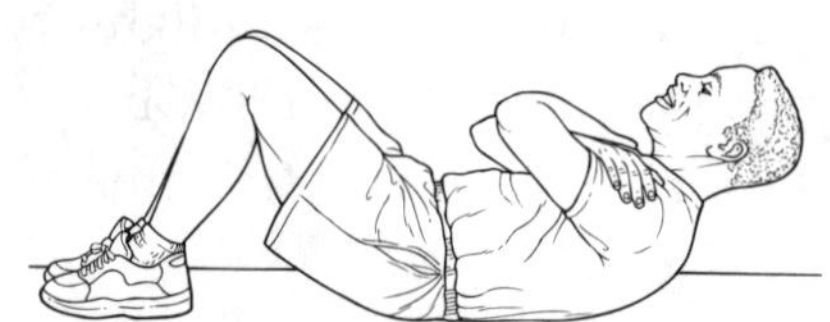

2. Curl-ups (keep neck straight and chin tucked in)

Extension Exercises

3. Press-Ups

- Lie facedown with your arms bent, palms flat on the floor.
- Lift yourself up on your elbows, keeping lower half of body relaxed. If it's comfortable, press your chest forward.
- Keep hips pressed to the floor. Feel the stretch in your low back.
- Lower your upper body to the floor. Repeat slowly 3 to 10 times.

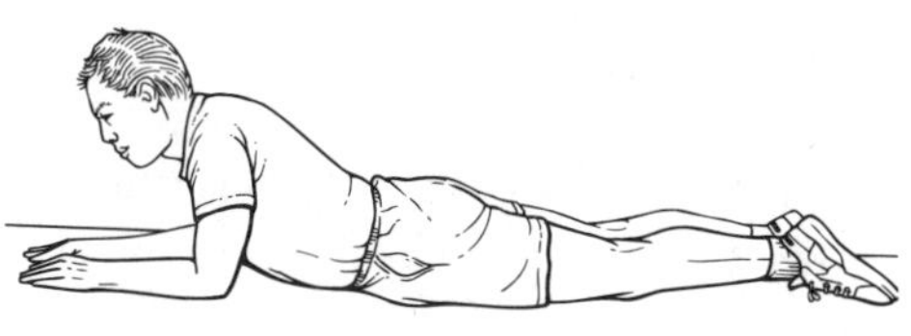

3. Press-ups

4. Backward Bend

Practice the backward bend at least once a day and do it frequently when you work in a bent-forward position.

- Stand upright with your feet slightly apart. Back up to a countertop for greater support and stability.
- Place your hands in the small of your back and gently bend backward. Keep your knees straight (not locked) and bend only at the waist. See illustration.
- Hold the backward stretch for 5 to 10 seconds.

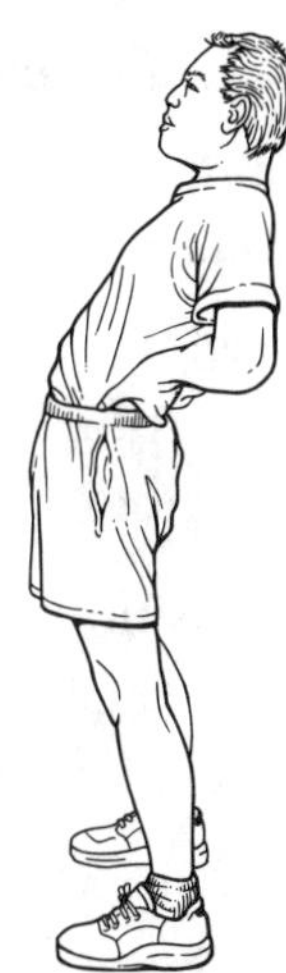

4. Backward bend (keep neck straight and chin down)

Additional Strengthening and Stretching Exercises

5. Prone Buttocks Squeeze

This exercise strengthens the buttocks muscles, which support the back and help you lift with your legs.

- Lie flat on your stomach with your arms at your sides.
- Slowly tighten your buttocks muscles and hold for 5 to 10 seconds (do not hold your breath). Relax slowly.
- You may need to place a small pillow under your stomach for comfort.

6. Hamstring Stretch

This exercise stretches the muscles in the back of your thigh, which will allow you to bend your legs while keeping your back in the neutral position.

- Lie on your back in a doorway with one leg through the doorway on the floor. Put the leg you want to stretch straight up with the heel resting on the wall next to the doorway.

- Keep the leg straight and slowly move your heel up the wall until you feel a gentle pull in the back of your thigh. Do not overstretch.
- Relax in this position for 30 seconds, then bend the knee to relieve the stretch. Repeat with the other leg.

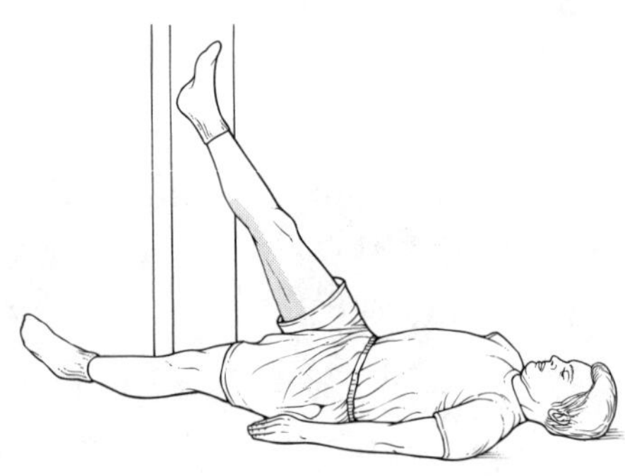

6. Hamstring stretch

7. Hip Flexor Stretch

This exercise stretches the muscles in the front of your hip, to avoid "swayback" caused by tight hip muscles.

- Kneel on one knee with your other leg bent and foot in front of you. Keep a natural curve in your back.
- Slowly shift your weight onto your front foot, maintaining a natural curve in your back. Hold for 10 seconds. You should feel a stretch in the groin of the leg you are kneeling on. Repeat with the other leg.

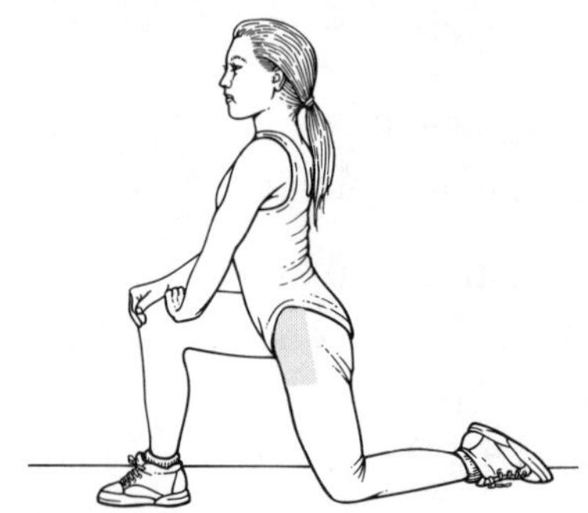

7. Hip flexor stretch

Exercises to Avoid

Many common exercises actually increase the risk of low back problems. Avoid the following:

- Straight-leg sit-ups
- Leg lifts (lifting both legs while lying on your back)
- Lifting heavy weights above the waist (military press, biceps curls while standing)
- Any stretching done while sitting with the legs in a V
- Toe touches while standing
- Fast, twisting movements

Home Treatment

It is important to stay as active as you can. The following tips may help you in your recovery:

- Use cold or moist heat on the injured area. See the icing guidelines on page 133. Ice your back until you feel numb, no more than 10 minutes every 2 hours. Always wrap the pack in a damp cloth to avoid harming your skin. Cold decreases inflammation, swelling, and pain.

Which Exercises for You?

- If you have no back problem now, try some of the prevention exercises on pages 107 to 110. *Do not* do the prevention exercises if you have just injured your back.
- If you have injured your back within the last 2 weeks, or you have more pain in your leg than in your back or buttocks, see Home Treatment on page 110 and When to Call Kaiser Permanente on page 112.
- Discontinue any exercise that increases pain.
- Gradually increase any exercise that helps you feel better.

- Moist heat often works well. Try taking warm showers, or use a warm, damp towel to apply heat. If you like, you can heat the towel in a microwave oven.
- If heat feels better, try a warm shower or use a warm towel. (Do not sit in the bathtub; this puts your back in the wrong position.) Use heat for no more than 20 minutes every 2 hours. Be careful not to irritate your skin. Be especially careful if you use electric heating pads, because people sometimes burn themselves by falling asleep on them.
- Avoid positions or activities that worsen your symptoms, such as sitting for long periods of time. Follow the posture and body mechanics guidelines discussed earlier.
- Keep a positive attitude. Most back injuries are temporary and heal. Healing improves when you keep active. Focus on what you *can* do rather than what you *can't* do.
- Keep moving, improving, and listening to your body. It hurts sometimes to move around, but hurt does not equal harm. Even for the first 2 to 3 days when it usually hurts the worst, it is important to stay as active as you can and gradually return to your usual activities. Soon you will be back to all your usual activities.
- The first few days you may need to take short breaks from your daily activities. If you lie down during your breaks, make sure you are on a firm surface.
- Medication can relieve pain and help you move around more easily. We recommend acetaminophen (Tylenol) because it has the fewest side effects. If Tylenol does not work for you, try coated aspirin (Ecotrin), ibuprofen (Advil, Motrin, Nuprin), naproxen (Aleve), or ketoprofen (Orudis KT). No matter which drug you use, it is important to follow the directions on the label.
- Take short walks for a few minutes every hour or 2, and work up to 20-minute walks.
- Relax your muscles frequently. See page 329 for progressive muscle relaxation.

After 2 to 3 days of home treatment:

- Because returning to work helps most people recover quickly, your goal is to get back to work or your usual activities as soon as possible. You may be able to go right back to your regular schedule. You may need to talk with your employer about how to modify your duties for the first few days or weeks.
- Continue frequent walks (increase as you can) and the exercises above.
- Try swimming, which is good for your back. It may be painful immediately after a back injury, but lap swimming, walking in water, or kicking with swim fins often helps prevent back problems from recurring. Using a snorkel and mask also helps, since you do not need to raise your head to breathe.
- When your back has improved, begin easy exercises that do not increase your back problem. One or two of the exercises in the Prevention section (pages 107 to 110) may be helpful. Start with 5 repetitions twice a day and increase to 10 repetitions as you are able.

Back Surgery

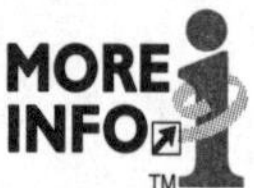

Very few people benefit from surgery for back problems. If you have serious weakness or loss of bladder or bowel control, then back surgery may be needed, and you may need to see a surgical specialist.

When to Call Kaiser Permanente

- If you have loss of bowel or bladder control. Although constipation and frequent or urgent urination are common in people with low back pain, any new problems with bowel or bladder control should be discussed with your physician.
- If you have new numbness in the genital or rectal area.
- If you have leg weakness that is not solely due to pain. Many people with low back pain say their legs feel weak. However, significant leg weakness should be evaluated, especially if you are unable to bend your foot upward, get up out of a chair, or climb stairs.
- If you have new or increased back pain with unexplained fever, painful urination, or other signs of urinary tract infection. See page 100.
- If you have a dramatic increase in your chronic back pain, especially if it is unrelated to a new or changed physical activity.
- If you have a history of cancer or HIV infection and develop new or increased back pain.
- If you have new back pain that does not show improvement after a few days of home treatment, contact your physician for advice.
- If you develop a new, severe pain in your low back that does not change with movement and is not related to stress or muscle tension.

- If you cannot walk or stand.
- If back pain does not improve after 2 weeks of home treatment.

Physicians or Nurse Practitioners

In addition to diagnosing the cause of back pain and evaluating back injuries, a physician (MD or DO) or nurse practitioner may also:

- Help you develop an individualized exercise and home care plan or modified work plan if needed.
- Prescribe muscle relaxants, anti-inflammatory drugs, and pain relievers. Note: If you do get a strong painkiller or muscle relaxer, avoid postures and activities that could reinjure your back.
- Refer you to physical therapy.
- Recommend back surgery.

Doctors of osteopathy (DO) may also do spinal manipulation.

Physical Therapists

After the initial first-aid actions, a physical therapist with training in orthopedic treatment can help you in either a group or individual setting by:

- Identifying specific muscle or disc problems.
- Providing other therapies, such as manual therapy, if you aren't improving.
- Helping you improve your posture and customizing an exercise program for recovery and long-term protection.

Other Professionals

Chiropractors can provide relief from some types of back pain through spinal manipulation. Acupuncturists, massage therapists, and others may also provide short-term relief.

Neck Problems

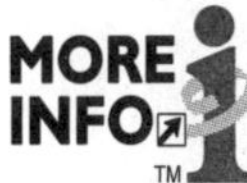

Neck pain and stiffness are usually caused by strain or spasm of the neck muscles or inflammation of the neck joints. They may occasionally be due to arthritis or damage to the discs between the neck (cervical) vertebrae. Neck movement may be limited, usually more to one side than the other. Neck problems often cause headaches or pain in the shoulder, upper back, or down the arm.

When you sit, stand, or move in a way that mistreats your neck, you may feel aches, pains, or discomfort in your neck, shoulders, upper back, head, ears, sinuses, jaw, chest, or arms. You may feel numbness, tingling, or weakness in your arms or hands. You may also feel dizzy.

Neck pain and headaches are sometimes related to tension in the trapezius muscles, which run from the back of the head across the back of the shoulder. When you have neck pain, these muscles may also feel tight and painful.

Neck muscle strain may be due to:

Forward head posture.

- Sleeping on a pillow that's too high, too flat, or doesn't support your head.
- Sleeping on your stomach or with the neck twisted or bent.
- Extended periods of the "thinker's pose" (resting your chin on your upright fist or arm).
- Watching TV or reading lying down with the neck in an awkward position.
- Stress.
- A workstation that puts the neck in an awkward position.
- Other pressures on the neck muscles.
- Injury that causes sudden movement of the head and neck (whiplash) or a direct blow to the neck.
- Strenuous activity with the upper body and arms.

Meningitis is a serious illness that causes a severe stiff neck with headache and fever (see page 160).

Prevention

Good posture, body mechanics, and exercise are important to preventing neck problems. Most neck problems that aren't due to arthritis or an injury are completely avoidable.

If pain is worse at the **end of the day**, evaluate your posture and body mechanics during the day.

- Sit straight in your chair with your low back supported. Avoid sitting for long periods without getting up or changing positions. Take mini-breaks several times each hour to stretch your neck muscles.

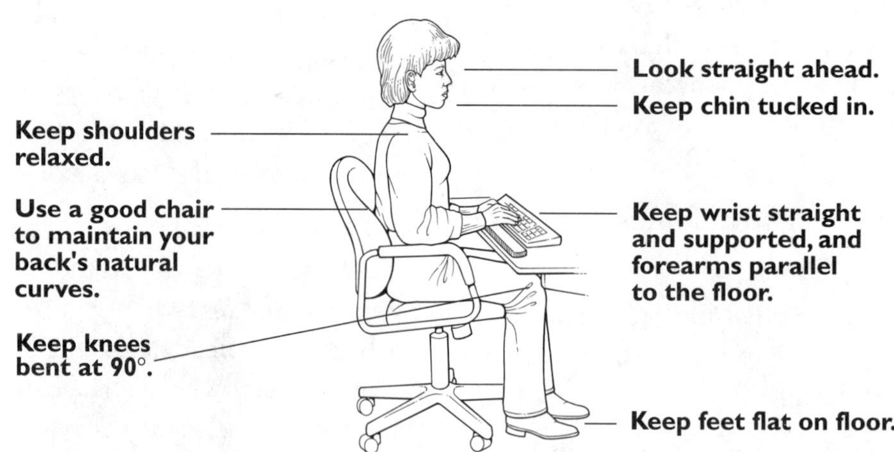

Good posture and support when you are seated can make any task more comfortable and will reduce strain on the eyes, neck, shoulders, arms, wrists, and back.

- If you work at a computer, adjust the monitor so that the top of the screen is at eye level. Use a document holder that puts the copy at the same level as the screen. The screen should be about an arm's length from your eyes.
- If you use the telephone a lot, consider a headset or speakerphone.
- Adjust your car seat to a more upright position that supports your head and low back.
- If neck stiffness is worse **in the morning**, check your sleeping posture (and your activities the day before).
- Improve your sleeping support. A hard mattress or special neck support pillow may solve the problem (try before buying). Or, you can fold a towel lengthwise into a 4-inch-wide pad, wrap it around your neck, and pin it for good support.

Neck Exercises

You do not need to do every exercise. Stick with the ones that help you the most. Stop any exercise that increases pain. Start with 5 repetitions twice a day. Do each exercise slowly.

1. Dorsal glide: Sit or stand tall, looking straight ahead (a "palace guard" posture). Slowly tuck your chin as you glide your head backwards over your body. Hold for a count of 5, then relax. Repeat 6 to 10 times. This stretches the back of the neck. If you feel pain, do not glide so far back. Some people find this exercise easier while lying on their back with ice on the neck.

2. Chest and shoulder stretch: Sit or stand tall and glide your head backward as in exercise 1. Raise both arms so that your hands are next to your ears. Relax your shoulders and, as you exhale, lower your elbows down toward your sides and backward. Feel your shoulder blades slide down and together. Hold for a few seconds. Relax and repeat.

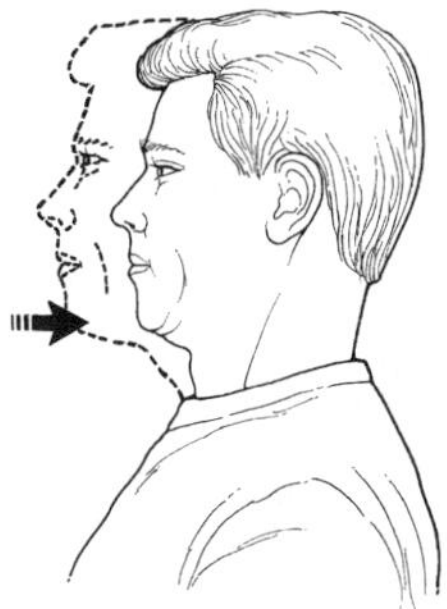

Dorsal glide

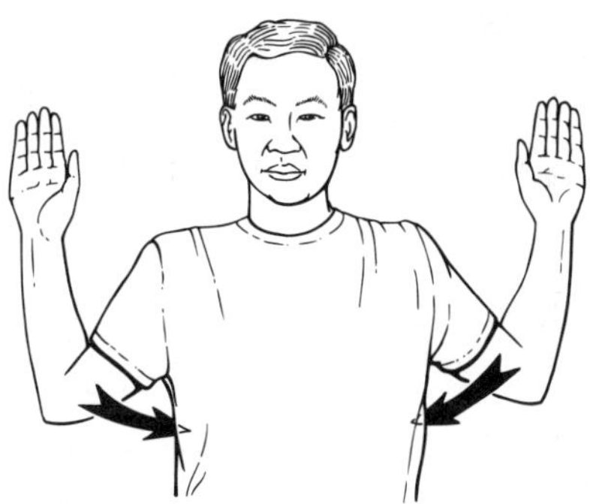

Chest and shoulder stretch: move elbows down toward your sides and backward.

- Avoid pillows that force your head forward when you are sleeping on your back.
- When sleeping on your side, make sure your nose is in line with the center of your body.
- If stress is a factor, practice the progressive muscle relaxation exercises on page 329.
- Strengthen and protect your neck by doing neck exercises once a day. See page 115.

Home Treatment

Much of the home treatment for back problems is also helpful for neck problems, including the guidelines on posture, body mechanics, ice, and moist heat. Also see page 110.

- If there has been a recent accident involving the neck, see page 69.
- Place a cold pack up to 10 minutes at a time or moist heat up to 20 minutes at a time over painful muscles, as often as once every 2 hours. It will help decrease any pain, muscle spasm, or swelling. If the problem is near the shoulder or upper back, it will usually help more to place ice or heat on the back of the neck.
- Keep your head and neck centered over your body. Avoid slouching or forward head posture.
- Use aspirin, ibuprofen, or acetaminophen to help relieve pain.
- Walking is also helpful in relieving and preventing neck problems. The gentle swinging motion of your arms often relieves pain. Start with short walks of 5 to 10 minutes, 3 to 4 times a day.
- If neck problems occur with headache, see Tension Headaches on page 194.
- Once the pain subsides, do the prevention exercises on page 115. Start with 5 repetitions twice a day. Gradually increase to 10 repetitions. Stop doing any exercise that causes pain.

When to Call Kaiser Permanente

Call immediately:

- If a stiff neck occurs together with headache and fever. Also see "Encephalitis and Meningitis" on page 160.
- If the pain extends or shoots down one arm, or you have numbness or tingling in your hands.
- If you develop new weakness in the arms or legs.
- If a blow or injury to the neck (whiplash) has caused new pain.
- If you are unable to manage the problem with home treatment.
- If the problem has lasted 2 weeks or longer without improvement despite home treatment.

I don't deserve this award, but then I have arthritis and I don't deserve that either.
Jack Benny

6

Bone, Muscle, and Joint Problems

This chapter covers pain from arthritis to ankle sprains. The focus is less on reducing pain and more on limiting its impact on our quality of life. We hope these guidelines will make your life more comfortable.

Arthritis

Arthritis refers to a variety of joint problems that cause pain, swelling, and stiffness. Simply put, arthritis means inflammation of a joint. Arthritis can occur at any age, but it affects older people the most.

There are over 100 different types of arthritis, each with its own specific symptoms. Little is known about what causes most types. Some seem to run in families; others seem to be related to imbalances in body chemistry or immune system problems.

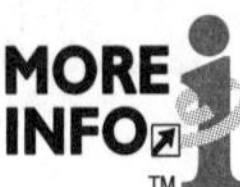

The chart on page 118 describes the 3 most common kinds of arthritis. Osteoarthritis is the most common type and can usually be successfully managed at home. Rheumatoid arthritis and gout will improve with a combination of self-care and professional care.

Prevention

It may not be possible to prevent arthritis, but you can prevent a lot of pain by being kind to your joints. This is especially important if you already have arthritis.

- Modify activities that cause repeated jarring, such as high-impact aerobic activities, to low-impact activities if they cause pain.
- Exercise regularly.
- If you are experiencing back, hip, knee, or foot problems, controlling your weight may help.

Common Types of Arthritis			
Type	**Cause**	**Symptoms**	**Comments**
Osteoarthritis	Breakdown of joint cartilage.	Pain, stiffness, and swelling; common in fingers, hips, and knees.	Most common type in women and men between the ages of 45 and 90.
Rheumatoid Arthritis	Inflammation of the membrane lining the joint (synovium).	Pain, stiffness, welling in multiple joints; joints may be "hot" and red; common in hands, wrists, and feet.	Occurs most often around age 30 to 40; more common in women.
Gout	Buildup of uric acid crystals in the joint fluid.	Sudden onset of burning pain, stiffness, and swelling; common in big toe, ankle, knee, wrist, and elbow.	Most common in men over 40; may be aggravated by drinking alcohol.

While repeated jarring activities can increase joint pain, regular exercise can relieve or prevent it. Exercise is needed to nourish the joint cartilage and remove waste products. It also strengthens the muscles around the joint. Strong muscles support the joint and reduce injuries caused by fatigue. Stretching maintains your range of pain-free motion.

Home Treatment

- A warm shower or bath may help relieve morning stiffness. Try to avoid sitting still after a warm shower or bath.
- If the joint is not swollen, apply moist heat for 20 to 30 minutes, 2 to 3 times a day. Do not apply heat to a swollen, inflamed joint.
- Gently move the joint through as full a range of motion as possible without pain, several times a day, to prevent stiffness.
- When a joint is hurting, avoid activities that put unusual strain on it for a few days. Take short rest breaks from your regular activities throughout the day.
- Apply cold packs to inflamed, swollen joints for up to 10 minutes, once an hour. Cold will help relieve pain and reduce inflammation (although it may be uncomfortable for the first few minutes).
- Regular exercise is important to help maintain strength and flexibility in the muscles and joints. Strengthening exercises prevent the muscle decline that leads to

loss of function. Try low-impact activities, such as swimming, water aerobics, biking, or walking.

- Acetaminophen can provide safe pain relief for osteoarthritis. Aspirin, ibuprofen, naproxen, or ketoprofen can also help ease pain but can cause stomach upset. Do not use more than one anti-inflammatory medication (aspirin, ibuprofen, naproxen, etc.) at the same time. See page 349 for the symptoms of aspirin overdose.
- Enroll in an arthritis self-management program. Participants usually have less pain and fewer limitations on their activities.
- Call your local Arthritis Foundation office for more information.

When to Call Kaiser Permanente

- If you have fever or a skin rash along with severe joint pain.
- If the joint is so painful that you cannot use it.
- If there is sudden, unexplained swelling, redness, or pain in any joint.
- If there is severe pain and swelling in multiple joints.
- If you experience sudden back pain that occurs with weakness in the legs or loss of bowel or bladder control.
- If joint pain continues for over 6 weeks and home treatment is not helping.
- If you experience side effects from aspirin or other arthritis medication (stomach pain, nausea, persistent heartburn, or dark, tarry stools). Do not exceed recommended doses of over-the-counter medications without your physician's advice.

Bunions and Hammer Toes

A bunion is a swelling of the joint at the base of the big toe. The big toe may bend toward and overlap the other toes. A hammer toe is a toe that bends up permanently at the middle joint. Both conditions are usually irritated by wearing shoes that are too short or narrow. These problems sometimes run in families.

Prevention

Tight or high-heeled shoes increase the risk of bunions and hammer toes and irritate them if they are already present. Wear shoes with no heel (or a low heel) and a roomy toe area. Tennis or basketball court shoes are often best. Make sure that your shoes fit properly.

Home Treatment

Once you have a bunion or hammer toe, there is usually no way to completely get rid of it. Home treatment will help keep it from getting worse.

- Wear low-heeled, roomy shoes that have good arch supports.

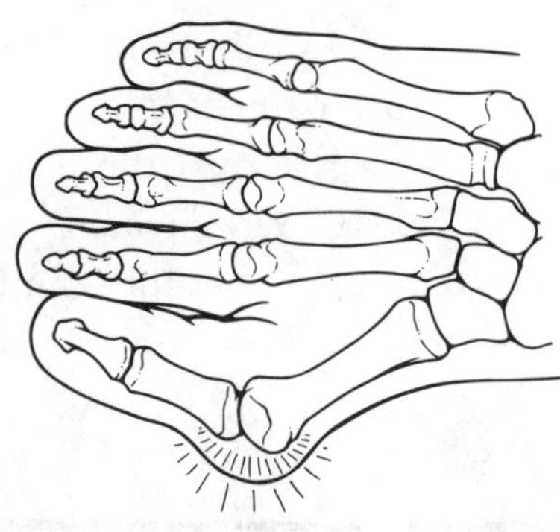

A bunion is a swelling caused by a misshapen joint at the base of the big toe.

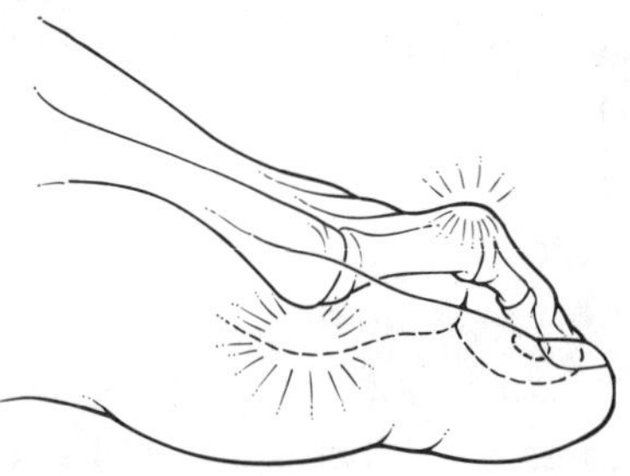

A hammer toe is a toe that bends up permanently at the middle joint.

- Cushion the bunion or hammer toe with moleskin or doughnut-shaped pads to prevent rubbing and irritation.
- Cut out the area over the bunion or hammer toe from an old pair of shoes to wear around the house, or wear comfortable sandals that don't press on the area.
- Try aspirin, ibuprofen, or acetaminophen to relieve pain. Ice or cold packs may also help.

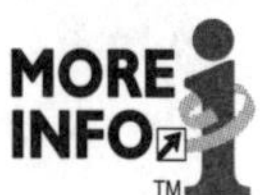

If severe pain or joint deformity interferes with walking or daily activities, you may want to consider surgical treatment. Surgery may not cure the problem completely. The more information you gather about the risks and benefits of surgery for bunions and hammer toes, the easier it will be for you to make a wise health decision.

When to Call Kaiser Permanente

- If severe pain in the big toe comes on suddenly, and you have not been diagnosed with gout.
- If severe pain interferes with walking or daily activities.
- If the big toe begins to overlap the second toe.
- If you have diabetes, poor circulation, or peripheral vascular disease. Irritated skin over a bunion or hammer toe can easily become infected in people with these conditions.
- If pain does not respond to home treatment in 2 to 3 weeks.

Bursitis and Tendinitis

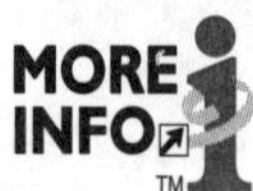

A bursa is a small sac of fluid that helps the muscles slide easily over other muscles or bones. Injury or overuse of a joint or tendon may result in pain, redness, heat, and inflammation of the bursa, a condition known as bursitis. Bursitis often develops quickly, over just a few days, often after a specific injury or overuse.

MORE INFO For more information, see the inside front cover.

Tendons are tough, rope-like fibers that connect muscles to bones. Injury or overuse may cause pain, tenderness, and inflammation in the tendons or the tissues surrounding them, a condition known as tendinitis. Both bursitis and tendinitis can also be related to job, sports, or household activities that require repeated twisting or rapid joint movements.

Bursitis and tendinitis can occur at several different places in the body and can occur together in one place. The same home treatment is good for both problems.

Prevention

Regular warm-ups and stretching may help prevent bursitis or tendinitis. Warm up well before exercising, gradually increase the intensity of the activity, and stretch afterwards. See pages 122 to 123 for additional, joint-specific prevention tips.

Home Treatment

Bursitis or tendinitis will usually go away or at least subside in a few days or weeks if you avoid the activity that caused it.

The most common mistake in recovery is thinking that the problem is gone when the pain is gone. Chances are, bursitis or tendinitis will recur if you do not take steps to strengthen and stretch the muscles around the joint and change the way you do some activities.

- When a joint or tendon is hurting, change the way you do the activity that causes pain so that you can do it without pain. See pages 122 to 123 for joint-specific guidelines. To maintain fitness, substitute activities that don't stress the inflamed area.
- As soon as you notice pain, apply ice or cold packs for periods of up to 10 minutes, once an hour for the first 48 hours. After 48 hours, use ice or heat, whichever brings more relief. See page 133. Although heating pads or hot baths may feel good, ice or cold packs will relieve inflammation and speed healing.
- Aspirin, ibuprofen, or naproxen may help ease pain and inflammation, but don't use medication to relieve pain while you continue overusing a joint.
- Gently move the joint through as full a range of motion as you can without pain several times a day to prevent stiffness. As the pain subsides, continue stretching and add exercises to strengthen the affected muscles.
- Warm up before and stretch after the activity. Apply ice to the injured area after exercise to prevent pain and swelling.
- Gradually resume the activity at a lower intensity. Increase slowly and only if pain does not recur.

In addition to the general prevention and home treatment information for bursitis and tendinitis above, the following tips will be useful if you have a specific joint problem.

Wrist pain may be due to tendinitis. Though this is not the same as carpal tunnel syndrome, the same home care may help. See page 125.

Elbow pain is often due to one of the following common types of tendinitis in the forearm muscle tendons. The inside or outside of the elbow is defined by holding the arm at your side with the palm facing forward.

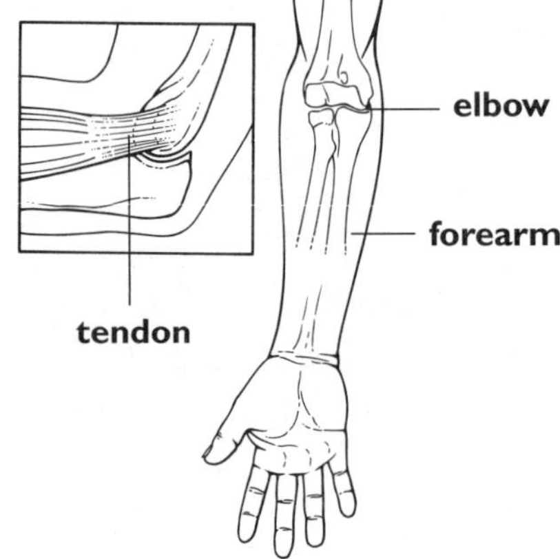

Elbow pain is often caused by inflammation of a tendon in the forearm.

Tennis elbow causes pain on the outside of the elbow where the muscles that bend the wrist back are attached.

Golfer's elbow causes pain on the inside of the elbow where the muscles that bend the wrist down are attached.

- Strengthen the wrist, arm, shoulder, and back muscles to help protect the elbow.
- A brace or elbow sleeve may help relieve pain.
- Use tools with larger handles.
- Use a 2-handed tennis backhand and a midsize, more flexible racquet.
- Avoid activities that put a strain on the elbow.
- Avoid sidearm pitching and throwing curve balls.

Shoulder pain that occurs on the outside of the upper arm is often due to impingement (caused by tendinitis or bursitis) in the shoulder joint. Pain on the top of the shoulder or in the neck is often due to tension in the trapezius muscles, which run from the back of the head across the back of the shoulders. See Neck Problems on page 113.

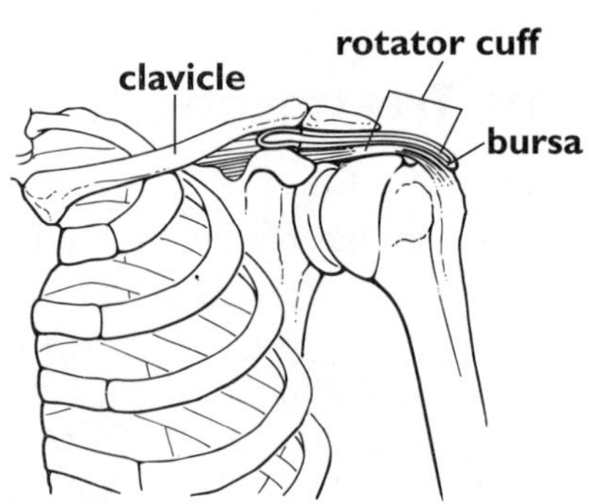

Common causes of shoulder pain are tendinitis, bursitis, and muscle tension.

Common symptoms of impingement are pain, pinching, and stiffness in your shoulder when you raise your arm. It is often caused by repeated overhead movements. Problems develop when the shoulder continues to be used without getting time to rest. This leads to further swelling and pain.

For home treatment of shoulder pain, see the information on page 121. In addition, keep the following tips in mind:

- Avoid overhead activities, but continue to use your shoulder.
- Practice the pendulum exercise to help prevent stiffness (see below).
- Use proper throwing technique for baseball and football.
- Use a different swim stroke: breast stroke or sidestroke instead of the crawl or butterfly.

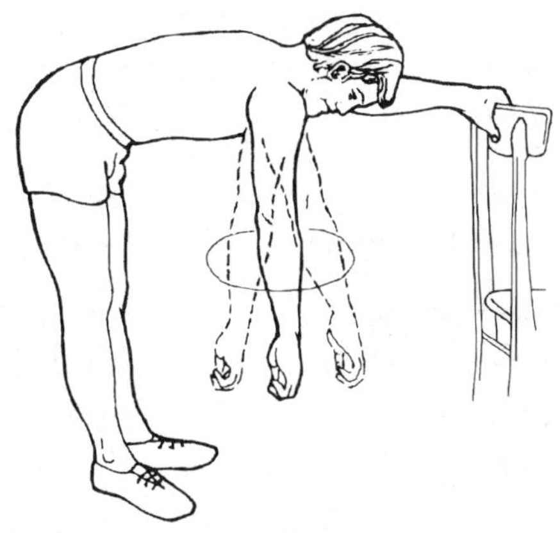

Pendulum exercise: Let your arm "dangle" freely. Move it clockwise and counterclockwise in increasingly large circles. Swing your arm forward, backward, and side to side.

Hip pain: Tendinitis or bursitis in the hip can cause pain at the side of the hip when rising from a chair and taking the first few steps, while climbing stairs, or while driving. If pain is severe, sleeping on your side may also be painful. Pain in the front of the hip may also be due to arthritis. See page 117.

- Wear well-cushioned shoes and avoid high heels.
- Walk up and down stairs one at a time, leading with your strong leg, until the pain is gone.
- Avoid activities that force one side of the pelvis higher than the other, such as running in only one direction on a track or working sideways on a slope. Keep the pelvis level.
- Sleep on your uninjured side with a pillow between your knees, or on your back with pillows beneath your knees.
- See the hip stretches on pages 110 and 295. Stretch after activity, when your muscles are warm.

Knee pain may be caused by bursitis or tendinitis. See Knee Problems on page 126.

Heel or foot pain may be due to plantar fasciitis or Achilles tendinitis. See page 130. Pain in the front of the lower leg may be due to shin-splints. See page 127.

When to Call Kaiser Permanente

- If there is fever, rapid swelling, redness, or an inability to use a joint.
- If severe pain continues when the joint is at rest and you have applied ice.
- If the problem is severe and you can think of no injury or activity that might have caused it.
- If the pain persists for 2 weeks or longer despite home treatment. Your physician or physical therapist can help you develop a specific exercise and home treatment plan.

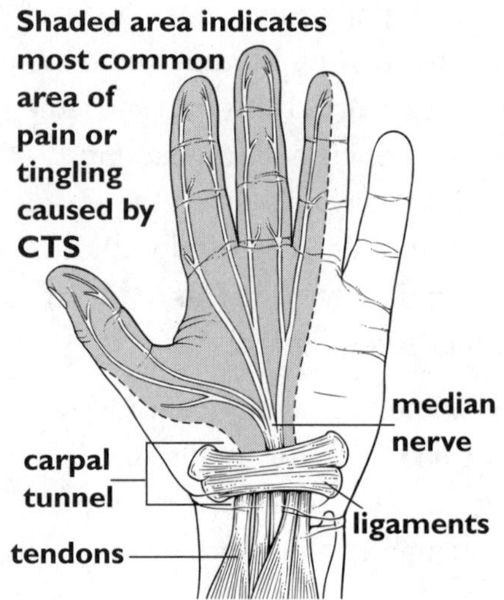

Pain and tingling in the hand may be caused by pressure on a nerve in the wrist.

Carpal Tunnel Syndrome

The carpal tunnel is a narrow passageway between the bones and ligaments in your wrist. The median nerve, which controls sensation in the fingers and some muscles in the hand, passes through this tunnel along with some of the finger tendons. Carpal tunnel syndrome (CTS) develops when there is pressure on the median nerve where it goes through the carpal tunnel.

Doing activities that use the same finger or hand movements over and over again can cause CTS. Other causes include being overweight, a cyst (ganglion) on the tendon sheath in the wrist, or rheumatoid arthritis. Previous wrist injuries, pregnancy, diabetes, thyroid disease, and taking birth control pills also may increase your risk for CTS.

Pressure on the median nerve causes the following symptoms of CTS:

- Numbness or tingling in the fingers of one or both hands, except for the little finger.
- Numbness or pain in your hand or wrist that wakes you up at night.
- Numbness or pain that gets worse when you use your hand or wrist, especially when you grip an object or bend (flex) your wrist.
- Occasional aching pain in your arm from your hand to your shoulder.
- A weak grip.

Prevention

- Stop any activity that you think may be causing finger, hand, or wrist numbness or pain. If your symptoms improve when you stop an activity, resume that activity gradually and with greater efforts to keep your wrist straight or only slightly bent.
- Use your whole hand (not just your fingers and thumb) to grasp objects.
- Reduce the speed and force of repetitive hand movements such as typing.
- Switch hands and change positions often when you are doing repeated motions.
- Take frequent breaks and rest your hands.
- If you are not able to change positions or equipment at work often enough to prevent numbness or pain, wear a wrist splint that will reduce the stress on your fingers, hand, or wrist.
- Pay attention to your posture. When you are typing, make sure your fingers are lower than your wrists (using a keyboard wrist support may help). When your forearms are hanging by your sides, keep your shoulders relaxed.
- Keeping your arm, hand, and finger muscles strong and flexible and maintaining good overall fitness will also help prevent the symptoms of carpal tunnel syndrome.
- Avoid using too much salt if you tend to retain fluid.

Home Treatment

- Follow the prevention tips above.
- Use aspirin, ibuprofen, or naproxen sodium to relieve pain and reduce swelling.
- Apply ice or a cold pack to the palm side of the wrist. See "Ice and Cold Packs" on page 133.
- Avoid sleeping on your hands. Wear a wrist splint at night to relieve pressure on your wrist.
- Do simple range-of-motion exercises with your fingers and wrist to prevent stiffening. Stop if you have pain.
- Other lifestyle changes such as losing weight, quitting smoking, reducing the amount of alcohol you drink, and controlling diabetes may help relieve symptoms of CTS that are related to swelling.
- Vitamin B_6 has not been shown to be an effective treatment for CTS.

When to Call Kaiser Permanente

- If tingling, numbness, weakness, or pain in your fingers and hand has not gone away after 2 weeks of home treatment.
- If you have little or no feeling in your fingers or hand.
- If you cannot do simple hand movements, or you accidentally drop things.

- If you cannot pinch your thumb and first finger together or your pinch is weak.
- If you cannot use your thumb (no thumb strength).
- If you have problems at work because of pain in your fingers or hand.

If you are considering surgery to treat carpal tunnel syndrome, gather as much information as possible about the risks and benefits of surgical treatment. Getting all the facts and thinking about your own needs and values will help you work with your physician to make a wise health decision.

Knee Problems

The knee is a vulnerable joint. It is basically just 2 long leg bones held together with ligaments and muscles. Problems develop when you put too much stress on the joint. The 3 most common knee problems are:

- Strained or sprained ligaments and muscles caused by a blow to the knee, forcing it in a direction that it does not normally bend. See Strains, Sprains, and Fractures on page 134.
- **Kneecap pain,** also known as patellofemoral pain. This problem causes pain around or behind the kneecap when running downhill, going up or down stairs, or after sitting for long periods of time.

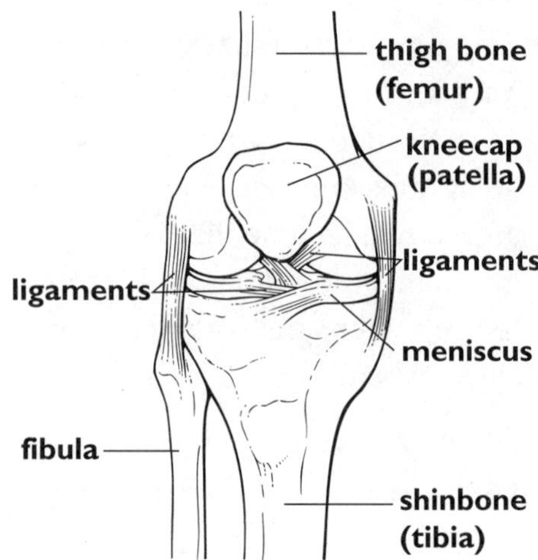

Knee problems can develop when too much stress is put on the joint.

- **Patellar tendinitis,** also known as jumper's knee, is an inflammation of the tendon that attaches the kneecap (patella) to the shinbone (tibia). It is common among basketball and volleyball players.

Prevention

- The best way to prevent knee problems is to stay active and strengthen and stretch the leg muscles, especially the front and back of the thigh (quadriceps and hamstring). See page 295.
- Avoid deep knee bends.
- Avoid running downhill unless you are fully conditioned.
- Avoid wearing shoes with cleats when playing contact sports.
- Wear shoes with good arch supports. Replace running shoes every 300 to 500 miles.

For more information, see the inside front cover.

- Avoid wearing high-heeled shoes.
- Also see Bursitis and Tendinitis on page 120.

Home Treatment

- Apply ice to your knee. See "Ice and Cold Packs" on page 133.
- Reduce by at least ½ the activities that cause pain.
- A brace or elastic or neoprene sleeve or a band with a hole for the kneecap that holds the kneecap in place may help ease pain during activity. You can buy one at a pharmacy or sporting goods store.
- Warm up well before vigorous activities.
- Stretch the front and back of your thigh (quadriceps and hamstring) muscles after exercise, when they are warm. See pages 110 and 295.
- Also see Strains, Sprains, and Fractures on page 134 and Bursitis and Tendinitis on page 120.
- If knee pain is not related to exercise or due to a recent or past injury, see Arthritis on page 117.

When to Call Kaiser Permanente

- If the knee wobbles from side to side or "gives out."
- If you felt or heard a "pop" during a knee injury that was followed by immediate swelling.
- If you are unable to straighten the knee, or if the joint "locks."
- If the knee is red, hot, swollen, or painful to touch.
- If pain is severe enough that you are limping, or if it does not improve substantially within 2 to 5 days.

Muscle Cramps and Leg Pain

Leg and muscle cramps ("charley horse" or "stitch") are common. They often occur during exercise, especially during hot weather, or at night. Dehydration or low levels of potassium in the body and using a muscle that is not stretched well may cause cramps.

Pain in the front of the lower leg may be due to shinsplints, especially if you have recently increased your exercise.

Arthritis can also cause leg pain (see page 117). Leg pain that runs from the buttocks down the back of the leg and into the foot may be due to sciatica. See page 105.

Phlebitis, an inflammation of a vein, also causes leg pain, usually in the calf of one leg. This condition can be serious if blood clots formed in the vein break loose and lodge in the lungs. It is most common after surgery or prolonged bed rest. Decreased blood flow to the leg muscles caused by narrowing of the arteries (called intermittent claudication) is another possible cause of leg cramps. Symptoms may include cramping pain in the calf that comes on with activity or exertion and is relieved by rest. Symptoms often occur after you walk a certain distance.

Prevention

- Warm up well and stretch before any activity. Stretch after exercise to keep hot muscles from shortening and cramping.
- Drink extra water before and during exercise, especially during hot or humid weather.
- Include plenty of potassium in your diet. Bananas, orange juice, and potatoes are good sources.
- To avoid stomach muscle cramps ("stitches") during exercise, do side stretches before exercising and learn to breathe with your lower lungs. See page 328.
- If cramps wake you at night, take a warm bath and do some stretching exercises before going to bed. Keep your legs warm while sleeping.

Growing Pains

Children age 6 to 12 often develop harmless "growing pains" in their legs at night. The cause is unknown. A heating pad, acetaminophen, or gentle massage of the legs may help.

Home Treatment

If there is pain, swelling, or heaviness in the calf of one leg only, or other symptoms that cause you to suspect phlebitis (see When to Call Kaiser Permanente), call your physician before attempting home treatment.

- Follow the prevention guidelines.
- Gently stretch the cramping muscle. Rub or massage the cramp.
- To stretch the calf, straighten your leg, grab your foot, and pull it toward you.
- Drink some extra water. Cramps are often related to dehydration.
- The best treatment for shinsplints is ice, aspirin, ibuprofen, or acetaminophen, and 1 to 2 weeks of rest followed by a gradual return to exercise. Try to identify the cause (shoes, exercise surface) and correct it.

When to Call Kaiser Permanente

- If you have the following symptoms :
  - Pain deep in the leg or calf
  - Heat, redness, or pain along the course of a leg vein
  - Swelling of one leg
  - Leg or foot is cold and looks white or blue
  - Shortness of breath, or chest pain

- If leg cramps worsen or persist in spite of prevention and home treatment.
- If cramps or leg pain occur repeatedly during even mild exercise, such as walking, even if relieved by rest.

Fibromyalgia

Fibromyalgia is a condition that causes chronic muscle and soft tissue pain and tenderness on both sides of the body, above and below the waist. Fibromyalgia does not damage the body, destroy the joints, or cause any internal organ problems, but the pain may be severe enough to interfere with work and other activities.

The cause of fibromyalgia is not known. People who have fibromyalgia have many tender spots in specific areas of their bodies (trigger points). They often have trouble sleeping because of the pain. There may also be stiffness, weakness, and fatigue. Fibromyalgia is more common in women than in men.

Regular exercise, such as walking, biking, or swimming, is the cornerstone of treatment for fibromyalgia. Physicians sometimes prescribe medications to help treat the symptoms. If stress makes your symptoms worse, see page 328.

Osteoporosis

Osteoporosis or "brittle bones" is a condition that affects 25 percent of women over age 60. It is much less common and not as severe in men. It is more common after menopause, when estrogen levels decline. Osteoporosis is caused by loss of bone mass and strength. Bones weakened by osteoporosis are easily broken. Risk factors for osteoporosis include:

- Current smoker
- Thin, small-boned frame
- Family history of osteoporosis (especially hip fracture)
- History of fracture (other than spine) after age 50

Osteoporosis is a silent disease; there may be no symptoms until a bone breaks and the condition is recognized after X-rays. The first sign may be back pain, or fracture of a wrist after a fall.

Prevention

It is best to start to build sturdy bones in childhood, but the steps given here will help anytime. Peak bone mass is reached during your twenties and thirties. These steps can help you build and keep strong bones throughout your life.

- Get regular weight-bearing exercise, such as walking. Exercise helps keep bones strong. See Chapter 16.

- Get plenty of calcium in your diet. The average American diet contains about 500 mg per day, but 1,300 mg are recommended for teenagers and 1,000 mg for adults until age 50. After age 50 both men and women need 1,200 mg of calcium daily. Pregnant women and breastfeeding mothers should get about 1,200 mg per day. The best source of calcium is low-fat dairy products. See page 304.
- If you are unable to get all the calcium you need from your diet, take 2 to 3 calcium carbonate tablets (Tums or other calcium supplements) each day with meals or with milk. Don't take more than 4 to 6 tablets per day, and drink lots of water, because they can cause constipation. Too much calcium also increases the risk for kidney stones.
- If you smoke or use other tobacco products, consider getting help to quit. See page 26 for tips on quitting.
- Drink alcohol only in moderation (1 drink per day), if at all.
- Getting enough vitamin D is also important. Children and adults need 200 IU per day. After age 50, 400 IU are recommended, and adults over age 65 need 600 to 800 IU daily.
- Most of the vitamin D we need comes from our skin absorbing sunlight and from drinking vitamin D fortified milk (each 8-ounce serving has 100 IU). Older adults may need to take supplemental vitamin D. A good way to do this is to take a multivitamin with vitamin D every day.

When to Call Kaiser Permanente

- If a fall causes hip pain or if you are unable to get up after a fall.
- If you have sudden, unexplained back pain that does not improve after 2 to 3 days of home treatment.

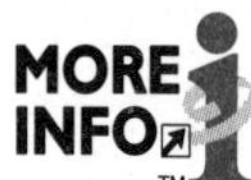

If you are at risk for osteoporosis and are nearing menopause, talk with your physician about whether you need medication.

Plantar Fasciitis

Plantar fasciitis is a condition that occurs when the thick, fibrous tissue that covers the bottom of your foot (plantar fascia) becomes inflamed and painful. Athletes (especially runners), middle-aged people, and those who are overweight tend to develop plantar fasciitis. Repetitive exercises such as running and jumping sports can lead to heel pain and plantar fasciitis.

An excessive inward rolling of the foot during walking or running (called pronation) can also cause heel pain and plantar fasciitis. Pronation can be due to poor arch support, worn-out shoes, tight calf muscles, or by running downhill or on uneven surfaces.

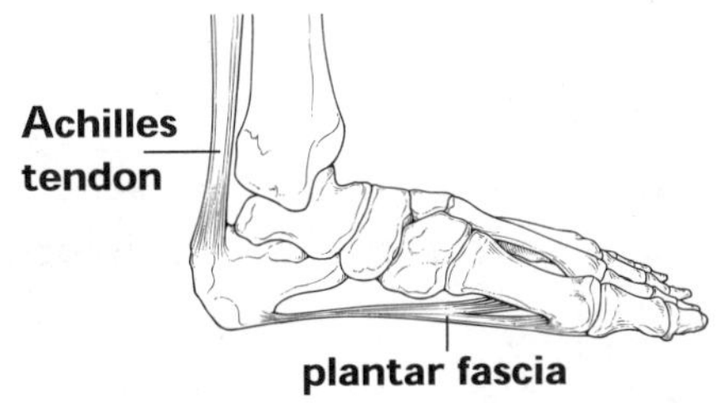

Foot or heel pain is often caused by inflammation of the Achilles tendon or the plantar fascia.

Achilles tendinitis can cause pain in the back of the heel.

A **heel spur** is a calcium buildup that may occur where the plantar fascia attaches to the heel. It does not change the treatment of plantar fasciitis.

Prevention

- Stretch your Achilles tendon and calf muscles several times a day (see page 295). Stretching is important for both athletes and nonathletes.
- Maintain a reasonable weight for your height.
- Wear shoes with well-cushioned soles and good arch supports. Replace athletic shoes every few months because padding wears out.
- Establish good exercise habits. Increase mileage slowly, limit your running and training on hilly terrain, and run on softer surfaces (grass or dirt) rather than concrete. Cross-train by alternating running with different sports.

Home Treatment

Treat heel pain when it first appears to keep plantar fasciitis or other problems from becoming chronic.

- Reduce all weight-bearing activities to a pain-free level.
- Apply ice to your heel. See "Ice and Cold Packs" on page 133.
- You may wish to try an over-the-counter arch support.
- Do not go barefoot until the pain is completely gone. Wear shoes or arch-supporting sandals during all weight-bearing activities, even going to the bathroom during the night.
- Take aspirin, ibuprofen, naproxen, or ketoprofen to relieve pain.
- Stretch your calf muscles. See page 295.
- For Achilles tendinitis, try putting heel lifts or heel cups in both shoes. Use them only until the pain is gone (continue other self-care).
- Avoid "running through the pain." Reduce your activity to a level that does not cause pain. Try low-impact activities such as cycling or swimming to speed healing.
- Do not return to high-impact activity until you have been pain-free for 1 week. When you do return, start slowly and ice your heel afterward. If the pain recurs, start home treatment again.

When to Call Kaiser Permanente

- If heel pain occurs with fever, redness, or heat in your heel, or if there is numbness or tingling in your heel.
- If pain continues when you are not standing or bearing any weight on your heel.
- If heel pain persists for 1 to 2 weeks despite home treatment.

Your physician may recommend other treatments for plantar fasciitis, such as taping, exercises, shoe inserts, or in some cases steroid injections. Surgery is usually done only as a last resort when other treatments fail to relieve pain.

Sports Injuries

Injuries are common among physically active people. Most sports injuries are due to either traumatic injury or overuse and can be avoided by proper conditioning, training, and equipment.

Prevention

- Warm up before exercise. Cold, stiff muscles and ligaments are more susceptible to injury. Cool down and stretch after activities. See page 295.
- Increase the intensity and duration of activities and exercise gradually. As your fitness level improves, you will be able to do increasingly strenuous exercise without injury.
- Use proper sports techniques and equipment. For example, wear supportive, well-cushioned shoes for running, aerobics, and walking; use a 2-handed tennis backhand stroke; wear protective pads for roller-skating. Make sure that your bicycle's seat and handlebars are adjusted properly for your body.
- Alternate hard workouts with easier ones to let your body rest. For example, if you run, alternate long or hard runs with shorter or easier ones. If you lift weights, don't work the same muscles 2 days in a row.
- Cross-train (do several activities regularly) to rest your muscles. Alternate days of walking with biking, running, or swimming.
- Don't ignore aches and pains. A few days of reduced activity or rest, ice, and other home treatment when you feel the first twinge of pain may help you avoid more serious problems.

Home Treatment

The biggest home treatment challenge for most sports injuries is to get enough rest to allow healing without losing overall conditioning. This approach is called relative rest.

- Keep the rest of your body fit by cross-training with activities that don't stress the injured area: swimming or biking for sore ankles or feet; walking or biking for sore shoulders or elbows. Don't hurry the return to the activity that caused the injury. Cross-training can maintain your level of fitness.
- Resume your regular activity gradually. Start with a slow, easy pace and increase only if you have no pain.
- Break your sport down into components. If you can throw a ball a short distance without pain, try increasing the distance. If you can walk comfortably, try jogging. If you can jog without pain, try running.

When to Call Kaiser Permanente

Information on specific injuries can be found on the following pages:

- Bursitis and Tendinitis, page 120.
- Tennis or golfer's elbow, page 122.
- Patellar tendinitis, page 126.
- Achilles tendinitis and plantar fasciitis, page 130.
- Strains, Sprains, and Fractures, page 134.

Ice and Cold Packs

Ice can relieve pain, swelling, and inflammation from injuries and other conditions such as arthritis. Apply ice consistently as long as you have symptoms. Use either a commercial cold pack or one of the following:

- Ice towel: Wet a towel with cold water and squeeze it until it is just damp. Fold the towel, place it in a plastic bag, and freeze it for 15 minutes. Remove the towel from the bag and place it on the affected area.
- Ice pack: Put about 1 pound of ice in a plastic bag. Add water to barely cover the ice. Squeeze the air out of the bag and seal it. Wrap the bag in a wet towel and apply to the affected area.
- Homemade cold pack: See instructions on page 339.

Ice the area at least 3 times a day. For the first 48 hours, ice for up to 10 minutes once an hour. After that, a good pattern is to ice for 10 minutes 3 times a day: in the morning, in the late afternoon after work or school, and about ½ hour before bedtime. Also ice after any prolonged activity or vigorous exercise.

Always keep a damp cloth between your skin and the cold pack, and press firmly against all the curves of the affected area. Do not apply ice for longer than 10 minutes at a time, and do not fall asleep with the ice on your skin.

Strains, Sprains, and Fractures

A **strain** is an injury caused by overstretching a muscle.

A **sprain** is an injury to the muscle and the ligaments, tendons, or soft tissues around a joint.

A **fracture** is a broken bone.

All 3 injuries cause pain and swelling. Unless a broken bone is obvious, it may be difficult to tell if an injury is a strain, sprain, or fracture. Injuries often involve all 3. Rapid swelling often indicates a more serious injury. If a bone is poking through the skin, or if a limb below the injury is white, cold, or numb, immediate medical care is needed.

Most minor strains and sprains can be treated at home, but severe sprains and fractures need professional care. Apply home treatment while you wait to see your physician.

You may have a severe sprain or broken bone if:

- The injured area is visibly swollen.
- The injured area is twisted or bent out of shape or a bone is poking through the skin.
- The injured area is black and blue.
- The pain from the injury prevents normal use of the limb, such as walking.

A **stress fracture** is a weak spot or small crack in a bone caused by repeated overuse. Stress fractures in the small bones of the foot are common during intensive training for basketball, running, and other sports. The main symptom is persistent foot pain and tenderness that increases during use. There may be no visible swelling.

Splinting

Splinting immobilizes a suspected fracture to prevent further injury. There are 2 ways to immobilize a fracture: tie the injured limb to a stiff object, or fasten it to some other part of the body. Do not tie too tight.

For the first method, tie rolled-up newspapers or magazines, a stick, a cane, or anything that is stiff to the injured limb with a rope, a belt, or anything else that will work.

Position the splint so the injured limb cannot bend. A general rule is to splint from a joint above the fracture to a joint below it. For example, splint a broken forearm from above the elbow to below the wrist.

For the second method, tape a broken toe to the next toe or immobilize an arm by tying it across the victim's chest.

Prevention

- Make sure you can always see where you are walking. To avoid falling, don't climb stairs with both hands full.
- To avoid falling, use a stepstool when reaching for high objects. Do not stand on chairs or other objects.
- Get help to carry heavy or awkward objects.
- See prevention tips for Sports Injuries on page 132.

Home Treatment

Generally speaking, if the injury is to a muscle, ligament, tendon, or bone, the basic treatment is the same. It is a 2-part process: **RICE** (rest, ice, compression, elevation) to treat the acute pain or injury; and **MSA** (movement, strength, alternate activities) to help the injury heal completely and to prevent further problems.

Begin the **RICE** process immediately for most injuries. If you suspect a fracture, splint the affected limb to prevent further injury (see page 134).

If the sprain is to a finger or part of the hand, remove all rings immediately. See "Removing a Ring" on page 70.

R. Rest. Do not put weight on the injured joint for at least 24 to 48 hours.

- Use crutches to support a badly sprained knee or ankle.
- Rest a sprained finger or toe by taping it to a healthy one next to it.

Injured muscle, ligament, or tendon tissue needs time and rest to heal. Stress fractures need rest for 2 to 4 months.

I. Ice. Cold will reduce pain and swelling and promote healing. Heat feels nice, but it may do more harm than good, since it may increase the swelling after an injury.

- Apply ice or cold packs immediately to prevent or minimize swelling. For difficult-to-reach injuries, a cold pack works best. See "Ice and Cold Packs" on page 133.

C. Compression. Wrap the injury with an elastic (Ace) bandage or compression sleeve to immobilize and compress the sprain. Don't wrap it too tightly, which can cause more swelling. Loosen the bandage if it gets too tight. A tightly wrapped sprain may fool you into thinking you can keep using the joint. With or without a wrap, the joint needs total rest for 1 to 2 days.

E. Elevation. Elevate the injured area on pillows while you apply ice and anytime you are sitting or lying down. Try to keep the injury at or above the level of your heart to help minimize swelling.

- Aspirin, ibuprofen, naproxen, or Orudis may help ease inflammation and pain. Do not use drugs to mask the pain while you continue to use the injured joint. Do not give aspirin to anyone younger than 20. Review aspirin guidelines on pages 349 and 350.

- The use of heat (hot water bottle, warm towel, heating pad) after 48 hours of cold treatments is controversial. Some experts think it will increase swelling; others think it may speed healing. If you use heat, do not apply anything that is uncomfortably warm.

Begin the **MSA** process as soon as the initial pain and swelling have subsided. This may be in 2 days or up to a week or longer, depending on the location and severity of the injury. Resume sports and activities slowly. Any increased pain may be a sign that you need to rest a while longer.

M. Movement. After 1 to 2 days of rest, begin moving the joint. Move your joint gently through its full range of motion. If an activity causes pain, stop it and give the joint more rest. Gentle stretching will prevent scar tissue (formed as the injury heals) from limiting movement later.

S. Strength. Once the swelling is gone and range of motion is restored, begin gradual efforts to strengthen the injured area. This may require specific exercises.

A. Alternate activities. After the first few days, but while the injury is still healing, phase in regular exercise using activities or sports that do not place a strain on the injured part. See page 132.

When to Call Kaiser Permanente

- If a bone is poking through the skin, or if a limb below the injury is white, cold, or numb.
- If you suspect a severe sprain or fracture (see page 134). After you have stopped weight-bearing activities, splinted the injury, and applied ice, a short delay in receiving professional care will not affect the outcome.
- If a sprained joint is very unstable, won't support your weight, or wobbles from side to side.
- If you cannot bear weight on a sprained ankle after 24 hours, or if it hurts to bear weight after 3 days.
- If pain is still severe after 2 days of home treatment.
- If a sprain does not improve after 4 days of home treatment.

Temporomandibular (TM) Disorder

The temporomandibular (TM) joint is the joint in front of the ear that connects the lower jawbone (mandible) to the skull. Pain and discomfort in the jaw muscles and TM joint is called temporomandibular disorder (TM disorder).

The symptoms of TM disorder can include:

- Pain in one or both jaws when chewing or yawning.

- Clicking, popping, or painful grating in the jaw joint.
- Locking of the jaw in an open or closed position, or inability to "open wide."
- Headache, neck pain, facial pain, or shoulder pain.

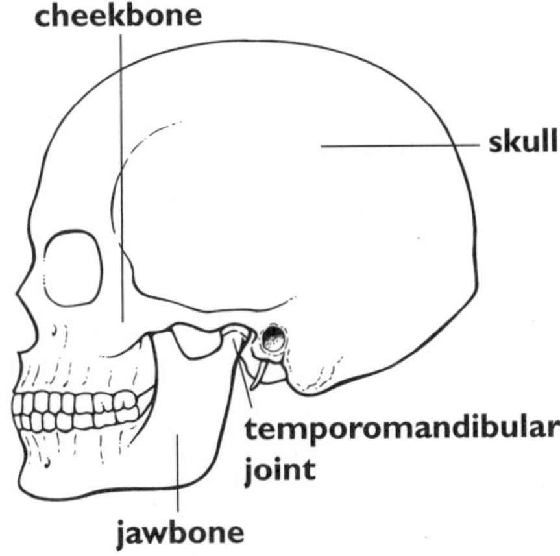

Pain and discomfort in the jaw muscles and jaw joint is called temporomandibular disorder.

The most common cause of TM disorder is tension in the jaw, neck, and shoulder muscles. This can be brought on by stress or by habits such as clenching or grinding your teeth. TM disorder can also occur when there is a problem, such as arthritis, in the joint itself.

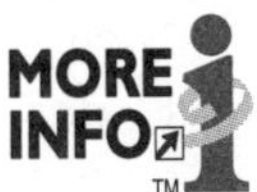
Home treatment and nonsurgical treatments will successfully relieve most symptoms of TM disorder. Your physician may recommend use of a plastic mouth plate (splint), physical therapy, or prescription pain relievers. Surgery is needed for a very small percentage of TM problems.

Prevention

The key to preventing TM disorder is to reduce muscle tension in your jaw. You can reduce muscle tension with these steps:

- Relax. If you have a lot of stress and anxiety in your life, try relaxation techniques (see page 328).
- Do not bite your nails or cradle the telephone receiver between your shoulder and jaw.
- Stop chewing gum or tough foods at the first sign of pain or discomfort in your jaw muscles.
- Change your diet. Eat softer foods, and use both sides of your mouth to chew your food.
- Maintain good posture. Poor posture may disturb the natural alignment between your facial bones and muscles and cause pain.
- Get regular dental checkups.

Home Treatment

- Continue the prevention tips.
- Avoid opening your mouth too wide.
- Rest your jaw, keeping your teeth apart and your lips closed. (Keep your tongue on the roof of your mouth, not between your teeth.)

- Put an ice pack on the joint for 8 minutes, 3 times a day. Gently open and close your mouth while the ice pack is on. If the jaw muscle is swollen, apply ice 6 times a day.
- Take aspirin or ibuprofen to reduce swelling and pain.
- If there is no swelling, use moist heat on the jaw muscle 3 times a day. Gently open and close your mouth while the heat is on. Alternate with the cold pack treatments.
- If you are under severe stress or suffer from anxiety or depression, see Chapter 18.

When to Call Kaiser Permanente

- If the pain is severe.
- If TM symptoms occur after an injury to the jaw.
- If your jaw locks in certain positions.
- If any jaw problem or pain continues more than 2 weeks without improvement.
- If you have noticed a change in the way your teeth fit together when you close your mouth.

Weakness and Fatigue

Weakness is a lack of physical or muscle strength and a feeling that extra effort is required to move your arms, legs, or other muscles.

Fatigue is a feeling of tiredness, exhaustion, or lack of energy.

Unexplained muscle weakness is usually more serious than fatigue. It may be caused by diabetes (see page 239), thyroid problems, stroke, or other problems related to the brain and spinal cord. Call your physician immediately if you have unexplained muscle weakness.

Fatigue, on the other hand, can usually be treated with self-care. Most fatigue is caused by lack of physical activity, stress or overwork, lack of sleep, depression, worry, or boredom. Colds and flu may sometimes cause fatigue and weakness, but the symptoms disappear as the illness runs its course.

Prevention

- Regular exercise is your best defense against fatigue. If you feel too tired to exercise vigorously, try a short walk.
- Eat a well-balanced diet. See Chapter 17.
- Make sure you are getting enough sleep. See page 317.
- Deal with emotional problems instead of ignoring or denying them. See page 307.
- Take steps to control your stress and workload. See page 326.

Chronic Fatigue Syndrome

Chronic fatigue syndrome (CFS) is a flu-like illness that causes severe fatigue lasting longer than 6 months. Other symptoms include mild fever, sore throat, painful lymph glands, confusion, irritability, and sleep problems. The fatigue and other symptoms usually develop quickly in a previously healthy person.

CFS is difficult to diagnose. There is no definitive lab test. Many other illnesses, such as depression, thyroid disorders, or mononucleosis, cause similar symptoms. A CFS diagnosis is made only after fatigue and other symptoms continue for at least 6 months and other possible causes have been ruled out.

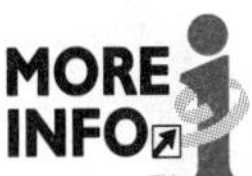

Treatment is focused on adequate rest, balanced diet, and moderate exercise. No medications are known to cure chronic fatigue syndrome. Treatment of the individual symptoms can be effective. For treatment of depression, which develops in about ½ of people with CFS, see page 313.

Call your physician if unexplained fatigue is severe, persistent, and interferes with your activities for more than 2 weeks despite home treatment.

Home Treatment

- Follow the prevention guidelines above and be patient. It may take a while before you feel energetic again.
- Listen to your body. Alternate rest with exercise.
- Limit medications that might contribute to fatigue. Tranquilizers and cold and allergy medications are particularly suspect.
- Reduce your use of caffeine and alcohol.
- If you smoke or use other tobacco products, consider getting help to quit. See page 26 for tips on quitting.
- Cut back on watching television. Spend that time with friends, try new activities, or travel to break the fatigue cycle.

When to Call Kaiser Permanente

- If you have unexplained muscle weakness in one area of your body.
- If severe fatigue causes you to limit your usual activities for longer than 2 weeks despite home treatment.
- If you experience sudden, unexplained weight loss.
- If you do not feel more energetic after 4 weeks of home treatment.
- If fatigue gets worse despite home treatment.

Life is made up of sobs, sniffles, and smiles,
with sniffles predominating.
O. Henry

7

Chest and Respiratory Problems

Chest and respiratory problems can be as simple as a minor cold or as life-threatening as a heart attack. For most respiratory problems, including allergies, colds, sore throats, sinusitis, and tonsillitis, this chapter will help you decide what to do at home and when to call your physician.

Start this chapter with a look at the chart on the next page. If you don't find what you're looking for, please check the index.

Allergies

Allergies come in many forms. The most common causes of allergies are particles in the air. Hay fever is the most common allergic disease. Allergy symptoms include itchy, watery eyes; sneezing; runny, stuffy, or itchy nose; and fatigue. The symptoms are a lot like cold symptoms, but they usually last longer. Dark circles under the eyes (allergic shiners) or postnasal drip may also accompany hay fever.

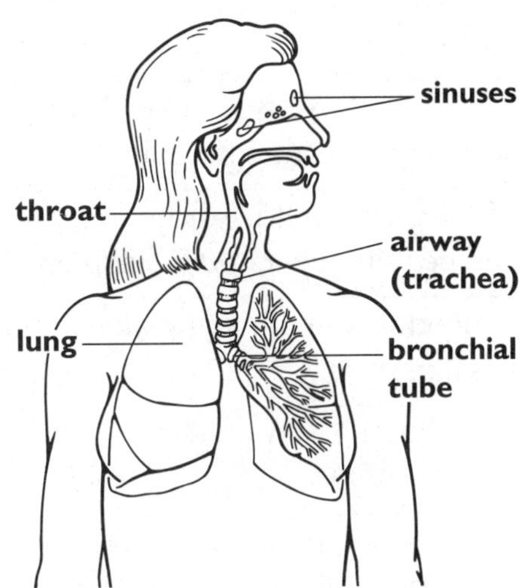

Respiratory problems can occur in the upper respiratory tract (nose, sinuses, throat, or trachea) or in the lower respiratory tract (bronchial tubes or lungs).

Chest, Respiratory, Nose, and Throat Problems

Symptoms	Possible Causes
Chest and Respiratory	
Wheezing or difficult (rapid, shallow, labored) breathing	Allergies, p. 141; Asthma, p. 146; Bronchitis (Chest Cold), p. 150.
Cough, fever, yellow-green or rusty sputum, and difficulty breathing (possibly with chest-wall pain)	Bronchitis (Chest Cold), p. 150; Pneumonia, p. 163.
Chest pain with sweating or rapid pulse	Possible heart attack. Call for help. See p. 54. Chest Pain, p. 151.
Burning, pain, or discomfort behind or below the breastbone	Heartburn, p. 83; Chest Pain, p. 151.
Coughing	Coughs, p. 157.
Pounding or racing heartbeat; heart skipping or missing a beat	Heart Palpitations, p. 160.
Nose and Throat	
Stuffy or runny nose with watery eyes, sneezing	Allergies, p. 141; Colds, p. 154.
Cold symptoms with fever, headache, severe body aches, fatigue	Influenza, p. 161.
Thick green, yellow, or gray nasal discharge with fever and facial pain	Sinusitis, p. 165.
Foul odor from nose; swollen, inflamed nasal tissue	Objects in the Nose, p. 63; Sinusitis, p. 165.
Sore throat	Sore Throat, p. 167; Tonsillitis, p. 170.
Sore throat with white spots on tonsils, swollen glands, fever of 101° or higher	Strep Throat, p. 167.
Swollen tonsils, sore throat, fever	Tonsillitis, p. 170.
Swollen lymph nodes in the neck	Swollen Lymph Nodes, p. 169; Tonsillitis, p. 170.
Hoarseness, loss of voice	Laryngitis, p. 163.

You can often discover the cause of an allergy by noting when symptoms occur. Symptoms that occur at the same time each year (especially during spring, early summer, or early fall) are often caused by tree, grass, or weed pollen. Allergies that persist all year long may be due to dust, mites in household dust, cockroaches, mold spores, or animal dander. An animal allergy is often easy to detect: symptoms clear up when you stay away from the animal or its bedding.

Allergies seem to run in families. Parents with hay fever often have children with allergies. Hay fever may develop in children but is more common in teens and adults.

Severe Allergic Reactions

A few people have severe allergies to insect stings or to certain foods or drugs, especially antibiotics such as penicillin. For these people, the allergic reaction is sudden and severe and may cause breathing difficulty and a drop in blood pressure (anaphylactic shock).

An anaphylactic reaction is a medical emergency, and prompt care is needed. If you have ever had a severe allergic reaction, your physician may suggest that you carry an epinephrine syringe (such as EpiPen or Ana-Kit) designed for giving yourself a shot that will decrease the severity of the reaction. If you

What About Allergy Shots?

Allergy shots (immunotherapy) are a series of shots given to desensitize your body to substances that trigger allergic reactions (allergens). You may need to receive shots for 3 to 5 years before you stop having allergic reactions.

Immunotherapy is effective only if skin sensitivity testing has identified the specific allergy trigger. It is very effective against allergies to bee stings and other insect venom. For most people, immunotherapy is effective against grass, tree, and weed pollens, as well as house dust and house dust mites.

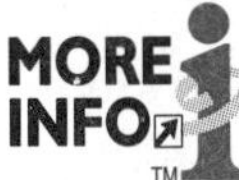

Because of the time and expense involved, you need a realistic idea of the benefits before you agree to the treatment. Discuss these with your physician. Allergy shots may be worthwhile for you if:

- You cannot avoid allergy triggers, or avoiding them has not helped.
- Your symptoms have bothered you a lot for at least 2 years.
- You have tried home treatment without success.
- Neither prescription nor nonprescription medications bring you relief.
- Immunotherapy has been shown to be effective for the allergens identified by your skin tests.

have had an allergic reaction to a drug, wear a medical identification bracelet that will tell health professionals about your allergy in case you cannot.

Prevention

- If practical, avoid the substance that causes allergy attacks. See page 145 for more information about food allergies.
- Allergy shots (immunotherapy) may help control symptoms of allergies and asthma or may reduce the risk of having an anaphylactic reaction. See page 143.

Home Treatment

If you can discover the source of your allergies, avoiding that substance may be the best treatment. Keep a record of your symptoms and the plants, animals, foods, or chemicals that seem to trigger them.

General information about avoiding irritants:

- Avoid yardwork (raking, mowing), which stirs up both pollen and mold. If you must do yard work, wear a mask and take an antihistamine beforehand.
- If you smoke or use other tobacco products, consider getting help to quit. See page 26 for tips on quitting.
- Avoid inhaling other people's smoke.
- Eliminate aerosol sprays, perfumes, room deodorizers, cleaning products, and other substances that may trigger allergy symptoms.

If your symptoms are seasonal and seem to be related to pollen:

- Keep your house and car windows closed. Keep bedroom windows closed at night.
- Limit the time you spend outside when pollen counts are high. Dogs and other pets may bring large amounts of pollen into your house.

If your symptoms are year-round and seem to be related to dust:

- Keep your bedroom and other places where you spend a lot of time as dust-free as possible.
- Avoid carpeting, upholstered furniture, and heavy draperies that collect dust. Vacuuming doesn't pick up house dust mites.
- Cover your mattress and box spring with dust-proof cases and wipe them clean weekly. Avoid wool or down blankets and feather pillows. Wash all bedding in hot water once a week.
- Consider using an air conditioner or air purifier with a special HEPA filter. Rent one before buying to see if it helps.

If your symptoms are year-round and are worse during damp weather, they may be related to mold or mildew:

- Keep your home well ventilated and dry. Keep the humidity below 50 percent. Use a dehumidifier during humid weather.
- Use an air conditioner, which removes mold spores from the air. Change or clean heating and cooling system filters regularly.
- Clean bathroom and kitchen surfaces often with bleach to reduce mold growth.

If you are allergic to a pet, especially one with feathers or fur:

- Keep the animal outside, or at least out of your bedroom.
- If your symptoms are severe, the best solution may be to find a new home for the pet.

Antihistamines and decongestants may relieve some allergy symptoms. Use caution when taking these drugs. See pages 346 and 348.

For more information about allergies, including immunotherapy, call LungLine, a service of the National Jewish Medical and Research Center at 1-800-222-LUNG (5864).

When to Call Kaiser Permanente

Call 911 or seek other emergency services immediately if you develop signs of a severe allergic reaction (anaphylaxis). The following severe symptoms may occur soon after you take a drug, eat a certain food, or are stung by an insect:

- Lightheadedness (feeling like you might pass out).
- Swelling around the lips, tongue, or face that is interfering with breathing or is getting worse.
- Wheezing or difficulty breathing.

Call Kaiser Permanente:

- If your lips, tongue, or face are swollen, even if you are not having difficulty breathing and the swelling is not getting worse.
- If there is significant swelling around the site of an insect sting (e.g., the entire arm or leg is swollen).
- If you develop a skin rash, itching, feeling of warmth, or hives.

Food Allergies

Less than 1 percent of adults have true food allergies. Most adverse reactions to foods are due to food intolerances, reactions to food additives, or food poisoning. Most true food allergies are to legumes, nuts, shellfish, eggs, wheat, and milk. An allergic reaction to a food can result in anaphylactic shock. See When to Call Kaiser Permanente on page 145.

By gradually introducing simple solid foods into your child's diet, you will be able to identify possible food allergies. Children often outgrow food allergies by age 6. If your child was allergic to a food when younger, try reintroducing it as he or she gets older (unless the reaction was severe).

Call your physician if allergy symptoms worsen over time and home treatment doesn't help. Your physician may recommend stronger medication or allergy shots (immunotherapy).

Asthma

Asthma is a condition that causes long-term inflammation of the airways. The inflammation makes the airways overreact to certain triggers. During an asthma flare-up, the muscles surrounding the tubes that carry air into the lungs (bronchial tubes) go into spasm; the mucous lining of the lungs swells; and secretions build up in the lungs, suddenly making breathing difficult.

A person who is having an asthma flare-up may make a wheezing or whistling sound while breathing. The person may cough a great deal and may spit up mucus. Sometimes a chronic, dry cough, especially at night or early in the morning, is the only symptom of asthma.

Many things can trigger asthma, including allergens such as dust, pollen, cockroaches, and animal dander. In general, viral respiratory infections, such as colds, are the most common triggers of asthma. Other triggers include exercise, cold air, cigarette or wood smoke, chemical vapors, pain relievers (especially aspirin), food preservatives and dyes, and emotional stress.

Asthma usually develops during childhood but may also begin later in life. The first flare-up often follows a cold or the flu. Asthma is more common in children who are exposed to cigarette smoke in the home. Many children appear to outgrow asthma symptoms as they get older, but the symptoms may return later in life.

Most children and adults can control their asthma by avoiding triggers that cause flare-ups and using medications to prevent and manage symptoms. Severe flare-ups can usually be treated with inhaled or oral medications. Asthma flare-ups are rarely fatal if they are treated promptly and appropriately.

Prevention

There is no way to prevent asthma. However, you may be able to limit the length and severity of asthma flare-ups if you can avoid or control your exposure to things that trigger asthma symptoms.

- Review home treatment for allergies on page 144.
- Control cockroaches. Do not leave food or garbage in open containers. Use poison bait and traps to kill cockroaches. Avoid chemical sprays, which can trigger an asthma flare-up.
- Avoid smoke of all kinds. If you smoke or use other tobacco products, consider getting help to quit. See page 26 for tips on quitting.

Avoid places where other people may be smoking. Parents should not smoke around children with asthma. Stay away from wood-burning stoves.

- Avoid irritants in the air. Stay indoors when the air pollution or pollen count is high. Try to avoid strong odors, fumes, and perfume.
- Avoid breathing cold air. In cold weather, breathe through your nose, and cover your nose and mouth with a scarf or a cold weather mask.
- Aspirin, ibuprofen, and similar pain medications can cause severe asthma flare-ups in some people. Discuss the use of these medications with your physician, and use them with caution. If these medications bother you, don't use them. Try acetaminophen instead.
- Do not use nonprescription cold and cough medications unless your physician tells you to do so.
- Stress may be a factor in triggering asthma flare-ups. Practice the relaxation exercises on page 328.
- Reduce your risk of colds and flu by washing your hands often and getting a flu shot each year.
- Build up the strength of your lungs and airways:
    - Get regular exercise. Swimming or water aerobics may be good choices because you are less likely to have an asthma flare-up when you breathe moist air. If vigorous exercise triggers asthma flare-ups, talk with your physician. Adjusting your medication and your exercise routine may help.
    - Practice belly breathing as described on page 328.
- Work with your physician to develop an asthma plan so you can manage your symptoms at home. Make sure family members and friends know about your plan so they can help you during an asthma flare-up. See page 148.
- When you aren't having symptoms, follow your plan to treat ongoing airway inflammation. Get regular checkups to make sure your asthma plan is working well for you.
- Learn to use a peak flow meter to monitor your ability to exhale. Used regularly, this device will give you an idea of how your lungs normally function. It also helps you tell when an asthma flare-up may be coming so you can take steps to prevent or treat it.

Since triggers for asthma flare-ups are often not known, you need to monitor your symptoms and peak flow so you can prevent or treat asthma flare-ups before they become severe. Using an asthma plan developed by a physician or other health care professional to guide your home treatment, you may be able to prevent emergency room visits or admissions to the hospital for asthma symptoms.

Asthma Action/Self-Management Plan

An asthma action/self-management plan is a written plan that you create with your physician that tells you how to manage your asthma symptoms at home. It helps take the guesswork out of treating your asthma. The plan will make clear the medication you will take to prevent and treat your asthma symptoms and when to take it, depending on the zone you are in (green, yellow, or red). In order to determine what zone you are in, you will have to know how to measure your ability to exhale using a peak flow meter or, for young children, how to understand their symptoms. The plan tells you when to talk to your physician about your asthma symptoms.

The asthma plan zones are:

- Green zone: Routine care to keep asthma symptoms from starting.
- Yellow zone: How to stop asthma symptoms and keep an asthma flare-up from getting worse. This may involve taking other medications in addition to the ones you usually take to control your asthma.
- Red zone: What to do for a severe asthma flare-up. This is a medical emergency.

Home Treatment

Once an asthma flare-up begins, prompt home treatment can provide relief.

- Learn to use a metered-dose inhaler. Inhalers help get the right amount of medication to your airways. A device called a spacer is now recommended for use with an inhaler. Ask your physician to watch you use your inhaler and spacer to make sure you are doing it right. With practice, most people can use an inhaler and spacer correctly.
- Drink extra fluids to thin the mucus in the bronchial tubes. Try to drink at least 2 quarts of water per day.
- Be confident that your home treatment will control the severity of the flare-up.
- Keep a diary outlining your asthma flare-up. After you've had a flare-up, write down what triggered it, what helped end it, and any concerns you have about your asthma plan. Take your diary when you see your physician for your regular checkups. Ask questions you may have about your plan or medication.

To get more information about managing asthma, contact the National Asthma Center at 1-800-222-5864, or your local chapter of the American Lung Association.

How to Use an Inhaler and Spacer

1. Shake the inhaler well for 5 seconds. Remove the protective cap and insert the mouthpiece of the inhaler into one end of the spacer. Hold the inhaler with your index finger on top and your thumb supporting the bottom.

2. Breathe out as much as possible to empty the lungs. Tilt your head back, place the mouthpiece of the spacer tube in your mouth, and close your lips around it.

3. Press down on the top of the inhaler to release a puff of medication. Breathe in slowly and deeply, filling your lungs with as much air as possible. If you hear a musical sound, you are inhaling too fast. Hold your breath for at least 10 seconds; then breathe out.

4. With your lips still closed around the mouthpiece, take 2 or 3 more deep breaths, holding each breath for 10 seconds. For maximum effectiveness, wait 1 or 2 minutes before taking the next puff.

5. Rinse out your mouth. Wash the inhaler mouthpiece, spacer, and protective caps weekly with mild soapy water and allow to air dry.

When to Call Kaiser Permanente

Always follow your asthma plan if you have one. **Call 911 or seek other emergency services immediately** if you are having severe asthma symptoms and:

- You are having severe difficulty breathing.
- Your medications have not helped after 20 minutes.

Call Kaiser Permanente:

- If you have symptoms that may indicate heart problems, such as chest pain or shortness of breath. See page 151.
- If you are having a severe asthma flare-up (peak flow is less than 50 percent of your best), even if your medications have relieved some symptoms.
- If your asthma symptoms don't get better after you follow your asthma plan.
- If you are coughing up yellow, dark brown, or bloody mucus.
- If acute asthma symptoms (wheezing, coughing, difficulty breathing) have happened for the first time.
- To discuss exactly what to do when a flare-up begins. Once you understand and have confidence in your asthma medication, you can often handle mild flare-ups without professional help.

- If you begin to use your asthma medication more often than usual. This may be a sign that your asthma is getting worse.
- If you or the people who live with you have not been educated about immediate treatment for asthma flare-ups.
- If the medication required to treat an asthma flare-up is not available.
- To talk about adjusting your medication. Your physician needs your feedback to figure out the best medicine and the right dosage for you.
- To assess allergies, which may worsen asthma flare-ups.
- To get a referral to a class. Talking with others who have asthma can give you information and boost your confidence in dealing with prevention and treatment.

Bronchitis (Chest Cold)

Bronchitis is an inflammation and irritation of the airways that lead to the lungs. Viruses are the usual cause of bronchitis, but it can also be caused by bacteria or by exposure to cigarette smoke or air pollution. The inflammation caused by acute bronchitis is not permanent. It goes away when the infection or irritation goes away.

Symptoms of bronchitis usually begin several days after an upper respiratory infection, such as a cold, goes away. Symptoms often include a dry cough that may become productive (produce sputum), mild fever, fatigue, discomfort or tightness in the chest, and wheezing.

Having bronchitis and another lung disease, such as asthma, may increase your risk for pneumonia.

Frequent lung infections, especially in a person who smokes, may lead to the development of chronic bronchitis. Tobacco smokers are also at high risk for developing emphysema. Chronic bronchitis, emphysema, and other lung conditions, such as asthma, are known as chronic obstructive pulmonary disease (COPD).

Prevention

Bronchitis usually cannot be prevented, but you can improve your body's ability to fight infection.

- Give proper home care to minor respiratory problems such as colds and flu. See pages 154 and 161.
- If you smoke or use other tobacco products, consider getting help to quit. See page 26 for tips on quitting. People who smoke or are around smokers have more frequent bouts of bronchitis.
- Avoid polluted air and don't exercise outdoors when the ozone concentration is high.

Home Treatment

Most cases of bronchitis can be managed with home treatment. Here is what you can do at home to prevent complications and feel better.

- Drink 8 to 12 glasses of water per day. Liquids help thin the mucus in the lungs so it can be coughed out.
- Get some extra rest. Let your energy go to healing.
- Take aspirin, ibuprofen, or acetaminophen to relieve fever and body aches. Do not give aspirin to anyone younger than 20.
- Use a nonprescription cough suppressant that contains dextromethorphan to help quiet a dry, hacking cough so you can sleep. Avoid cough preparations that contain more than 1 active ingredient. See Cough Preparations on page 347.
- Breathe moist air from a humidifier, hot shower, or a sink filled with hot water. The heat and moisture will thin mucus so it can be coughed out.
- If you have classic flu symptoms, try home treatment and reassess your symptoms in 48 hours. See Influenza (Flu) on page 161.

When to Call Kaiser Permanente

Call if you develop any of the following symptoms. They may mean that your lung infection is getting worse or that you are developing a bacterial lung infection.

- A cough with wheezing or difficulty breathing that is new or different.
- A cough that:
  - Brings up bloody sputum.
  - Lingers more than 10 to 14 days after other symptoms have cleared, especially if it is productive (brings up sputum). A dry, hacking cough may last several weeks after a viral illness such as a cold.
- A fever that fits the description on page 159.
- If you are unable to drink enough fluids to avoid becoming dehydrated or if you are unable to eat.
- If the sick person is an infant, an older adult, or someone who is chronically ill, especially with lung problems.
- If any cough lasts longer than 4 weeks.

Chest Pain

Call 911 or seek other emergency services immediately if you think you may be having a heart attack (see page 152).

Call Kaiser Permanente if chest discomfort or pain lasts longer than 30 minutes and there is no obvious cause.

If the person who is having heart attack symptoms loses consciousness, follow the Rescue Breathing and CPR guidelines on page 36.

Chest pain is a key warning sign of a heart attack, but it may also be caused by other problems.

If chest pain increases when you press your finger on the painful site, or if you can pinpoint the spot that hurts, it is probably chest-wall pain, which may be caused by strained muscles or ligaments or by a fractured rib. An inflammation of the cartilage in the chest wall (called costochondritis) can also cause chest-wall pain. Chest-wall pain usually lasts only a few days. Aspirin or ibuprofen may help. Do not give aspirin to anyone younger than 20.

A shooting pain that lasts a few seconds, or a quick pain at the end of a deep breath, is usually not a cause for concern. Hyperventilation (see page 56) can also cause chest pain.

Chest pain caused by pleurisy (inflammation of the membrane that surrounds the lungs) or pneumonia (see page 163) will get worse when you take a deep breath or cough. An ulcer (see page 95) can cause chest pain, usually below the breastbone, that is worse when your stomach is empty. Gallstones (see page 88) may cause pain in the right side of the chest or around the shoulder blade. The pain may worsen after a meal or in the middle of the night. Heartburn (see page 83) can also cause chest pain. Shingles (page 208) may cause a sharp, burning, or tingling pain that feels like a tight band around one side of the chest.

Am I Having a Heart Attack?

You may be having a heart attack if you feel **any** of these symptoms:

Chest discomfort or pain that:

❑ Lasts longer than 20 minutes AND is not relieved by rest or nitroglycerin AND feels like:

- Pressure
- Tightness
- Squeezing
- Crushing
- Intense burning
- Aching

In addition to the symptoms above, you may also have:

❑ Pain radiating to your:

- Back
- Shoulder
- Neck
- Jaw/teeth
- Arm
- Wrist

❑ Sweating

❑ Shortness of breath

❑ Dizziness

❑ Fainting

❑ Nausea (feeling sick to your stomach)

❑ Vomiting (throwing up)

❑ Unusual weakness

❑ Rapid and/or irregular heartbeat

❑ Sense of doom

The more boxes you check, the more likely it is that you are having a heart attack. There may be other explanations for chest pain, but it is important to get medical help **immediately**.

Angina is pain, pressure, heaviness, or numbness behind the breastbone or across the chest. It occurs when there is not enough oxygen reaching the heart muscle. It is a symptom of coronary artery disease. The pain caused by angina may radiate to the upper back, neck, jaws, shoulders, or arms. Angina may be brought on by stress or exertion and is relieved by rest and use of prescribed medication.

A **heart attack** (myocardial infarction) is caused by blocked blood flow to the heart muscle. The pain of a heart attack is usually more severe than angina, lasts longer, and does not go away with rest or by taking medication that was previously effective for angina. Other symptoms that may be present include sweating, nausea, shortness of breath, weakness, or indigestion.

Lifestyle and other factors that may increase your risk of a heart attack include:

- Previous heart disease.
- Current smoker.
- Family history of heart disease.
- Diabetes.
- High blood pressure.
- High total cholesterol and high LDL (bad) cholesterol.
- Low HDL (good) cholesterol.
- Lack of physical activity.
- High stress levels.

Home Treatment

For chest-wall pain caused by strained muscles or ligaments or a fractured rib:

- Use pain relievers such as aspirin, ibuprofen, or acetaminophen. Do not give aspirin to anyone younger than 20.
- Use an ice pack for up to 10 minutes every 1 to 2 hours to help relieve pain the first few days after an injury.
- After applying ice during the first 48 hours (or until the swelling has gone down), apply heat (a hot water bottle, warm towel, or heating pad) to help relieve pain. Use heat that is no warmer than bath water or the low setting on a heating pad. To prevent burns, do not go to sleep with a heating pad turned on.
- Using products such as Ben-Gay or Icy-Hot may soothe sore muscles.
- Avoid any activity that strains the chest area. As your pain gets better, slowly return to your normal activities.

When to Call Kaiser Permanente

Call 911 or seek other emergency services immediately if symptoms of a heart attack are present (see page 152).

If a physician has diagnosed the cause of your chest pain and prescribed a home treatment plan, follow it. **Call 911 or seek other emergency services immediately** if the pain worsens and may be caused by a heart problem, or if you develop any of the heart attack symptoms listed on page 152.

Call Kaiser Permanente:

- If you suspect that you have angina and your symptoms have not been diagnosed.
- If symptoms of angina do not respond to your prescribed treatment, or if the pattern of your angina changes.
- If minor chest pain occurs without the symptoms of a heart attack and any of the following apply:
  - You have a history of heart disease or blood clots in the lungs.
  - Chest pain is constant, nagging, and not relieved by rest.
  - Chest pain occurs with symptoms of pneumonia. See page 163.
  - Chest pain lasts longer than 2 days without improvement.

Colds

The common cold is brought to you by any one of 200 viruses. The symptoms of a cold include runny nose, red eyes, sneezing, sore throat, hoarseness, dry cough, headache, and general body aches. There is a gradual 1- or 2-day onset. As a cold progresses, the nasal mucus may thicken and turn yellow or green. This is the stage just before a cold dries up. A cold usually lasts about 1 or 2 weeks, but some symptoms may last 2 to 3 weeks.

Colds occur throughout the year but are most common in late winter and early spring. The average child has 6 colds a year; adults have fewer.

Using a mouthwash will not prevent a cold, and antibiotics will not cure a cold. There is no cure for the common cold. If you catch a cold, treat the symptoms.

If a person seems to have a cold all the time, or if cold symptoms last 2 weeks or longer, suspect allergies (see page 141) or sinusitis (see page 165).

Prevention

- Eat well and get plenty of sleep and exercise to keep up your resistance.
- Try to avoid people who have colds.
- Keep your hands away from your nose, eyes, and mouth, but cover your mouth when you cough or sneeze.
- Wash your hands often, particularly when you are around people who have colds.
- Humidify your bedrooms or your whole house if possible.
- If you smoke or use other tobacco products, consider getting help to quit. See page 26 for tips on quitting.

Home Treatment

Home treatment for a cold will help relieve symptoms and prevent complications.

- Get extra rest. Slow down just a little from your usual routine. It isn't necessary to stay home in bed, but take care not to expose others to your cold.
- Drink plenty of liquids. Hot water, herbal tea, or chicken soup will help relieve congestion.
- Take aspirin, ibuprofen, or acetaminophen to relieve aches. Do not give aspirin to anyone younger than 20.
- Humidify your bedroom and take hot showers to relieve nasal stuffiness.
- Check the back of your throat for postnasal drip. If you see streaks of mucus, gargle with warm water to prevent a sore throat.
- Use disposable tissues, not handkerchiefs, to reduce the chance of spreading the cold virus to others.
- If your nose is red and raw from rubbing it with tissues, put a dab of petroleum jelly on the sore area.
- Avoid cold remedies that contain a combination of drugs to treat many different symptoms. Treat each symptom separately. Take a decongestant for stuffiness, a cough medicine for a cough. See Home Treatment for coughs on page 158.
- Do not use nasal decongestant sprays for more than 3 days in a row. Continued use may lead to a "rebound" effect, causing the mucous membranes to become more swollen than they were before you used the spray. See page 346 to learn how to make nose drops at home.
- Avoid antihistamines. They are not an effective treatment for colds.

When to Call Kaiser Permanente

If you have or develop the following:

- Signs of a bacterial infection (see "Viral or Bacterial?" on page 156).
- Facial pain, fever, and other signs of sinusitis (see page 165).
- A cough that lasts more than 3 weeks.
- Difficulty breathing, wheezing, or shortness of breath.
- A very sore throat with difficulty swallowing.
- Severe ear pain, sudden hearing loss, or discharge from the ear.
- If hoarseness persists for 3 to 4 weeks (see page 163).
- You seem to get better and then get worse again.
- A fever that fits the description on page 159.

Viral or Bacterial?

Viral infections

- Usually produce symptoms in several parts of the body at once: sore throat, runny nose, headache, hoarseness, cough, dizziness, fever, fatigue, muscle aches. In the digestive system, viruses cause nausea, vomiting, or diarrhea.
- Typically include colds, flu, chest colds (bronchitis), and stomach flu.
- Are often cured by the body's immune system.
- Cannot be cured by antibiotics.

Bacterial infections

- Usually involve a single complaint affecting one area of the body: sinuses, throat, lungs, an ear.
- Sometimes follow a viral infection.
- May be cured by antibiotics.

Antibiotics won't usually help a cold, flu, or chest cold (bronchitis) because they only kill bacteria—not viruses—and colds and flu are caused by viruses. Yellow or green mucus is common when you have a cold or the flu. This does *not* mean that you have a bacterial infection or need antibiotics.

Our communities face a growing problem—infections caused by resistant bacteria that antibiotics won't kill. This is mostly due to repeated and unnecessary use of antibiotics. Taking antibiotics when you don't need them (even antibiotics you have used safely before) can hurt you by:

- Increasing your chances of having infections later that antibiotics can't treat. (This is called bacterial resistance.)
- Causing side effects like upset stomach, diarrhea, vaginal infections, rashes, and rarely, life-threatening allergic reactions.

If you used antibiotics before for a cold, flu, or chest cold and they seemed to work, the chances are your body would have recovered as quickly on its own. Antibiotics often get the credit that your body's own immune system deserves! Antibiotics won't help you get better faster or shorten the time you have symptoms. Antibiotics also do not prevent pneumonia or sinus or ear infections in otherwise healthy children or adults.

You can protect yourself from unnecessary antibiotics and stop the spread of drug-resistant bacteria if you:

- Give your body time enough to clear the infection naturally (sometimes 2 to 3 weeks).
- Understand that if your physician says antibiotics aren't needed, this is in your best interest.
- If an antibiotic *is* prescribed for you, take the medication until it is all gone, even after you begin to feel better. Do not keep or use antibiotics "left over" from a previous illness.

Coughs

Coughing is the body's way of removing foreign material or mucus from the lungs.

Productive coughs produce phlegm or mucus (sputum) that comes up from the lungs. This kind of cough generally should not be suppressed. It is needed to clear mucus from the lungs.

Nonproductive coughs are dry coughs that do not produce sputum. A dry, hacking cough may develop toward the end of a cold or after exposure to an irritant, such as dust or smoke. Dry coughs that follow viral illnesses may last up to several weeks and often get worse at night.

A chronic, dry cough, especially at night or early in the morning, may be the only sign of mild asthma. See page 146.

Long-term (chronic) coughs are sometimes caused by the backflow (reflux) of stomach acid into the lungs and throat. If you suspect that problems with stomach acid reflux may be causing your cough, see Heartburn on page 83.

Prevention

- If you smoke or use other tobacco products, consider getting help to quit. See page 26 for tips on quitting. Avoid other people's smoke. A dry, hacking "smoker's cough" means your lungs are constantly irritated.

Description and Treatment of Coughs

Type of Cough	Possible Causes
Loud cough like a seal's bark	Croup, p. 226.
Dry cough in the morning that gets better as the day goes on	Dry air; cigarette smoking. Increase fluids. Humidify the bedroom. Stop smoking. Also see Coughs, p. 157.
Hacking, dry, nonproductive cough; may be worse at night	Common for several weeks following a viral illness. May be due to postnasal drip, smoking, or mild asthma. Increase fluids. Try a decongestant. Stop smoking. Also see Coughs, p. 157; Asthma, p. 146.
Productive cough following a cold or flu	Bronchitis (Chest Cold), p. 150; Pneumonia, p. 163; Sinusitis, p. 165.
Dry, sudden-onset cough after a choking flare-up, most often in an infant or toddler	Foreign object in the throat. See Choking, p. 44.

- Drink 8 to 10 glasses of water every day. You are drinking enough if you are urinating more often than usual.

Home Treatment

- Drink lots of water. Water helps loosen phlegm and soothe an irritated throat. Also try drinking hot tea or hot water with honey and/or lemon juice in it. Do not give honey to children younger than 1 year of age.
- Cough drops can soothe an irritated throat. Expensive, medicine-flavored cough drops are not any better than inexpensive, candy-flavored ones or hard candy.
- Elevate your head with extra pillows at night to ease a dry cough.
- Use cough suppressants wisely. Avoid cold remedies that combine drugs to treat many symptoms. It is generally better to treat each symptom separately. See Cough Preparations on page 347.
- Coughing is useful because it brings up mucus from the lungs and helps prevent bacterial infections. People with asthma and other lung diseases need to cough. If you have a dry, hacking cough that does not bring anything up, ask your health professional about an effective cough suppressant medication.
- Do not take anyone else's prescription cough medication.
- Avoid exposure to dust, smoke, and other irritants, or wear an appropriate mask to protect yourself from the irritant.
- If you have classic flu symptoms, try home treatment and reassess your symptoms in 48 hours. See Influenza (Flu) on page 161.

When to Call Kaiser Permanente

- If a cough lingers more than 10 to 14 days after other symptoms have cleared, especially if the cough is productive (brings up sputum). A dry, hacking cough may last several weeks after a viral illness such as a cold.
- If any cough lasts longer than 3 weeks.
- If you develop a fever that fits the description on page 159.

Fever

A fever is a high body temperature. It is a symptom, not a disease. A fever is one way your body fights illness. A temperature of up to 102° can be helpful because it helps the body respond to infection. Most healthy adults can tolerate a fever as high as 103° to 104° for short periods of time without problems.

For specific fever guidelines for children younger than 4 years of age, see page 231.

Home Treatment

- Drink 8 to 12 glasses of water a day. You are drinking enough if you are urinating more often than usual.
- Take and record your temperature every 2 hours and whenever symptoms change.
- Take acetaminophen, aspirin, or ibuprofen to lower fever. Do not give aspirin to anyone younger than 20.
- Take a sponge bath with lukewarm water if a fever causes discomfort.
- Watch for signs of dehydration. See page 80.
- Dress lightly.
- Eat light, easily digested foods, such as soup.
- If you have classic flu symptoms, try home treatment and reassess your symptoms in 48 hours. See Influenza (Flu) on page 161.

When to Call Kaiser Permanente

For Adults and Children 3 Years and Older

- Fever of 104° or higher that does not go down after 2 hours of home treatment.
- Persistent fever. Many viral illnesses cause fever of 102° or higher for a day or 2. Call if the fever stays high:
  - 102° or higher for 2 full days
  - 101° or higher for 3 full days
  - 100° or higher for 4 full days

For Children Younger Than 3 Years

- If an infant younger than 3 months of age has a fever of 100.4° or higher (rectal).
- If a child age 3 months to 3 years has a fever that is:
  - 104° or higher
  - 102° to 104° and does not come down after 12 hours
  - 100° to 102° and does not come down after 24 to 48 hours
- See page 231 for additional information on fever in children.

For Adults and Children

- If fever occurs with any of the following symptoms:
  - Very stiff neck and headache (see "Encephalitis and Meningitis" on page 160).
  - Shortness of breath and cough (see Bronchitis on page 150 and Pneumonia on page 163).
  - Pain above the eyes or the cheekbones (see Sinusitis on page 165).
  - Pain or burning when urinating (see Urinary Tract Infections on page 100).
  - Abdominal pain, nausea, and vomiting (see Stomach Flu and Food Poisoning on page 93, or Appendicitis on page 77).
- If the fever occurs in someone with chronic medical conditions such as immune disorders or serious heart or lung disease.

- If a fever is accompanied by disturbing or unexplained symptoms.
- If you develop a fever after you start taking a new medication.

Encephalitis and Meningitis

Encephalitis is an inflammation of the brain that may occur after a viral infection, such as chickenpox, flu, measles, mumps, mononucleosis, or cold sores. Mosquitoes in the eastern and southeastern U.S. can spread encephalitis.

Meningitis is a viral or bacterial illness that causes inflammation in the tissues that surround the brain and spinal cord. It may follow an infection, such as an ear or sinus infection, or a viral illness.

Encephalitis and meningitis are serious illnesses that have similar symptoms. Call a health professional immediately if the following symptoms develop, especially after a viral illness or after you are bitten by mosquitoes:

- Severe headache with stiff neck, fever, nausea, and vomiting
- Drowsiness, lack of energy, confusion, memory problems, or unusual behavior

Heart Palpitations

Heart palpitations are an uncomfortable sensation that your heart is beating rapidly and/or irregularly. Heart palpitations can feel like:

- A pounding or fluttering feeling in your chest.
- A feeling that your heart is doing a "flip-flop," or that it is skipping or missing a beat.
- Your heart is racing, or there is an extra heartbeat.
- Your heart is beating in your neck.

Although palpitations may be caused by a heart problem, they often occur because of stress, fatigue, or overuse of alcohol or stimulants (caffeine, nicotine). People who experience severe anxiety may have heart palpitations. See Anxiety on page 312. Many medications, including diet pills, antihistamines, and decongestants, can cause heart palpitations.

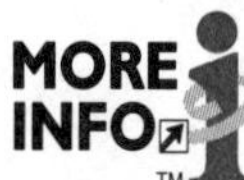

Nearly everyone has heart palpitations from time to time. There is usually no cause for concern. However, if you have heartbeat changes that are new and different, or you have risk factors for heart disease (smoking, high blood pressure, high cholesterol, inactive lifestyle, and/or high stress levels), see your physician to have your condition evaluated.

Prevention

- If you smoke or use other tobacco products, consider getting help to quit. See page 26 for tips on quitting.
- Avoid caffeine and alcohol or limit your intake.
- If you take prescription or non-prescription medications regularly, ask your pharmacist if the drugs you take can cause heart palpitations.
- If anxiety or stress may be causing heart palpitations, see Anxiety on page 312 and try the relaxation exercises on page 328.
- Make physical activity a daily habit. (If you frequently have heart palpitations, talk to your physician before starting an exercise program.)
- See your physician for regular checkups if you have risk factors for heart attack (see page 153). Early detection and management of heart problems is the best way to prevent serious illness.

Home Treatment

- Take deep breaths and try to relax. This may slow a racing heart.
- If you start to feel lightheaded (like you might pass out), lie down to avoid injuries that might result if you pass out and fall down.
- Keep a record of the date and time; your activities when the irregular heartbeat happened; how long the irregular beats lasted; and any other symptoms.
- Check your pulse (see page 57) and record how fast and how many "skipped" beats per minute.
- Follow the prevention guidelines.

When to Call Kaiser Permanente

- **Call 911 or seek other emergency services immediately** if symptoms of a heart attack are present (see page 152).
- If heart palpitations occur with any of the following symptoms:
  - Weakness or fatigue.
  - Lightheadedness (feeling like you might pass out).
  - Confusion.
  - Feeling as if something bad is going to happen.
  - If it seems as if your heart beats irregularly all the time.
- If heart palpitations are new or different than before and are not relieved by home treatment.

Influenza (Flu)

Influenza, or flu, is a viral illness that commonly occurs in the winter and affects many people at once. Flu is not the same as the common cold—the symptoms of flu are usually more severe and come on quite suddenly. Symptoms include fever (101° to 104°), shaking chills, body aches, muscle pain, headache, pain when you move your eyes, fatigue, weakness, and runny nose. Symptoms may last up to 10 days. Most other viral illnesses have milder symptoms that don't last as long.

Although a person with the flu feels very sick, the illness seldom leads to more serious complications. Flu can be dangerous for infants, older adults, and people with chronic conditions.

Antiviral medications may be recommended for people at high risk for complications from the flu. These drugs may slightly reduce the severity and duration of some types of influenza if they are taken soon after symptoms develop. These medications work best if taken no more than 48 hours after symptoms first appear.

Prevention

- Get a flu shot each autumn if you are age 50 or over; if you have a chronic illness, such as asthma, heart disease, or diabetes; or if you live in a nursing home.
- Consider annual flu shots if you or your family members are likely to be exposed to the disease through work (for example, if you are a health care worker) or by being around other children, or if you just want to reduce the chance that you and your family will catch the disease. The vaccine can be given to anyone over 6 months of age.
- Keep up your resistance to infection by eating a healthful diet, getting plenty of rest, and exercising regularly.
- Avoid exposure to the flu virus. Wash your hands often and keep your hands away from your nose, eyes, and mouth.
- If you smoke or use other tobacco products, consider getting help to quit. See page 26 for tips on quitting.

Home Treatment

- Get plenty of rest.
- Drink extra fluids to replace fluids lost from fever, to ease a scratchy throat, and to keep the nasal mucus thin. Hot tea with lemon, plain water, fruit juice, and soup are all good choices.
- Take acetaminophen, aspirin, or ibuprofen to relieve fever, headache, and muscle aches. Do not give aspirin to anyone younger than 20.

When to Call Kaiser Permanente

It is common for adults with influenza to have high fevers (up to 104°) for 3 to 4 days. When trying to decide if you need to see a physician, consider the likelihood that you have the flu versus a possible bacterial infection. If it is the flu season and many people in your community have similar symptoms, it is likely that you have the flu. Call your health professional:

- If you want to consider antiviral medication for a baby, older adult, or person with chronic health problems. Medication may be of limited help in reducing severity or duration of the flu.

- If you develop a fever that fits the description on page 159.
- If you seem to get better, then get worse again.

Laryngitis

Laryngitis is an infection or irritation of the voice box (larynx). The most common cause is a viral infection such as a cold. Other causes include allergies; excessive talking, singing, or yelling; cigarette smoke; and the backflow (reflux) of stomach acid into the throat. Heavy drinking or smoking can lead to chronic laryngitis.

Symptoms include hoarseness or loss of voice, the urge to clear your throat, fever, tiredness, throat pain, and cough.

Prevention

To prevent hoarseness, stop shouting as soon as you feel minor pain. Give your vocal cords a rest.

Home Treatment

- Your voice box will usually heal in 5 to 10 days. Medication does little to speed recovery.
- If hoarseness is caused by a cold, treat the cold (see page 154). Hoarseness may last up to 1 week after a cold goes away.
- Rest your voice. Talk as little as possible. Don't shout or whisper, and avoid clearing your throat.
- If you smoke or use other tobacco products, consider getting help to quit. See page 26 for tips on quitting. Avoid inhaling other people's smoke.
- Humidify your bedrooms or your whole house if possible.
- Drink 8 to 12 glasses of water a day. You are drinking enough if you are urinating more often than usual.
- To soothe the throat, gargle with warm salt water (1 teaspoon of salt in 8 ounces of water), or drink weak tea or hot water with honey and/or lemon juice in it. Do not give honey to children younger than 1 year of age.
- If you suspect that problems with stomach acid reflux may be contributing to your laryngitis, see Heartburn on page 83.

When to Call Kaiser Permanente

- If you develop a fever that fits the description on page 159.
- If hoarseness persists for 3 to 4 weeks.

Pneumonia

Pneumonia is an infection or inflammation that affects the bronchial tubes and lungs. Pneumonia is usually caused by bacteria, but viruses and other organisms can cause it as well. Pneumonia may also develop as a complication of another viral illness, such as measles or chickenpox.

Pneumonia sometimes follows a viral upper respiratory infection, such as a cold or bronchitis. A person who has bacterial pneumonia is usually very sick. Symptoms may include:

- Productive cough with yellow, green, rust-colored, or bloody sputum (mucus coughed up from the lungs).
- Fever and shaking chills (see page 159).
- Rapid, shallow breathing.
- Chest-wall pain that is often made worse by coughing or taking a deep breath.
- Rapid heartbeat.
- Fatigue that is worse than you would expect from a cold.

Prevention

- Get a pneumococcal vaccination if you are over 65, or if you are younger than 65 and have a chronic disease. (If you are younger than 65 and you have asthma, talk to your physician about whether you should receive the pneumococcal vaccine). See page 19.
- Keep up your resistance to infection by eating a healthful diet, getting plenty of rest, and exercising regularly.

Tuberculosis (TB)

Tuberculosis is a contagious disease caused by organisms that usually infect the lungs (pulmonary TB). When a person who has pulmonary TB coughs, sneezes, or laughs, TB-causing organisms are released into the air where other people can inhale them. This is how TB is spread. Children and people with weak immune systems are particularly prone to TB.

Most people who are exposed to TB never develop symptoms because their immune systems are able to stop the disease. People who develop symptoms of TB, such as persistent cough, weight loss, fatigue, night sweats, and fever, need drug treatment to stop the disease from progressing and to reduce the risk of spreading TB to others. Treatment, which consists of several medications, may last from 6 months to 2 years.

People who have weak immune systems, abuse alcohol and drugs, or have a chronic lung disease called silicosis are at high risk for developing progressive TB, which can damage the lungs or spread to other parts of the body.

To prevent TB infection, avoid close contact with people who have TB if possible. If you live with someone who has TB, ask your physician what you can do to protect yourself from TB infection and whether you need to be tested for TB.

Home Treatment

Call Kaiser Permanente if you suspect you have pneumonia. If pneumonia is diagnosed:

- Take the entire course of all prescribed medications.
- Drink 8 to 12 glasses of water a day. You are drinking enough if you are urinating more often than usual. Extra fluids help thin the mucus in the lungs.
- Get lots of rest. Don't try to rush your recovery.
- Take acetaminophen or aspirin to reduce fever and make you feel more comfortable. Do not give aspirin to anyone younger than 20.

When to Call Kaiser Permanente

- If you develop symptoms of pneumonia.
- If your breathing becomes rapid or labored during any respiratory illness.
- If you have new chest pain that gets worse whenever you take a deep breath.

Sinusitis

Sinusitis is an inflammation or infection of the sinuses. The sinuses are hollow spaces in the head that are lined with mucous membranes. The sinuses usually drain easily unless inflammation or infection is present. Sinusitis most often follows a cold and may also be associated with allergies, an infected tooth (dental abscess), or air pollution. Sinusitis can occur in infants and children, but it is more common in adults.

The key symptom of sinusitis is pain over the cheekbones and upper teeth; in the forehead over the eyebrows; or around and behind the eyes. There may also be headache, swelling around the eyes, fever, stuffy nose, coughing, or mucus draining down the back of the throat (postnasal drip). In children, coughing and nasal discharge that last more than 7 to 10 days along with complaints of headache and facial pain are signs that the problem may be sinusitis, not just a cold.

If your symptoms are severe or continue for more than 10 to 14 days, you may need to take antibiotics.

Prevention

- Promptly treat nasal congestion caused by colds. See page 154.
- Avoid cigarette, cigar, and pipe smoke in your home and workplace. Smoke irritates inflamed membranes in your nose and sinuses. If you smoke or use other tobacco products, consider getting help to quit. See page 26 for tips on quitting.
- If you have allergies, avoid the things that trigger your allergy attacks.

Home Treatment

Home treatment can often relieve early symptoms of sinusitis, such as facial pressure and stuffiness, and get your sinuses draining normally again so that you may not need antibiotic treatment.

- Drink extra fluids to keep mucus thin. Drink at least 8 to 10 glasses of water or juice per day.
- Apply moist heat (a warm towel or gel pack) to your face several times a day for 5 to 10 minutes at a time.
- Breathe warm, moist air from a steamy shower, a hot bath, or sink filled with hot water.
- Increase the humidity in your home, especially in the bedrooms. Avoid cold, dry air.
- Take an oral decongestant, use a decongestant nasal spray, or use a mucus-thinning agent (see page 346). Do not use a nasal spray for more than 3 days in a row. Avoid products that contain antihistamines unless your symptoms may also be related to allergies.
- Take aspirin, acetaminophen, or ibuprofen to relieve facial pain and headache. Do not give aspirin to anyone younger than 20.
- Check the back of your throat for postnasal drip. If you see streaks of mucus, gargle with warm water to prevent a sore throat.
- Blow your nose gently. Do not close one nostril when blowing your nose.
- Salt water (saline) irrigation helps wash mucus and bacteria out of the nasal passages. Use nonprescription saline nose drops or a homemade solution (see page 346):
  - Use a bulb syringe and gently squirt the solution into your nose, or snuff the solution from the palm of your hand, one nostril at a time.
  - The salt water should go in through your nose and come out your mouth.
  - Blow your nose gently afterward. Repeat the salt water wash 2 to 4 times a day.

When to Call Kaiser Permanente

- If cold symptoms or an ongoing daytime cough last longer than 10 to 14 days without improvement.
- If you have a severe headache that is different from a "normal" headache and is not relieved by acetaminophen, aspirin, or ibuprofen.
- If you have facial swelling or facial pain.
- If facial pain (especially in one sinus area or along the ridge between the nose and lower eyelid) persists after 2 to 4 days of home treatment. If you also have a fever over 102°, call in 1 to 2 days.
- If sinusitis symptoms persist after you have taken a full course of antibiotics.

Sore Throat and Strep Throat

Most sore throats are caused by viruses and may occur with a cold or may follow a cold. A mild sore throat may be caused by dry air, smoking, air pollution, or yelling. People who have allergies or stuffy noses may breathe through their mouths while sleeping, which can cause a mild sore throat.

Strep throat is a sore throat caused by streptococcal bacteria. It is more common in children from 3 to 15 years of age. A person can get strep throat even if his or her tonsils have been removed.

In general, the more coldlike your symptoms are, the less likely it is that you have strep throat. Strep throat causes some or all of these symptoms:

- Severe and sudden sore throat
- Fever of 101° or higher
- Swollen lymph nodes in the neck
- White or yellow coating on the tonsils

Strep throat is treated with antibiotics to prevent rheumatic fever. Antibiotics are effective in preventing rheumatic fever if started within 9 days of the onset of the sore throat.

Another cause of persistent sore throat is mononucleosis (mono, or "the kissing disease"), which is caused by the Epstein-Barr virus. Mono is most common in older teens and young adults. In addition to a severe sore throat, fever, and fatigue, mono symptoms often include weakness, body aches, and swollen lymph nodes in the neck. Another less common symptom is pain in the upper left part of the abdomen caused by enlargement of the spleen. Mono is diagnosed with a blood test.

Most people recover from mono after several weeks. However, for some people it may take several months to get their normal energy level back, and it is normal for the lymph nodes to remain enlarged for up to 1 month (see Swollen Lymph Nodes on page 169). There is no specific treatment for mono except rest, plenty of fluids, salt water gargles for throat pain, and aspirin or acetaminophen for body aches. Do not give aspirin to anyone younger than 20.

A less common cause of sore throat is the backflow (reflux) of stomach acid into the throat. Although reflux is often associated with heartburn or an "acid" taste in the mouth, sometimes a sore throat is the only symptom. If you think stomach acid reflux may be causing your throat pain, see Heartburn on page 83.

Prevention

- Drink 8 to 12 glasses of water a day.
- Identify and avoid irritants that cause sore throat (such as smoke, fumes, or yelling).
- If you smoke or use other tobacco products, consider getting help to quit. See page 26 for tips on quitting.

- Avoid contact with people who have strep throat.
- If you have mono, try to keep from spreading the virus: don't share eating or drinking utensils; avoid kissing; and do not donate blood until your symptoms are gone and you are feeling better.

Home Treatment

Home care is usually all that is needed for viral sore throats. If you are taking antibiotics for strep throat, these tips will also help you feel better.

- Gargle with warm salt water (1 teaspoon of salt in 8 ounces of water). The salt reduces swelling and discomfort.
- If you have postnasal drip, gargle often to prevent more throat irritation.
- Drink more fluids to soothe your sore throat. Honey and lemon in hot water or in weak tea may help. Do not give honey to children younger than 1 year of age.
- If you smoke or use other tobacco products, consider getting help to quit. See page 26 for tips on quitting.
- Avoid inhaling other people's smoke.
- Acetaminophen, aspirin, or ibuprofen will relieve pain and reduce fever. Do not give aspirin to anyone younger than 20.
- Some nonprescription throat lozenges (such as Sucrets Maximum Strength, Spec-T, and Tyrobenz) are safe, effective, and have a local anesthetic to soothe pain. Regular cough drops or hard candy may also help.

When to Call Kaiser Permanente

- If any one of the following symptoms develops:
  - Difficulty swallowing
  - Excessive drooling caused by inability to swallow
  - Labored or difficult breathing
- If you develop a severe sore throat after being exposed to strep throat.
- If a sore throat occurs with 2 of these 3 symptoms of strep throat:
  - Fever of 101° or higher
  - White or yellow coating on the tonsils
  - Swollen lymph nodes in the neck
- If a rash occurs with sore throat. **Scarlet fever** is a rash that may occur when there is a strep throat infection. Like strep throat, scarlet fever is treated with antibiotics.
- If you cannot trace the cause of a sore throat to a cold, allergy, smoking, overuse of your voice, or other irritation.
- If a mild sore throat lasts longer than 2 weeks.

Snoring

Up to ½ of adults snore occasionally, and ¼ of adults are habitual snorers. Snoring is caused by blockage of the airways in the back of the mouth and nose. These airways can be blocked for many reasons, such as excess neck tissue caused by being overweight or a stuffy nose caused by allergies or a cold. Some people who snore have sleep apnea. Sleep apnea is present when a person repeatedly stops breathing for 10 to 15 seconds or longer during sleep.

Snoring can disrupt a person's sleep patterns, so he or she may be sleepy and less alert during the day. A person's snoring can also disrupt the sleep of other family members or roommates. Here are some tips for people who snore:

- Exercise daily to maintain a healthful body weight and improve muscle tone. Avoid exercise within 2 hours of bedtime, because exercise may make it harder to fall asleep.
- Avoid heavy meals, alcohol, sleeping pills, and antihistamines before bedtime.
- Sleep on your side rather than your back. (Sew a pocket onto the back of your pajama top, and put a tennis ball inside the pocket. This will keep you from sleeping on your back.)
- Establish regular sleeping patterns. Go to bed at the same time every night, even on weekends.
- Let the person who doesn't snore fall asleep first.

If snoring becomes a problem for you and affects your family life, see a health professional. An examination of the nose, mouth, and neck may be needed. A physician may also want to do a sleep study to see if sleep apnea is one of the reasons why you snore. Treatment will depend on what is causing you to snore.

Swollen Lymph Nodes

The lymph nodes are small glands located throughout the body. The most noticeable lymph nodes are those in the neck. The lymph nodes swell as the body fights minor infections from colds, insect bites, or small cuts. More serious infections can cause the lymph nodes to greatly enlarge and become very firm and tender.

Swelling in the lymph nodes on either side of the neck is common with a cold or sore throat. The lymph nodes in the groin may swell if there is a vaginal or other pelvic infection, or if there is a cut or sore on the leg or foot.

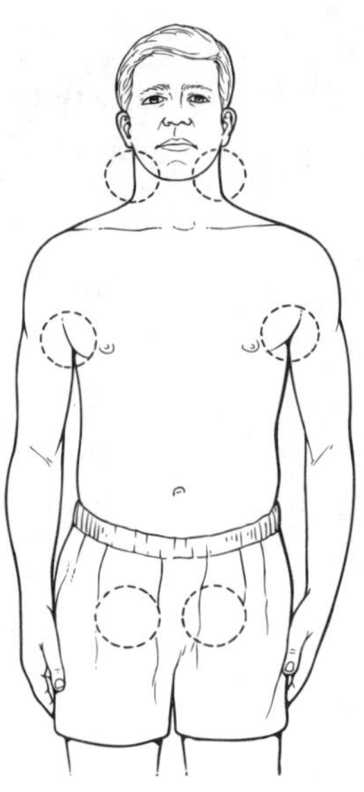

Swollen lymph nodes may be felt in the areas shown.

Lymph nodes may remain hard long after the initial infection goes away. This is especially true in children, whose lymph nodes may get smaller but remain hard and visible for several weeks.

Home Treatment

- There is no specific home treatment for swollen lymph nodes. Continue treating the cold or other infection that is causing the lymph nodes to swell.
- Your child may develop hard, swollen lymph nodes following a cold or minor infection. If the lymph nodes near the site of the infection are not tender and are not getting larger, you can monitor them at home and report them at the child's next regular physician visit.

When to Call Kaiser Permanente

- If the lymph nodes are large, very firm, red, and very tender.
- If swollen lymph nodes are associated with other signs of infection in a nearby cut or sore:
  - Fever of 100° or higher with no other cause.
  - Swelling and tenderness.
  - Discharge from the cut or sore.
  - Red streaks extending from the area.
- If you develop swollen lymph nodes after traveling outside the U.S. or in wilderness areas.
- If swollen lymph nodes continue to get bigger, or appear without apparent cause and persist for 2 weeks or longer.
- If swollen lymph nodes appear in areas other than the ones shown on page 170.

Tonsillitis

The tonsils and adenoids are tissues in the throat that assist in making antibodies to help fight infections. The tonsils can be seen on either side of the throat at the back of the mouth. The adenoids are above the roof of the mouth and usually cannot be seen.

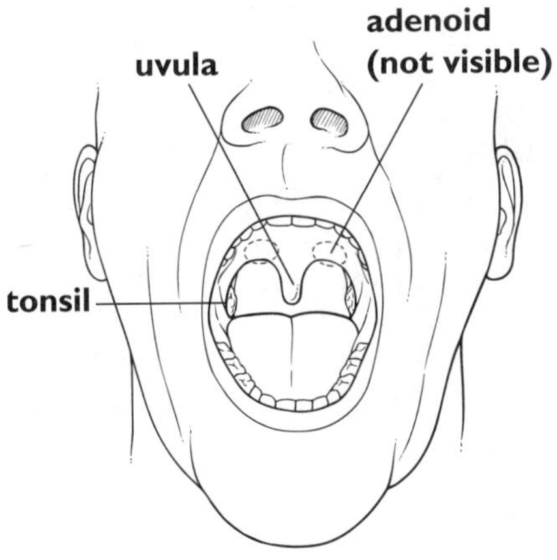

Location of tonsils and adenoids

Inflammation of the tonsils (tonsillitis) or adenoids (adenoiditis) is common in children, and the two conditions may occur separately or together. Tonsillitis and adenoiditis are usually caused by a virus. Symptoms of tonsillitis or adenoiditis are sore throat, fever, and tiredness along with cold symptoms, such as runny nose and a cough. It may be painful to swallow, and the tonsils are often bright red, spotted with pus, and swollen. The lymph nodes in the neck may also swell. Adenoiditis can also cause headache and vomiting.

A severe sore throat with very swollen tonsils, fever, and swollen lymph nodes in the neck can be caused by a strep or other bacterial throat infection. See page 167 for symptoms of strep throat. Strep throat must be treated with antibiotics.

A child with chronically inflamed adenoids may breathe through his or her mouth, snore, and have a nasal- or muffled-sounding voice. In children, inflamed adenoids can block the passageway between the ears and the throat (eustachian tubes), contributing to ear infections. See page 180.

Surgical removal of the tonsils (tonsillectomy) or adenoids (adenoidectomy) used to be common operations for children who had frequent sore throats. Now it is thought that these lymph tissues may be helpful in fighting infection and should not be removed unless it is necessary.

Home Treatment

Home treatment is usually all that is needed for mildly swollen and painful tonsils that accompany other cold symptoms. See page 154.

When to Call Kaiser Permanente

- If sore throat occurs with 2 of these 3 signs of a bacterial infection in the tonsils:
  - Fever of 101° or higher.
  - White or yellow coating on the tonsils or swollen, tender tonsils.
  - Swollen lymph nodes in the neck.
- If you develop a sore throat or tonsillitis after being exposed to strep throat.

- If a child has at least 4 to 6 bouts of tonsillitis in 1 year despite antibiotic treatment.
- If a child persistently breathes through his or her mouth, snores, or has a very nasal- or muffled-sounding voice.

Tonsillectomy and Adenoidectomy

It was once common to remove children's tonsils and adenoids. Today, in recognition of the risks, costs, and limited benefits, tonsillectomy and adenoidectomy are done less often, and only when the benefits greatly outweigh the risk, inconvenience, and pain.

Tonsillectomy may be recommended if at least 1 of the following criteria is met:

- There have been at least 4 to 6 severe tonsillitis infections caused by strep bacteria in the past year despite treatment with at least 2 different antibiotics.
- The enlarged tonsils cause severe breathing difficulty or sleep disturbance.
- There are deep pockets of infection in the tonsils that haven't responded to drug treatment.

Adenoidectomy may be recommended if at least 1 of the following criteria is met:

- The enlarged adenoids are blocking the airway, causing breathing difficulty and sleep disturbance.
- The adenoids are believed to cause persistent ear infections, despite antibiotic treatment.

If your physician recommends surgery but none of the above criteria are met, it may be wise to get a second opinion. See page 14.

You can observe a lot just by watching.
Yogi Berra (naturally)

8

Eye and Ear Problems

From dry eyes to pinkeye and earaches to earwax, your eyes and ears can cause you trouble. With home care and patience, most of these problems will clear up. This chapter will explain what you can do at home and when to get professional help.

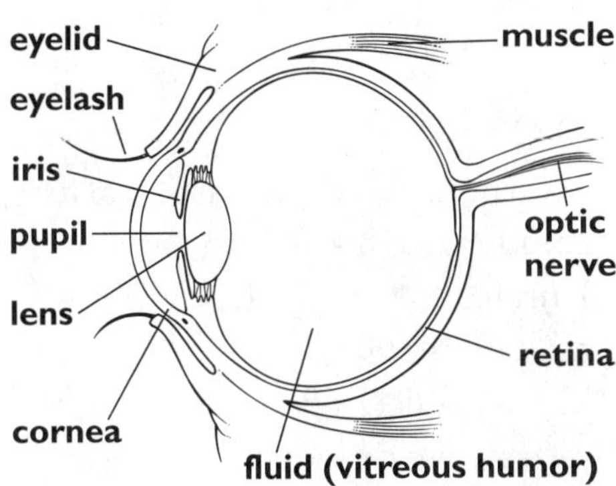

The structures at the front of the eye (lens, pupil, cornea, iris) let light into the eye. Light hits the back of the eye (retina) and is changed into nerve signals that are carried to the brain by the optic nerve. The brain reads the signals from the optic nerve as images that you "see."

Blood in the Eye

Sometimes blood vessels in the whites of the eyes break and cause a red spot or speck. This is called a subconjunctival hemorrhage. The blood may look alarming, especially if the spot is large, but it is usually not a cause for concern. The red spot will go away in 2 to 3 weeks.

However, if your eye is bloody and painful; if there is blood in the colored part of the eye; or if the bleeding followed a blow to the eye, call a health professional immediately. Also call if bleeding in the eye occurs often; occurs after you begin taking blood thinners (anticoagulants); or covers more than ¼ of the white of the eye.

Eye Problems	
Symptoms	**Possible Causes**
Red, itchy, watery eyes	Allergies, p. 141. Think about allergy to eye care products, makeup, or smoke. Possible contact lens problem, p. 176.
Excessive discharge from eye; red, swollen eyelids; sandy feeling	Eye Infections, p. 175. Possible contact lens problem, p. 176.
Pimple or swelling on eyelid	Styes, p. 177.
Pain in the eye	Chemical Burns, p. 43; Migraine Headaches, p. 192; Cluster Headaches, p. 193; Objects in the Eye, p. 62; Possible contact lens problem, p. 176; Eye Infections, p. 175.
Severe eye pain, blurred vision, reddened eyeball	Possible iritis or acute glaucoma, p. 179. **See a physician now!**
Red spot on white of eye	Blood in the Eye, p. 173.
Blow to the eye	Bruises (black eye), p. 40.
Dry, scratchy eyes	Dry Eyes, p. 174.

Dry Eyes

Eyes that don't have enough moisture in them may feel dry, hot, sandy, or gritty. Low humidity, smoke, the natural aging process, certain diseases, and medications (such as antihistamines, decongestants, or birth control pills) may cause dry eyes.

Home Treatment

- Give your eyes a rest. While reading, watching television, or using a computer, take frequent breaks and close your eyes. If you can, blink your eyes more often.
- If possible, avoid smoke and other eye irritants.
- Try a nonprescription artificial tear solution, such as Akwa Tears, Duratears, or HypoTears. These are different from drops like Visine, which reduce eye redness rather than dryness.

When to Call Kaiser Permanente

Call if dry eyes are persistent and artificial tears do not help.

Floaters and Flashes

Floaters are spots, specks, and lines that "float" across your field of vision. They are caused by stray cells or strands of tissue that float in the vitreous humor, the gel-like substance that fills the eyeball. Floaters can be annoying but are not usually serious. However, if you see floaters or flashes of light for the first time, call your eye physician or family physician. If you have had floaters for some time, or if you have occasional flashes, mention it at your next routine eye exam.

Eye Infections

Conjunctivitis, or pinkeye, is an inflammation of the delicate membrane (conjunctiva) that lines the inside of the eyelid and the surface of the eye. Bacteria and viruses (which can be very contagious), allergies, pollution, or other irritants can cause pinkeye.

The symptoms of pinkeye are redness in the whites of the eyes, red and swollen eyelids, lots of tears, and a sandy feeling in the eyes. There may be a discharge that causes the eyelids to stick together during sleep.

Prevention

- Do not share towels, handkerchiefs, or washcloths with a person who has pinkeye.
- If a chemical or object gets into your eye, immediately flush the eye with water. See page 43 or page 62.

Home Treatment

Although most cases of pinkeye will clear up on their own in 5 to 7 days, viral pinkeye can last many weeks. Pinkeye caused by allergies or pollution will last as long as you are exposed to the irritating substance. Good home care will speed healing and bring relief.

- Apply cold or warm compresses several times a day to relieve discomfort.
- Gently wipe the edge of the eyelid with moist cotton or a clean, wet washcloth to remove encrusted matter.
- Don't wear contact lenses or eye makeup until the infection or inflammation is gone. Discard eye makeup after an eye infection.

Eye Twitches

Eye twitches or muscle spasms around the eye are most often associated with fatigue or stress. Twitches will usually stop on their own in a short time, and they will improve with rest or reduced stress.

Call a health professional if twitches occur with redness, swelling, discharge from the eye, or fever, or if eye twitches last longer than 1 to 2 weeks.

Contact Lenses

If you wear contact lenses, these tips will help you avoid problems.

Follow the cleaning instructions for your lenses. Keep your lenses and anything that touches them (hands, storage containers, solution bottles, makeup) very clean. Wash your hands before handling your contacts.

Use a commercial saline solution. (Generic brands are just as good as name brands.) Homemade solution is easily contaminated with bacteria.

Insert your contacts before applying eye makeup. Do not apply makeup to the inner rim of the eyelid. Replace eye makeup every 3 to 6 months to reduce the risk of contamination.

When worn for long periods of time, extended-wear lenses are more likely to cause severe eye infections. If you choose to wear them, follow the wearing and cleaning schedule your eye care professional recommends.

Symptoms of a possible problem with your contacts include unusual redness, pain, or burning in the eye; discharge; blurred vision; or extreme sensitivity to light. Remove your lenses and disinfect them. If symptoms last longer than 2 to 3 hours after you remove your contacts, call your eye care professional.

Visit your eye care professional once a year to check the condition of your lenses and the health of your eyes.

- If eyedrops are prescribed, insert them as follows:
  - For older children and adults: Pull the lower lid down with 2 fingers to create a little pouch. Put the drops there. Close the eye for several minutes to let the drops move around.
  - For younger children: Ask the child to lie down with eyes closed. Put a drop in the inner corner of the eye. When the child opens the eye, the drop will run in.
  - Be sure the dropper is clean and does not touch the eye, eyelid, or the eyelashes.

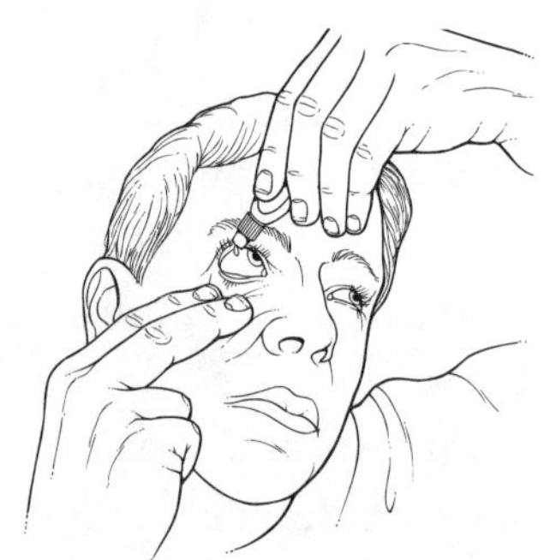

Inserting eyedrops

- Putting antibiotic ointment in the eye can be tricky, especially with children. If you can get it on the eyelashes, it will melt and get into the eye.
- Make sure any nonprescription medicine you use is ophthalmic (for eyes), not otic (for ears).
- Wash your hands thoroughly after treating pinkeye.

When to Call Kaiser Permanente

- If there is pain in the eye (rather than irritation), blurring, or loss of vision that is not cleared even momentarily by blinking.
- If the eye is painfully sensitive to light.
- If the skin around the eye or the eyelid is red.
- If it feels like there is a foreign object in the eye.
- If the eye is red and there is a greenish yellow discharge that does not begin to go away in 24 hours.
- If there is an abnormal difference between the sizes of the pupils.
- If symptoms of an eye infection last longer than 7 days.

Styes

A sty is a noncontagious infection of the eyelash follicle. It looks like a small, red bump, much like a pimple, either in the eyelid or on the edge of the lid. It comes to a head and breaks open after a few days.

Styes are very common and are not a serious problem. Most will go away on their own with home treatment and don't require removal.

Home Treatment

- Do not rub the eye, and do not squeeze the sty.
- Apply warm, moist compresses for 10 minutes, 5 to 6 times a day, until the sty comes to a head and drains.

PRK and LASIK

PRK and LASIK are two different surgical procedures that can correct vision problems such as nearsightedness, farsightedness, and astigmatism. For each procedure, a surgeon uses laser instruments to reshape the cornea (the clear tissue that covers the iris and pupil) in a way that allows improved vision. These procedures take only a few minutes to complete. If both eyes need correction, they can be treated at the same time.

Some people may still need to wear glasses or contact lenses after the surgery, especially when light is dim and at night (usually the prescription is not as strong). A person may see halos around lights for up to 6 months after having corrective eye surgery.

PRK and LASIK cannot restore vision loss caused by cataracts or macular degeneration; nor can they prevent these age-related eye changes from happening.

These services are provided on a fee-for-service basis, separate from and not covered under your Health Plan benefits, and may not be available in all Kaiser Permanente service areas.

When to Call Kaiser Permanente

- If the sty interferes with your vision.
- If the sty gets worse despite home treatment.
- If the redness centered on the sty spreads to involve the entire eyelid.

Dizziness and Vertigo

Dizziness is a word that is often used to describe 2 different sensations: lightheadedness and vertigo. It is important to know exactly what you mean when you say, "I feel dizzy," because it can help you and your health professional narrow down the list of possible problems.

Lightheadedness is a feeling that you are about to pass out (faint). Although you may feel unsteady, there is no sensation of movement.

Lightheadedness usually goes away or improves when you lie down. If lightheadedness gets worse, it can lead to a fainting spell with nausea or vomiting.

Lightheadedness usually does not indicate a serious problem. It is common to feel lightheaded occasionally. Lightheadedness is often caused by a momentary drop in blood pressure and reduced blood flow to the head when you get up too quickly from a seated or lying position. This is called **orthostatic hypotension**. It may be caused by dehydration or medications such as water pills (diuretics).

Lightheadedness is common when you have flu, a cold, or allergies. Vomiting, diarrhea, and fever can cause dehydration and lightheadedness. Other common causes of lightheadedness include side effects of medication, hyperventilation, stress, anxiety, drinking alcohol, or using illegal drugs. A more serious cause of lightheadedness is bleeding. If a person is bleeding internally, lightheadedness and fatigue may be the first noticeable symptoms of blood loss.

An uncommon cause of lightheadedness is an abnormality in your heart rhythm. This can cause recurrent spells of lightheadedness and can lead to a fainting spell (cardiac syncope). Unexplained fainting spells need to be evaluated by a health professional. See Fainting on page 73.

Vertigo is a sensation that your body or the world around you is spinning or moving. Vertigo is usually related to inner ear problems. It may occur with nausea and vomiting. It may be impossible to walk when you have severe vertigo.

The most common form of vertigo is triggered by changes in the position of your head, such as when you move your head from side to side or bend your head back to look up. This is called **benign positional vertigo**.

Cataracts and Glaucoma

Cataracts are cloudy areas in the lens of the eye. They may cause vision problems such as cloudy, foggy, or filmy vision; glare from lamps, sunlight, or car headlights; and double vision. Cataracts are common in older adults.

Glaucoma is an eye disorder that results when there is excess pressure in the eyeball. If the pressure is not relieved, the optic nerve may be damaged, causing blindness. Glaucoma rarely has symptoms and develops slowly over several years.

Cataracts and glaucoma are easy to detect during routine eye exams. Both respond well to medical treatment. Talk with your physician about the best schedule of eye exams for you, based on your age and risk factors for these eye problems.

Call your health professional immediately if you have sudden blurry vision, loss of vision, or pain in the eye.

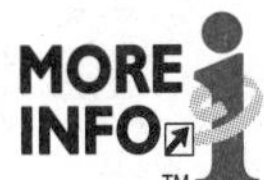

If you are considering cataract surgery, gather as much information as possible about the risks and benefits of surgery. Getting all the facts and thinking about your own needs and values will help you work with your physician to make a wise health decision.

Vertigo also may be caused by labyrinthitis, an inflammation in the part of the inner ear that controls balance. Labyrinthitis is usually caused by a viral infection and sometimes follows a cold or the flu.

Other underlying problems that can contribute to vertigo are Meniere's disease (a balance problem believed to be caused by a buildup of fluid in the inner ear), multiple sclerosis, and, in rare cases, a brain tumor.

Home Treatment

Lightheadedness is usually not a cause for concern unless it is severe, persistent, or occurs with other symptoms such as an irregular heartbeat or fainting. The greatest danger of lightheadedness is the injuries that might result if you fall.

- When you feel lightheaded, lie down for 1 or 2 minutes. This will allow more blood to flow to your brain. After lying down, sit up slowly and remain sitting for 1 to 2 minutes before slowly standing up.
- Viral illnesses, such as colds or the flu, may cause lightheadedness. Resting will help prevent it. Also, drink extra fluids to prevent dehydration, which can cause or increase lightheadedness.
- Do not drive, operate machinery, or put yourself in any other potentially dangerous situation while you are having vertigo.

- When you are having vertigo, avoid lying flat on your back. Propping yourself up slightly may relieve the spinning sensation.

When to Call Kaiser Permanente

Call 911 or seek other emergency services immediately:

- If vertigo is accompanied by headache, confusion, loss of speech or sight, weakness in the arms or legs, or numbness in any part of the body.
- If lightheadedness occurs with chest pain that is squeezing or crushing, and/or occurs with any other symptoms of a heart attack (see page 54).
- If someone who is feeling dizzy loses consciousness and you are unable to arouse the person.
- If severe and persistent lightheadedness is accompanied by a sudden change in your normal heart rate.

Call Kaiser Permanente:

- If vertigo occurs with other signs of serious illness, such as headache with severe stiff neck, fever, irritability, confusion, or a seizure. (See "Encephalitis and Meningitis" on page 160.)
- If lightheadedness or vertigo develops after an injury.
- If you have vertigo that is severe (may cause vomiting) or that occurs with hearing loss.
- If you suspect dizziness may be a side effect of a medication.
- If you experience vertigo that:
  - Has not been diagnosed.
  - Lasts longer than 5 days.
  - Is significantly different from other episodes.
- If you have repeated spells of lightheadedness over a few days.
- If you feel lightheaded and your pulse is less than 50 or more than 130 beats per minute. See page 57 to learn how to take your pulse.

Ear Infections

Ear infections can occur in the middle ear or the ear canal. For information about infections in the ear canal, see Swimmer's Ear on page 186.

A middle ear infection (otitis media) usually develops during a cold. Colds can cause the eustachian tube (which connects the middle ear to the throat) to swell and close. When the eustachian tube is closed, air cannot reach the middle ear. This creates a vacuum that draws fluid into the middle ear. Bacteria or viruses then grow in the fluid, causing a middle ear infection.

The infected fluid that is trapped in the middle ear puts pressure on the eardrum. If the ear infection is not treated, the pressure may continue to build until the eardrum ruptures. A single **eardrum rupture** usually is not serious and rarely causes hearing loss. However, repeated eardrum ruptures can lead to permanent hearing loss. See "Recurrent Ear Infections and Persistent Effusion" on page 185.

Symptoms of a middle ear infection include ear pain, dizziness, ringing or a feeling of fullness in the ear, hearing loss, fever, headache, and runny nose. Children who can't yet talk may tug on their painful ears. Drainage from the ear that is bloody or looks like pus may indicate a ruptured eardrum. Ear pain usually improves once an eardrum ruptures.

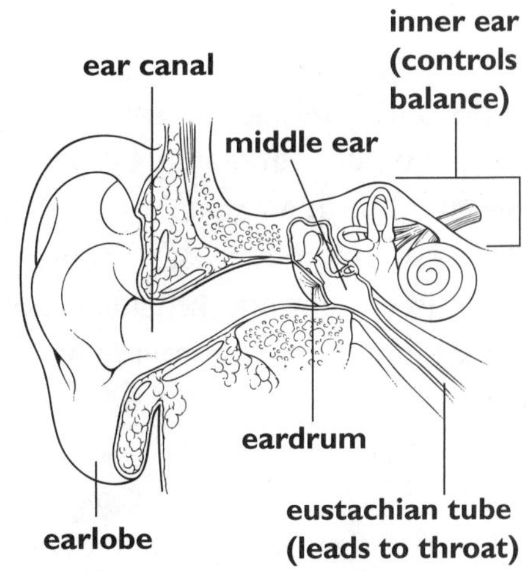

Ear infections can occur in the ear canal or middle ear. Dizziness can be caused by an inflammation of the inner ear.

Ear Problems

Symptoms	Possible Causes
Earache and fever; pulling at ears by infants and small children, especially with inconsolable crying	Ear Infections, p. 180.
Pain while chewing; headache	TM Disorder, p. 136.
Pain when ear is wiggled or while chewing; itching or burning in ear	Swimmer's Ear, p. 186.
Discharge from ear	Swimmer's Ear, p. 186; eardrum rupture, p. 180.
Feeling of fullness in ear, with runny or stuffy nose, cough, fever	Colds, p. 154; Ear Infections, p. 180.
Feeling of something moving or "bumping around" in ear	Objects in the Ear, p. 61.
Hearing loss; inattentiveness	Hearing Loss, p. 184; Earwax, p. 183; serous otitis, p. 182.
Ringing or noise in the ears	Tinnitus, p. 188.

When a person has fluid buildup in the middle ear, it is called **serous otitis** or effusion. Effusion generally occurs after a middle ear infection has cleared up. There may be no symptoms, or there may be a muffling of sound, minor hearing loss, and mild discomfort. Effusion is not a cause for concern and may not require treatment unless it lasts longer than 3 months or causes significant hearing loss in both ears. See "Recurrent Ear Infections and Persistent Effusion" on page 185.

Prevention

- If you can, breastfeed your baby. Breastfed babies have fewer ear infections. If you bottlefeed your baby, hold the baby in an upright position to prevent milk from getting into the eustachian tubes. Do not allow infants to fall asleep with a bottle (however, it is all right to let a nursing baby fall asleep at the breast).
- Avoid exposing children to cigarette smoke, which is associated with more frequent ear infections.
- If you smoke or use other tobacco products, consider getting help to quit. See page 26 for tips on quitting.
- If possible, limit your child's contact with other children who have colds.
- Wean your child from his or her pacifier at about 6 months of age. Babies who continue to use their pacifiers after 12 months of age are more likely to develop ear infections.
- Wash your hands often if you have a cold or other upper respiratory infection to prevent spreading the infection.
- Make sure your child is up to date with his or her immunizations.

Home Treatment

- Apply heat to the ear to ease the pain. Use a warm washcloth or a heating pad set on low. Don't use a heating pad on an infant, and never leave a child alone with a heating pad.
- Acetaminophen, aspirin, or ibuprofen will help relieve earache. Do not give aspirin to anyone younger than 20 years of age.
- Rest. Let your energy go to fighting the infection.
- Drink more clear liquids.
- If dizziness occurs, see page 178.
- If an ear infection has caused the eardrum to rupture, avoid getting water in the ear until the eardrum heals (about 3 to 4 weeks).

When to Call Kaiser Permanente

- If your child has a severe earache and cannot be quieted even after you apply home treatment for several hours.
- If ear pain occurs with other signs of serious illness, such as headache with severe stiff neck, fever,

irritability, or confusion. (See "Encephalitis and Meningitis" on page 160.)

- If your baby pulls or rubs his or her ear and appears to be in pain (crying, screaming).
- If ear pain increases despite home treatment.
- If your child has a fever over 102° with other signs of an ear infection.
- If you suspect that the eardrum has ruptured or there is drainage from the ear that looks like pus or contains blood.
- If symptoms do not improve after 48 hours of treatment with an antibiotic.
- If your child has ear tubes and develops an earache or has drainage from the ear.
- If mild ear pain continues for longer than 3 to 4 days.
- If there is redness or swelling behind the ear.
- If you suspect your child has a problem hearing after being sick or having a cold.

Earwax

Earwax is a protective secretion that filters dust and keeps the ear clean. Normally, earwax is liquid, self-draining, and does not cause problems. Children have a lot of earwax, but earwax production seems to taper off as children grow older.

Occasionally, the wax will build up, harden, and cause some hearing loss or discomfort. Poking at the wax with cotton swabs, fingers, or other objects will only further compact the wax against the eardrum. When wax is tightly packed, professional help is needed to remove it. You can handle most earwax problems by avoiding cotton swabs and following the home treatment tips. You should be concerned only if the earwax causes ringing in the ears, a full feeling in the ears, some hearing loss, or vertigo (see When to Call Kaiser Permanente on page 184).

Home Treatment

Home treatment is not appropriate if you suspect that the eardrum is ruptured or there is drainage from the ear that looks like pus or contains blood.

- Soften and loosen the earwax with warm (body temperature) mineral oil. Place 2 drops of mineral oil in the ear twice a day for 1 or 2 days.
- Once the wax is loose and soft, all that is usually needed to remove the wax from the ear canal is the spray from a warm, gentle shower. Direct the water into the ear, and then tip the head to let the earwax drain out.
- If the warm mineral oil and shower do not work, use a nonprescription wax softener, followed by gentle flushing with a bulb ear syringe each night for 1 to 2 weeks. Make sure the flushing solution is body

temperature. Putting cool or hot fluids in the ear may cause dizziness.

When to Call Kaiser Permanente

- If home treatment does not work and the wax buildup is hard, dry, and compacted.
- If earwax is causing ringing in your ears, a full feeling in your ears, or hearing loss.
- If earwax buildup occurs with other problems such as nausea or difficulty with balance.
- If an earwax problem develops in a person who has a ruptured eardrum or ear tubes (tympanostomy tubes).

Hearing Loss

More than 28 million Americans cope with some degree of hearing loss. Most hearing loss is caused by problems in the inner ear or in the acoustic nerve, which sends sound signals to the brain. This is called **sensorineural hearing loss**. The damage to the inner ear that causes sensorineural hearing loss can be the result of exposure to loud noise, certain medications (including high doses of aspirin), or changes that come with age. In some cases, children are born with this type of hearing loss. People with sensorineural hearing loss are usually not totally deaf. They may have trouble understanding the speech of others yet be very sensitive to loud sounds. They may also hear ringing, hissing, or clicking noises.

Hearing loss that develops when something prevents sound from reaching the inner ear is called **conductive hearing loss**. The most common cause is packed earwax in the ear canal, which can be easily treated (see page 183). Infection, abnormal bone growth, and excess fluid in the ear are other causes of conductive hearing loss.

People who have conductive hearing loss often say that their own voice sounds loud while other voices sound muffled. There may be a low level of ringing in the ear (tinnitus). Depending on the underlying problem, conductive hearing loss is usually treated by ear flushing, medication, or surgery.

A rare form of hearing loss is caused by damage to the hearing centers in the brain. This is called **central deafness**, and it can occur after a head injury or stroke. The person's ear works normally, but his or her brain has difficulty interpreting sounds.

Some hearing loss may be the result of decreased blood flow to the inner ear. If you have circulatory problems caused by heart disease, high blood pressure, or diabetes, be sure to follow your care plan for keeping those conditions under control.

Recurrent Ear Infections and Persistent Effusion

If your child has at least 3 ear infections in a 6-month period, or 2 ear infections before the age of 6 months, talk to your pediatrician about preventive antibiotic treatment. This is a low dose of antibiotics given daily throughout the season when your child is prone to ear infections. Daily antibiotic treatment may reduce the frequency of ear infections, but it may not always prevent fluid buildup (effusion) in the middle ear.

Daily antibiotic treatment is prescribed less often than it used to be. This is because there is growing concern that routine use of antibiotics may cause bacteria to change so that common antibiotics cannot kill them.

If your child has repeated ear infections (3 in 6 months, or 4 to 6 in a year), your physician may suggest inserting ear tubes (tympanostomy tubes) through your child's eardrums to help prevent ear infections. The tubes remain in the child's eardrums for 6 to 12 months.

In some children, fluid remains in the middle ear more than 3 months after an ear infection clears up. If this occurs in your child, he or she should be given a hearing test because long-lasting effusion can cause hearing loss. If your child has effusion and significant hearing loss in both ears at the same time for more than 3 months, your physician may recommend ear tubes.

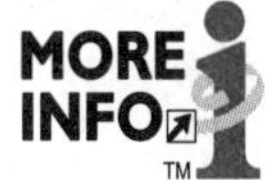

Ask your physician about the long-term risks and benefits of all the available treatment options for recurrent ear infections.

Prevention

- Avoid loud noise if possible. If you know you are going to be exposed to loud noise (at work, the shooting range, while snowmobiling, etc.), wear earplugs or protective earmuffs.
- Keep your ears clean and periodically check for wax buildup. Do not use cotton swabs or other objects to clean your ears. See page 183.
- Ask your pharmacist if any medications you are taking can affect your hearing. For example, the use of certain antibiotics, blood pressure medications, ibuprofen, and large doses of aspirin (8 to 12 tablets per day) is linked to hearing impairment.

When to Call Kaiser Permanente

- If hearing loss develops suddenly (within a matter of days or weeks).
- If you have hearing loss in one ear only.
- If you are thinking about wearing hearing aids. Make an appointment with a hearing specialist (otolaryngologist or audiologist) if:
  - You often ask people to repeat themselves or have difficulty understanding words.
  - You have difficulty hearing when someone speaks in a whisper.
  - You cannot hear soft sounds, such as a dripping faucet, or high-pitched sounds.
  - You continuously hear a ringing or hissing background noise.
  - A hearing problem is interfering with your life.

Swimmer's Ear

Swimmer's ear (otitis externa) is inflammation or infection of the ear canal (the passage leading from the external ear to the eardrum). It often develops after water has gotten into the ear, especially after swimming. Sand or other debris that gets into the ear canal may also cause swimmer's ear.

A scratch inside the ear or injury from a cotton swab or other object can cause inflammation in the ear canal.

Symptoms include pain, itching, and a feeling of fullness in the ear. The ear canal may be swollen. A more severe inflammation or infection can cause increased pain, discharge from the ear, and possibly some hearing loss. Unlike a middle ear infection (otitis media), the pain of ear canal inflammation or infection is worse when you chew, when you press on the "tag" in front of the ear, or when you wiggle your earlobe.

Prevention

- Keep your ears dry. After swimming or showering, shake your head to remove water from the ear canal. Gently dry your ears with the corner of a tissue or towel, or use a blow dryer on its lowest setting, held several inches from your ear.
- Put a few drops of rubbing alcohol or alcohol mixed with an equal amount of white vinegar in the ear after swimming or showering. Wiggle the outside of the ear to let the liquid enter the ear canal; then tilt your head and let it drain out. You can also use nonprescription drops (Star-Otic, Swim-Ear) to prevent swimmer's ear.
- Earwax actually helps protect your ear canals. Avoid cotton swabs and earplugs, and never put any other objects into your ears. Trying to remove wax can push it further into the ear and damage the eardrum or canal. See page 183.

- Avoid getting soap and shampoo in the ear canal. Remove dirt or sand that gets into the ear while swimming by using a bulb syringe. Or try directing a gentle stream of warm water from the shower into your ear; then tip your head to let the water drain out.
- Follow any instructions your health professional has given you to treat skin problems (eczema, psoriasis, seborrhea) that may cause ear canal irritation.

Home Treatment

- Make sure there isn't an object or insect in the ear. See Objects in the Ear on page 61.
- If the eardrum may be ruptured or there is drainage from the ear that looks like pus or contains blood, do not insert anything into the ear unless a health professional has told you to do so.
- Gently rinse the ear using a bulb syringe and a solution of 1 part white vinegar and 1 part rubbing alcohol. Make sure the flushing solution is at body temperature. Putting cool or hot fluids in the ear may cause dizziness.
- Avoid getting water in the ear until the irritation clears up. Cotton coated with petroleum jelly can be used as an earplug. Do not use plastic earplugs.
- If your ear is itchy, try nonprescription swimmer's eardrops (see Prevention). Use them before and after swimming or getting your ears wet.
- To insert eardrops, have the person lie down, ear facing up. Warm the drops first by rolling the container between your hands. Place drops on the wall of the ear canal in small quantities so air can escape and drops can get into the ear. Wiggling the outer ear will help. See illustration.

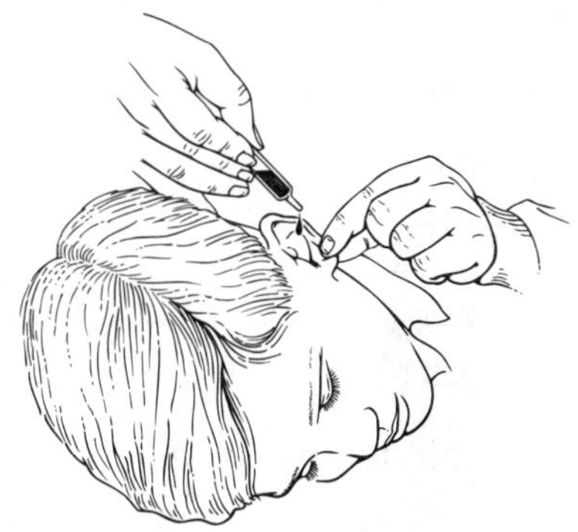

Never stick a dropper into the ear canal. Put drops on the outer ear near the opening of the ear canal, and gently wiggle the ear until the drops flow into the canal.

- You may find it easier to put eardrops in a small child's ear if you have the child lie down on your lap with his or her legs wrapped around your waist.
- To ease ear pain, apply a warm washcloth or a heating pad set on low. (Don't use a heating pad on an infant, and never leave a child alone with a heating pad.) There may be some drainage when the heat melts earwax. As long as the drainage does not contain pus or blood, it is not of concern.

- Acetaminophen or aspirin may also help relieve pain. Do not give aspirin to anyone younger than 20.

When to Call Kaiser Permanente

- If ear pain and itching persist or worsen after 3 days of home treatment.
- If the ear canal is swollen, red, and very painful.
- If redness extends to the outer ear.
- If there is redness or swelling behind the ear.
- If there is discharge from the ear that does not look like earwax.
- If ear pain follows a cold. See page 154.

Tinnitus

Most people experience occasional ringing (or roaring, hissing, buzzing, or tinkling) in their ears. The sound usually lasts only a few minutes. If it becomes persistent, you may have tinnitus.

Tinnitus is usually caused by damage to the nerves in the inner ear resulting from prolonged exposure to loud noise. Other causes include excess earwax, ear infection, dental problems, head or ear injuries, and medications, especially antibiotics and large amounts of aspirin. Excessive alcohol or caffeine intake can also cause tinnitus. In rare cases, tinnitus can be caused by a brain tumor.

Most intermittent tinnitus does not require medical treatment. However, if tinnitus is accompanied by other symptoms, becomes persistent, or starts to localize to one ear, a visit to a health professional usually is needed. Often there is no cure for tinnitus, but your health professional can help you learn how to live with the problem.

Prevention

Follow the prevention tips for Hearing Loss on page 185.

Home Treatment

- Cut back on or eliminate alcohol and beverages containing caffeine.
- Limit your use of aspirin, ibuprofen, and naproxen sodium.
- If you think earwax may be the cause of tinnitus, see Earwax on page 183.
- Soft background noise or music may make tinnitus less noticeable.

When to Call Kaiser Permanente

- If you have new tinnitus with other symptoms such as significant hearing loss, vertigo (see page 178), loss of balance, nausea, or vomiting.
- If tinnitus develops after an injury to the head or ear.
- If tinnitus lasts longer than 4 weeks despite home treatment.

I'm very brave generally, only today I happen to have a headache.
Tweedledum in Alice in Wonderland

9

Headaches

Headaches are one of the most common health complaints. Some possible causes include tension, infection, allergy, injury, hunger, changes in the flow of blood in the vessels of the head, or exposure to chemicals.

Most headaches that occur without other symptoms will respond well to self-care. The majority of headaches—more than 90 percent—are caused by tension and respond well to prevention and home treatment. See page 194.

An unusual headache that is very different from any you have had before, or a change in the usual pattern of your headaches, is a cause for concern. See "Headache Emergencies." However, if you have had similar headaches before and your physician has recommended a treatment plan for them, emergency care may not be needed.

Headaches that routinely occur during or after physical exertion, sexual activity, coughing, or sneezing may be a sign of a more serious disease and should be discussed with a health professional.

Headache Emergencies

Call your physician now if you have:

- A very sudden "thunderclap" headache.
- A sudden, severe headache unlike any you have had before.
- Headache with stiff neck, fever, nausea, vomiting, drowsiness, or confusion.
- A sudden, severe headache with a stiff neck that develops soon after the headache starts.
- Headache with weakness, paralysis, numbness, visual disturbances, slurred speech, confusion, or behavior changes.
- Headaches following a recent fall or blow to the head. See page 52 for information on head injuries.

Possible Headache Causes

If headache occurs:	Possible causes include:
On awakening.	Tension Headaches, p. 194; Allergies, p. 141; Sinusitis, p. 165; Neck Pain, p. 113; TM Disorder, p. 136.
In jaw muscles or in both temples.	TM Disorder, p. 136; Tension Headaches, p. 194.
Each afternoon or evening; after hours of desk work; with sore neck and shoulders.	Tension Headaches, p. 194; Neck Pain, p. 113.
On one side of the head, with visual disturbances or runny nose.	Migraine Headaches, p. 192; Cluster Headaches, p. 193.
After a blow to the head.	Head Injuries, p. 52.
After exposure to chemicals (paint, varnish, insect spray, cigarette smoke).	Chemical headache. Get into fresh air. Drink water to flush poisons.
With fever, runny nose, or sore throat.	Flu, p. 161; Sore Throat, p. 167; Colds, p. 154.
With fever, stiff neck, nausea, and vomiting.	Encephalitis and Meningitis, p. 160.
With runny nose, watery eyes, and sneezing.	Allergies, p. 141.
With fever and pain in the cheekbones or over the eyes.	Sinusitis, p. 165.
On mornings when you drink less caffeine than usual.	Caffeine-withdrawal headache. Cut back slowly, p. 194.
Following a stressful event.	Tension Headaches, p. 194.
At the same time during the menstrual cycle.	Premenstrual Syndrome, p. 264.
With new medication.	Drug allergy. Contact your physician.
With severe eye pain.	Possible acute glaucoma, p. 179. **See a physician now!**

Headaches in Children

Migraine headaches (see page 192) often begin during childhood or adolescence and are the most common form of headache in children.

Children's headaches can also be related to stress about school, sports, relationships, or peer pressure. Even fun activities can be overdone and cause fatigue and headaches. Many times, just talking about a problem with your child may help. Encourage your children to talk openly about problems and stress at school.

Hunger can also cause headaches in children. A daily breakfast and a nutritious after-school snack may prevent headaches. Eyestrain and lack of sleep are other possible headache causes. Children will often have headaches along with sore throats, colds, sinus problems, or other infections.

For the many children and teens who get headaches, treatment is based on the same factors as adult headache treatment: how often the headaches occur; how severe the pain is and how long it lasts; and how much the headaches disrupt normal activities. However, in children there is an increased emphasis on nondrug treatments.

Although migraines in children can be managed in much the same way as migraines in adults, less is known about the long-term effects of migraine medications in children. Some medications are not recommended for young children.

Home Treatment

- If your child's physician has prescribed a specific treatment for the child's headaches, begin treatment as soon as your child complains of pain.
- For headaches that are mild and occur only occasionally, let your child rest quietly in a darkened room with a cool compress on his or her forehead. If rest does not relieve your child's headache, try a nonprescription medication such as acetaminophen or ibuprofen. Follow the dosage directions on the package for your child's age group. Do not give aspirin to anyone younger than 20.
- If your child tends to have mild headaches that occur frequently, encourage him or her to go on with normal activities. Do not allow your child to avoid chores or other activities unless his or her headache pain is moderate or severe. It is useful to "practice what you preach" in this area. When you have a headache, deal with it in a matter-of-fact way. Try to maintain your own usual activities when you have a headache, and adopt a calm approach to managing the

pain. If your children see you successfully managing the impact of headaches on your life, they will be likely to do the same for themselves.

- Talk to your child. Let him or her know you care. Extra attention and quiet time may be all that are needed to relieve the pain.

When to Call Kaiser Permanente

- If a severe headache occurs with signs of encephalitis or meningitis (see page 160), especially if your child recently had a viral illness.
- If a headache is severe and is not relieved by relaxing or taking a nonprescription pain reliever.
- If a headache occurs with other symptoms, such as abdominal pain, nausea, or vomiting, and is not relieved by home treatment and taking a nonprescription pain reliever.
- If a child's headaches occur 2 times a week or more, or if you are using pain relievers to control a child's headaches more than once a week.
- If you cannot discover a reasonable cause for your child's headaches.
- If headaches awaken your child at night or are worse early in the morning.
- Also see "Headache Emergencies" on page 189.

Migraine Headaches

Migraine headaches are severe, usually one-sided headaches that often occur with nausea, vomiting, and extreme sensitivity to light or sound. People often describe the headache as throbbing or piercing. The pain may range from mild to terribly severe.

Although the headaches are usually one-sided, some people have pain on both sides of the head. In some people, the pain may switch sides each time they have a migraine.

Ten to 30 percent of migraines occur with an aura, a collection of symptoms that usually occur 15 to 30 minutes before a migraine headache begins. The most common symptom of an aura is visual disturbances, such as flashing lights, distortion in the size or shape of objects, or blind or dark spots in the field of vision. An aura may also include symptoms that affect the nervous system, such as numbness or tingling in the face or arm, strange smells or sounds, or weakness on one side of the body.

Migraines are more common in females than in males. The headaches may begin during childhood, but most begin during the teens and early 20s.

Cluster Headaches

Cluster headaches are sudden, very severe, sharp, stabbing headaches that occur on one side of the head, usually in the temple or behind the eye. The eye and nostril on the affected side may be runny, and the eye may also be red.

The pain often begins at night and may last from 30 minutes to a few hours. The headache may recur several times a day. Attacks may last 4 to 12 weeks, then disappear for months or years. Cluster headaches are 5 times more common in men than in women. Many men who get them are heavy smokers and drinkers. Avoid alcohol and tobacco products during an attack.

See your physician if you think you have cluster headaches or if you have persistent, severe headaches with no apparent cause. Also see "Headache Emergencies" on page 189.

Prevention

- Keep a diary of your headache symptoms. See "Tracking Your Headaches" on page 195. Once you know what events, foods, medications, or activities bring on your headaches, you may be able to prevent or limit their recurrence.
- Do what you can to manage stress. See Chapter 18 for tips.

Home Treatment

- At the first sign of a headache, try to go to a quiet, dark place and relax. Sleeping can relieve migraines.
- Some people find that taking a pain reliever such as aspirin, acetaminophen, or ibuprofen at the first sign of a headache brings relief. However, frequent use of pain relievers can cause rebound headaches (headaches that occur all the time unless you take pain relievers).
- Apply a cold pack to the painful area or put a cool cloth on your forehead. Do not apply heat, since it may make a migraine worse.
- Have someone gently massage your neck and shoulder muscles, or give yourself a massage.
- Practice a relaxation exercise such as progressive muscle relaxation or belly breathing. See page 328.
- If a physician has prescribed medication for your migraines, take the recommended dose at the first sign that a migraine is starting.

When to Call Kaiser Permanente

- If you suspect that your headaches are migraines.
- If headaches are becoming more frequent or more severe.
- Also see "Headache Emergencies" on page 189.

Professional diagnosis and treatment, combined with your self-care, can help decrease the impact of migraines on your life. Discuss relaxation and biofeedback techniques with your physician. They help many people prevent migraines. If nondrug treatments are not effective, there are many new prescription drugs available that can help you cope with migraines.

Tension Headaches

More than 90 percent of headaches are tension headaches, which become more frequent and severe during times of emotional or physical stress. Tightness or pain in the muscles of the neck, back, and shoulders may accompany a tension headache. A previous neck injury or arthritis in the neck can also cause tension headaches.

A tension headache may cause pain all over your head, pressure, or a feeling like having a tight band around your head. Your head may feel like it is in a vise. Some people feel a dull, pressing, burning sensation above the eyes.

The pain may also affect the jaw, face, neck, and upper back. You can rarely pinpoint the center or source of pain.

Prevention

- Reduce emotional stress. Take time to relax before and after you do something that has caused a headache in the past. Try the progressive muscle relaxation or belly breathing exercises on page 328.
- Reduce physical stress. When sitting at a desk, change positions often, and stretch for 30 seconds each hour. Make a conscious effort to relax your jaw, neck, shoulder, and upper back muscles.
- Evaluate your neck and shoulder posture at work and make adjustments if needed. See page 114.
- Exercise daily. It will help relieve tension.
- Treat yourself to a massage. Some people find regular massages very helpful in relieving tension. See page 336.
- Limit your caffeine intake to 1 to 2 cups per day. People who drink a lot of caffeinated beverages often develop a headache several hours after they have their last caffeinated beverage or may wake with a headache that is relieved by drinking caffeine. Cut down slowly to avoid caffeine-withdrawal headaches.

Home Treatment

- Stop whatever you are doing and sit quietly for a moment. Close your eyes and inhale and exhale slowly. Try to relax your head and neck muscles.

- Take a stretch break or try a relaxation exercise. See page 328.
- Gently and firmly massage your neck muscles. See page 115 for neck exercises.
- Apply heat to the painful area with a heating pad, hot water bottle, or a warm shower.
- Lie down in a dark room with a cool cloth on your forehead.
- Taking aspirin, acetaminophen, or ibuprofen often helps relieve a tension headache. However, using nonprescription or prescription headache medications too often may make headaches more frequent or severe.

When to Call Kaiser Permanente

- If a headache is severe and cannot be relieved with home treatment.
- If unexplained headaches continue to occur more than 3 times a week.
- If headaches become more frequent and severe.
- If headaches occur during or after physical exertion, sexual activity, coughing, or sneezing.
- If headaches awaken you out of a sound sleep or are worse first thing in the morning.
- If you need help discovering or eliminating the source of your tension headaches.
- Also see "Headache Emergencies" on page 189.

Tracking Your Headaches

If you have recurring headaches, keep a record of your symptoms. This record will help your physician if medical evaluation is needed. Write down:

1. The date and time each headache started and stopped.
2. Any factors that seem to trigger the headache: food, smoke, bright light, stress, activity.
3. The location and nature of the pain: throbbing, aching, stabbing, dull.
4. The severity of the pain.
5. Other physical symptoms: nausea, vomiting, visual disturbances, sensitivity to light or noise.
6. If you are a woman, note any association between headaches and your menstrual cycle or use of birth control pills or hormone replacement therapy.

I have a simple philosophy...
scratch where it itches.
Alice Roosevelt Longworth

10

Skin, Hair, and Nail Problems

Skin problems can be a nuisance, but they are rarely life-threatening. Diagnosing skin problems may require a physician's help, especially the first time you have a particular ailment. Use the chart on the next page and the index to find the skin problem you're interested in. Also see "Childhood Rashes" on page 218.

Acne

Acne is the term for pimples or blackheads that commonly form on the face, chest, upper back, or shoulders. A pimple forms when an oil gland in the skin is blocked, and secretions and bacteria build up under the skin. Acne usually starts during the teens and often persists into adulthood.

Many women get a few pimples just before their menstrual periods. Stress and some birth control pills may make acne worse. Fatty foods, such as chocolate and nuts, are not considered to be a cause of acne.

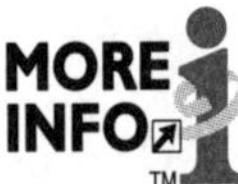

Many cases of acne will respond to home treatment, especially if they are mild. For severe or persistent cases, your physician can prescribe stronger topical medication, antibiotics, or other drugs.

Prevention

- Wash your face with a mild soap, such as Dove, or one that contains benzoyl peroxide, such as Oxy Sensitive. Wash as often as necessary to keep your face clean, but do not scrub or overdry.
- While foods are no longer considered a significant cause of acne, eat a healthful diet and avoid any food that seems to cause pimples.

Skin Problems	
Symptoms	**Possible Causes**
Raised, red, itchy welts or fluid-filled bumps after an insect bite or taking a drug	Hives, p. 209; Insect and Spider Bites and Stings, p. 59.
Red, painful, swollen bump under the skin	Boils, p. 202.
Red, flaky, itchy skin	Dry Skin, p. 206; Atopic Dermatitis, p. 200; Fungal Infections, p. 207; Rashes, p. 211.
Crusty, honey-colored rash between nose and upper lip	Impetigo, p. 235.
Rash that develops after you wear new jewelry or clothing, are exposed to poisonous plants, eat a new food, or take a new drug	Rashes, p. 211; Allergies, p. 141.
Red, itchy, blistered rash	Possible poison ivy, oak, sumac. See Rashes, p. 211; Chickenpox, p. 222.
Painful blisters in a band around one side of the body	Shingles, p. 208.
Change in shape, size, or color of a mole, or persistently irritated mole; sore that does not heal	Skin Cancer, p. 212.
Cracked, blistered, itchy, peeling skin between the toes	Fungal Infections (athlete's foot), p. 207.
Red, itchy, weeping rash on the groin or thighs	Fungal Infections (jock itch), p. 207; Impetigo, p. 235.
Scaly, itchy, bald spots or sores on scalp	Fungal Infections (ringworm), p. 207.
Flaky, silvery patches of skin, especially on knees, elbows, or scalp	Psoriasis, p. 199.
Sandpapery skin rash with sore throat, "raspberry" tongue	Scarlet fever, p. 168.
Sores on lip or in mouth	Canker Sores, p. 203; Cold Sores (fever blisters), p. 204.

Home Treatment

- Cleanliness is essential. Wash your face, shoulders, chest, and back with a very gentle soap, such as Aveeno, Neutrogena, or Basis. Avoid drying soaps, such as deodorant soaps. Always rinse well.
- Keep long hair off your face and shoulders, and wash it daily.
- Don't squeeze pimples and blackheads. This can cause infection and scarring.
- Benzoyl peroxide gel or cream, a nonprescription medication, is one of the best treatments for acne. Start with the lowest strength, and increase the strength if your skin is able to tolerate it. Apply the medication sparingly once a day, half an hour after washing. It may take several weeks to work and may cause mild redness and dryness. Never use more than 5 percent benzoyl peroxide unless a physician recommends that you do so.
- Use only water-based lotions and cosmetics that do not clog skin pores (noncomedogenic), and only if they don't aggravate acne.
- Controlling stress may help reduce acne flare-ups. See page 326.

When to Call Kaiser Permanente

- If acne gets worse despite several months of home treatment.
- If you have severe red or purple inflammation, cysts, or nodules under the skin.
- If scars develop as acne heals.

Psoriasis

Psoriasis is a chronic skin condition that causes raised red patches topped with silvery, scaling skin, usually on the knees, elbows, scalp, and back. The fingernails, palms, and soles of the feet may also be affected. Psoriasis is not contagious.

The patches, called plaques, are made up of dead skin cells that accumulate in thick layers. Normal skin cells are replaced every 30 days. In people who have psoriasis, skin cells are replaced every 3 to 4 days.

Small patches of psoriasis can often be treated with regular use of hydrocortisone cream. Tar products (lotions, gels, shampoos) may also be useful, although they may increase your skin's sensitivity to the sun. Limited exposure to the sun may also help (protect unaffected skin with sunscreen).

Stress may contribute to psoriasis. Stress reduction may help in some cases. See page 326.

Call your physician if psoriasis covers much of your body or is very red. Extensive or severe cases often need professional care.

Atopic Dermatitis

Atopic dermatitis (AD), or eczema, is a chronic skin disorder that often develops in people who have asthma, hay fever, and other allergies. It causes an itchy, red, raised rash that may weep or ooze clear fluid. The rash may develop as tiny blisters, which break and crust over. The blisters are prone to infection, especially if scratching is not controlled.

In children, AD appears most often on the face, scalp, buttocks, thighs, and torso. AD is often worse during infancy. It improves in many children by age 5 or 6.

In adults, it usually appears on the neck and in the bend of the elbows and knees. Adults whose hands or feet are often exposed to irritating substances, such as chemicals, develop AD on those areas.

Home Treatment

Helping the skin retain moisture is important to successful treatment of AD.

- Take brief, daily baths or showers with lukewarm (not hot) water. Use a gentle soap (such as Dove, Oil of Olay, or Neutrogena) or non-soap cleanser (such as Cetaphil or Aveeno). If possible, bathe without soap.
- After bathing, pat skin dry and apply a moisturizing cream (Lubriderm, Moisturel). The cream may help keep your skin from drying out. Reapply cream often.
- Use a humidifier in the bedroom.
- Taking an oral antihistamine (such as Benadryl) may help relieve itching and relax you enough to allow sleep. Avoid antiseptic and antihistamine creams and sprays, because they irritate the skin.
- Avoid contact with any irritants or allergens that cause problems. Wear gloves when working with irritating substances.
- Wash clothes and bedding in mild detergent and rinse at least twice. Do not use fabric softener if it irritates your skin.
- For more tips on relieving itching, see page 206.

When to Call Kaiser Permanente

- If crusting or weeping sores appear, because a bacterial infection may be present.
- If itching interferes with sleep, and home treatment is not working.
- If you cannot control atopic dermatitis with home treatment.

Rosacea

Rosacea causes the nose, cheeks, chin, and forehead to develop acne and become reddened and oily. Tiny blood vessels become visible on the skin's surface. The skin of the nose may become very red and bumpy if the condition is severe. Sometimes called "adult acne," rosacea most often affects young and middle-aged adults.

People who blush easily or whose facial flushing produces a redness that lasts longer than is typical may be more likely to develop rosacea. The condition tends to run in families.

Symptoms of rosacea may get worse in response to spicy foods; alcohol; exposure to sun, heat, or very cold temperatures; strenuous exercise; or certain skin care products, perfumes, or sunscreens.

If you have rosacea, try to identify and avoid things that trigger your symptoms and cause you to flush. Medications can help control pimples and redness. Laser treatment can be used to treat the blood vessels on the surface of the skin and reduce redness.

Laser skin care services are provided on a fee-for-service basis, separate from and not covered under your Health Plan benefits, and may not be available in all Kaiser Permanente service areas.

Blisters

Blisters are usually the result of persistent or repeated rubbing against the skin. Some illnesses, such as shingles, cause blister-like rashes (see page 208). Burns can also blister the skin. See page 41.

Prevention

- Avoid shoes that are too tight or that rub on your feet.
- Wear gloves to protect your hands when doing heavy chores.

Home Treatment

- If a blister is small and closed, leave it alone. Protect it from further rubbing by applying a loose bandage. Avoid the activity or shoes that caused the blister to form.
- If a small blister is in a weight-bearing area, protect it with a doughnut-shaped moleskin pad. Leave the area over the blister open.
- If a blister is larger than 1 inch across, it is usually best to drain it. The following is a safe method:
    - Sterilize a needle with rubbing alcohol.
    - Gently puncture the blister at the edge.
    - To drain the blister, press the fluid in the blister toward the hole you have made.

- Once you have opened a blister, or if it has torn open:
  - Wash the area with soap and water.
  - Do not remove the flap of skin covering a blister unless it is very dirty or torn, or if pus is forming under the skin flap. Gently smooth the skin flap flat over the tender skin underneath.
  - Apply an antibiotic ointment and a sterile bandage. Do not use alcohol or iodine. They will delay healing.
  - Change the bandage once a day to reduce the chance of infection.
  - Remove the bandage at night to let the area dry.

When to Call Kaiser Permanente

- If blisters form often and you do not know the cause.
- If signs of infection develop:
  - Increased pain, swelling, redness, or tenderness.
  - Heat or red streaks extending from the blister.
  - Discharge of pus.
  - Fever of 100° or higher with no other cause.
- If you have diabetes or peripheral vascular disease and blisters are forming on your hands, feet, or legs.

Calluses and Corns

Calluses are hard, thickened skin on parts of the foot that are exposed to friction. Corns are caused by pressure on the skin from the inside, such as from a bone.

Soak your feet in warm water, and rub the callus or corn with a pumice stone. You may need to do this for several days until the thickened skin is gone.

Do not try to cut or burn off corns or calluses. If you have diabetes or peripheral vascular disease, talk with your physician before attempting to remove troublesome corns or calluses.

Boils

A boil is a red, swollen, painful bump under the skin, similar to an overgrown pimple. Boils are often caused by infected hair follicles. Bacteria from the infection form an abscess or pocket of pus. The abscess can become larger than a ping-pong ball and may be extremely painful.

Boils occur most often in areas where there is hair and chafing. The face, neck, armpits, breasts, groin, and buttocks are common sites.

Prevention

- Wash boil-prone areas with soapy water. An antibacterial soap may help. Dry thoroughly.
- Avoid clothing that is too tight.

Home Treatment

- Do not squeeze, scratch, drain, or lance the boil. Squeezing can push the infection deeper into the skin. Scratching can spread the bacteria to other parts of the body.
- Wash yourself well with an antibacterial soap to keep the infection from spreading.
- Apply hot, wet washcloths to the boil for 20 to 30 minutes, 3 to 4 times a day. Do this as soon as you notice a boil. The heat and moisture can help bring the boil to a head, but it may take 5 to 7 days. Applying a hot water bottle or a waterproof heating pad over a damp towel may also help.
- Continue using warm compresses for 3 days after the boil opens. Apply a bandage to keep draining material from spreading, and change the bandage daily.

When to Call Kaiser Permanente

If needed, your health care professional can drain the boil and treat the infection. Call Kaiser Permanente:

- If the boil is on your face, near your spine, or in the anal area.
- If signs of worsening infection develop:
    - Increased pain, swelling, heat, redness, or tenderness.
    - Red streaks extending from the boil.
    - Continued discharge of pus.
    - Fever of 100° or higher with no other cause.
- If any other lumps, particularly painful ones, develop near the infected area.
- If the pain limits your normal activities.
- If you have diabetes.
- If the boil is as large as a ping-pong ball.
- If the boil has not improved after 5 to 7 days of home treatment.
- If many boils develop over several months.

Canker Sores

Canker sores are painful, open sores that form on the inside of the mouth. Possible causes of canker sores include injury to the inside of the mouth, infection, certain foods, stress, genetic tendency to get canker sores, and female hormones. The sores usually heal in 7 to 10 days.

Prevention

- Avoid injuring the inside of your mouth:
    - Chew food slowly and carefully.
    - Use a soft-bristle toothbrush, and brush your teeth thoroughly but gently.
- Avoid foods that seem to cause sores.

Home Treatment

- Avoid coffee, spicy and salty foods, and citrus fruits when you have open sores in your mouth.
- Apply a nonprescription canker sore medication to protect the sore, ease pain, and speed healing.
- Rinse your mouth with a mixture of 1 tablespoon of hydrogen peroxide in 8 ounces of water.
- Applying a thin paste of baking soda and water to the sore may relieve pain.

When to Call Kaiser Permanente

- If mouth sores develop after you start taking a medication.
- If a canker sore, or any sore, does not heal in 14 days.
- If a sore is very painful or recurs frequently.
- If white spots that are not canker sores appear in the mouth and are not improving after 1 to 2 weeks.

Cold Sores

Cold sores (fever blisters) are small, red blisters that usually appear on the lip and outer edge of the mouth. They often weep a clear fluid and scab over after a few days. They are sometimes confused with impetigo (see page 235), which usually develops between the nose and upper lip. The fluid that weeps from impetigo is cloudy and honey-colored, not clear.

Cold sores are caused by a herpes virus. Herpes viruses (chickenpox is another kind) stay in the body after the first infection. Later, something triggers the virus to become active again. Cold sores may appear after colds, fevers, exposure to the sun, stressful times, or during menstruation. Sometimes they develop for no apparent reason.

Prevention

- Avoid kissing a person who has a cold sore. Also avoid direct skin contact with genital herpes sores (see page 283) and herpes sores elsewhere on the body.
- Use sunscreen on your lips and wear a hat if exposure to the sun seems to trigger cold sores.
- Reducing stress may help in some cases. Practice relaxation exercises often. See page 328.

Home Treatment

- At the first sign of a cold sore (tingling or prickling at the site where the sore will appear), apply ice to the area. This may help reduce the severity of the sore.
- Apply petroleum jelly to ease cracking and dryness.
- Apply a paste made of cornstarch and a little water to the sore.
- Products such as Blistex or Campho-Phenique may ease the pain. If you apply these products by touching the container to your lips, don't let anyone else use the container.

- Be patient. Cold sores usually go away in 7 to 10 days.

When to Call Kaiser Permanente

Call if sores last longer than 2 weeks or you have frequent outbreaks of cold sores. A prescription medication may reduce the frequency and severity of outbreaks.

Dandruff

Dandruff occurs when the skin cells of the scalp flake off. This flaking is natural and occurs all over your body. On the scalp, however, flakes can mix with oil and dust to form dandruff. Dandruff cannot be cured, but it can be controlled.

Home Treatment

- Try frequent and energetic shampooing with any shampoo. Wash hair daily if it controls dandruff.
- If dandruff is excessive and itchy, try a dandruff shampoo (such as Head & Shoulders, Sebulex, T-Gel, or Tegrin). Work the dandruff shampoo into your scalp and leave it on for several minutes before rinsing.

When to Call Kaiser Permanente

Call if frequent shampooing or shampooing with a dandruff shampoo doesn't control dandruff.

Birthmarks

Birthmarks are relatively common. Those that are pigmented generally do not go away. Those due to blood vessels usually fade as the child grows.

Salmon patches ("angel kisses") are light pink birthmarks that may appear on the upper lip, eyelids, forehead, and back of the neck. They usually fade within a few months.

Strawberry birthmarks are soft, red lumps formed by clusters of blood vessels. They may be present at birth or appear during the first few months. They may grow for up to 6 months, stabilize for a short time, and then usually begin to recede and fade. Sixty percent are gone by age 5; nearly all disappear by age 9. No treatment is necessary unless they continue to grow.

Port-wine stains are light pink or wine-colored birthmarks that appear most often on the head and face. They are permanent, become darker as the child grows, and may need to be treated by a dermatologist to stop them from expanding.

Report any changes in birthmarks to your health professional. Birthmarks need to be removed if they interfere with breathing or vision, or if they disfigure the face. If surgery is desired for cosmetic reasons, it is best to talk with your health professional about the best timing for surgery.

Dry Skin

Dry, itchy, flaky skin is the most common skin problem, especially in the winter. It develops when the skin loses water (not oil) to the air. Dry indoor air is a common cause, as is excessive bathing in hot water.

Prevention

- Avoid showers. They strip the skin's natural oil, which helps hold in moisture. Baths are much kinder to the skin than showers are.
- Use bath oils in the tub.
- Use mild soaps (such as Dove or Cetaphil), especially under the arms and in the genital area.
- Use a moisturizing lotion after your bath.

Home Treatment

- Follow the prevention guidelines above.
- For very dry hands, try this for a night: Apply a thin layer of petroleum jelly and wear thin cotton gloves to bed. (Dry feet may benefit from similar treatment.)
- Avoid scratching, which damages the skin. If itching is a problem, see "Relief From Itching" on page 206.

When to Call Kaiser Permanente

- If you itch all over your body but there is no obvious cause or rash.
- If itching is so bad that you cannot sleep, and home treatment is not helping.
- If your skin is badly broken due to scratching.

Relief From Itching

- Keep the itchy area well lubricated. Be careful not to dry out the skin, because doing so will increase the itching.
- An oatmeal bath may help relieve itching: Wrap 1 cup of oatmeal in a cotton cloth and boil as you would to cook it. Use this as a sponge and bathe in tepid water without soap. Or try an Aveeno colloidal oatmeal bath.
- Calamine lotion is helpful for poison ivy or poison oak rashes.
- Try a nonprescription 1 percent hydrocortisone cream for small itchy areas. Use very sparingly on the face or genitals. If itching is severe, your physician may prescribe a stronger cream.
- Try a nonprescription oral antihistamine (Chlor-Trimeton, Benadryl).
- Cut nails short or wear gloves at night to prevent scratching.
- Wear cotton clothing. Avoid wool and acrylic fabrics next to the skin.

Fungal Infections

Fungal infections of the skin most commonly affect the feet, groin, scalp, or nails. Fungi grow best in warm, moist areas of the skin, such as between the toes, in the groin, and in the area beneath the breasts.

Athlete's foot is the most common fungal skin infection. Symptoms include cracked, blistered, and peeling areas between the toes; redness and scaling on the soles of the feet; and itching. Athlete's foot often recurs and must be treated each time.

Jock itch causes severe itching and moistness on the skin of the groin and upper thighs. There may be red, scaly, raised areas on the skin that weep or ooze pus or clear fluid.

Ringworm is a fungal infection that grows on the outer layer of skin, hair, or nails. It is more common in children than in adults.

On the skin, ringworm appears as patches that are clear in the center and have edges that are red, peeling, or have blister-like bumps. The skin is often very itchy. The rash can spread quickly.

On the scalp and beard, ringworm appears as round or oval patches of baldness, which may be scaly, red, crusty, or swollen with little blister-like bumps. The hair on the scalp and beard may have flakes that look like dandruff.

Fungal infections of the **fingernails** and **toenails** cause discoloration, thickening, and often softening of the nails. They are difficult to treat and often cause permanent damage to the nails.

Thrush is a yeast infection that occurs in the mouth, especially in babies. It causes a white coating inside the mouth, often on the cheeks, that may look like milk but is hard to remove. (Yeast infections also develop in the vagina. See page 268.)

Prevention

- Keep your feet clean, cool, and dry. Dry well between the toes after swimming or bathing.
- Wear leather shoes or sandals that allow your feet to "breathe," and wear cotton socks to absorb sweat. Use powder on your feet and in your shoes. Give shoes 24 hours to dry between wearings.
- Wear thongs or shower sandals in public pools and showers.
- Keep your groin area clean and dry. Wash and dry well, especially after exercising, and apply talcum powder to absorb moisture. Wear cotton underclothes and avoid tight pants and panty hose.
- Teach children not to play with dogs or cats that have bald or mangy spots on their coats.
- Don't share hats, combs, or brushes.

Home Treatment

- Follow the prevention guidelines.
- For athlete's foot and jock itch, use a nonprescription antifungal powder or lotion, such as Micatin or Lotrimin AF. Use the medication for 1 to 2 weeks after the symptoms clear up to prevent recurrence. Do not use hydrocortisone cream on a fungal infection.
- Ringworm on the body can be treated with one of the antifungals listed above.

When to Call Kaiser Permanente

- If signs of infection are present:
  - Increased pain, swelling, heat, redness, or tenderness.
  - Red streaks extending from the affected area.
  - Continued discharge of pus.
  - Fever of 100° or higher with no other cause.
- If you have diabetes and develop athlete's foot. People with diabetes are at increased risk for infection and may need professional care.
- If you experience a sudden loss of patches of hair associated with flaking, broken hairs, and inflammation of the scalp; or if several members of your household are experiencing hair loss.
- If ringworm is severe and spreading or is present on the scalp. Prescription medicine may be needed.

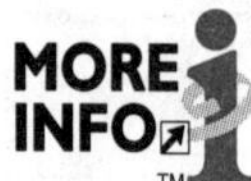
If home treatment fails to improve a fungal infection after 2 weeks or clear it up after 1 month, you may want to consider prescription medication. Discuss your options with your physician.

Shingles

Shingles (herpes zoster) is caused by the reactivation of the chickenpox virus in the body years after the initial illness. The virus usually affects one of the large nerves that spreads outward from the spine, causing pain and a rash in a band around one side of the chest, abdomen, or face. The rash will blister and scab, then clear up over the course of a few weeks.

No one knows what makes the virus active again. Shingles can affect anyone who has had chickenpox. However, older adults and people with weakened immune systems are more likely to get shingles. People with weakened immune systems include those who have had a bone marrow or an organ transplant; have cancer, especially of the lymph system; or are infected with HIV.

Exposure to the shingles rash can cause chickenpox in a person who has not had chickenpox before.

If you suspect shingles, call your physician or advice nurse to discuss medication that can limit the pain and rash. If possible, call within 1 day after the rash starts.

Hives

Hives are raised, red, itchy, often fluid-filled patches of skin (wheals or welts) that may appear and disappear at random. They range in size from less than ¼ inch to 1 inch or more, and they may last a few minutes or a few days.

A single hive commonly develops after an insect sting. Multiple hives often develop in response to a drug, food, or infection. Other possible causes of hives include plant allergies, inhaled allergens, stress, cosmetics, and exposure to heat, cold, sunlight, or pressure of clothing. Often a cause cannot be found.

Home Treatment

- Avoid the substance that causes hives.
- Apply cool water compresses to help relieve itching. Also see page 206.
- Take an oral antihistamine (such as Benadryl or Chlor-Trimeton) to treat the hives and relieve itching. Once the hives have disappeared, decrease the dose of the medication slowly over 5 to 7 days.

When to Call Kaiser Permanente

- **Call 911 or seek other emergency services immediately** if spreading hives occur with dizziness, wheezing, difficulty breathing, tightness in the chest, or swelling of the tongue, lips, or face.
- If hives develop soon after you take a new drug.
- If hives persist for several days despite home treatment.

Ingrown Toenails

Ingrown toenails usually develop when an improperly trimmed toenail cuts into the skin at the edge of the nail or when you wear shoes that are too tight. Because the cut can easily become infected, prompt care is needed.

Prevention

- Cut toenails straight across and leave the nails a little longer at the corners so that the sharp ends don't cut into the skin.
- Wear roomy shoes, and keep your feet clean and dry.

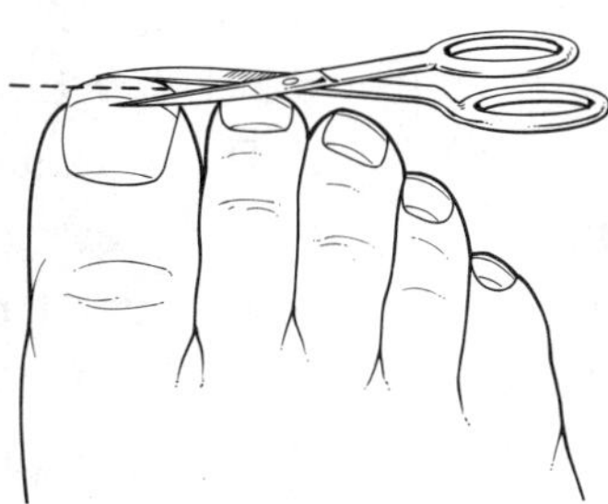

Cut toenails straight across.

Home Treatment

- Soak your foot in warm water.
- Wedge a small piece of wet cotton under the corner of the nail to cushion the nail and lift it slightly to keep it from cutting the skin. Repeat daily until the nail has grown out and can be trimmed.

- Soaking the feet in warm water for 15 minutes, 3 to 4 times a day, will help relieve swelling or tenderness while toenails grow out.

When to Call Kaiser Permanente

- If signs of infection develop:
  - Increased pain, swelling, redness, or tenderness.
  - Heat or red streaks extending from the area.
  - Discharge of pus.
  - Fever of 100° or higher with no other cause.
- If you have diabetes or circulatory problems.

Lice and Scabies

Lice are tiny, white, wingless insects that may live on the skin, hair, or clothing. They feed by biting the skin and sucking blood. The bites itch and may cause an allergic rash. Head lice live in the hair on the head; body lice live on clothing; and pubic lice (also called crabs) live in the groin, underarms, and eyelashes.

Lice are spread by close physical contact or contact with the clothing, bedding, brushes, or combs of an infected person. Pubic lice can be spread through sexual contact.

Scabies are tiny mites that burrow under the skin and lay eggs. This burrowing causes a rash that itches intensely. Scabies are often found between folds of skin on the fingers and toes, wrists, underarms, and groin. The scabies mites are spread through close contact with an infected person, such as sleeping in the same bed. Scabies are usually treated with a medication that is applied over the entire body and left on overnight. Itching may last for several weeks after treatment.

Prevention

Be alert for signs of lice: itching and lice or tiny eggs (nits) attached to the hair shafts of the head. Prompt treatment can help prevent spreading lice to others.

People who have lice or scabies should avoid close contact with others to prevent spreading the insects or mites that cause these conditions.

Home Treatment

- Nix and RID are nonprescription medications for lice. Follow the manufacturer's directions for use exactly. For head lice, comb the hair well with a fine-toothed comb after treatment to remove all nits.
- On the day you start treatment, wash all dirty clothing, bedding, and towels in hot water to help get rid of lice, nits, and mites. Iron things that cannot be washed.
- Some schools have a "no nits" policy stating that children may not return to school until they are free of lice nits. Children who have been treated for scabies can return to school after treatment is completed.

- Contact your pharmacist or health department for more information about treatment and preventing reinfestation.

When to Call Kaiser Permanente

Call if treatment with nonprescription medication is not successful. Stronger prescription drugs are available.

Rashes

A rash (dermatitis) is any irritation or inflammation of the skin. Rashes can be caused by illness, allergy, or heat, and sometimes by emotional stress. For rashes related to childhood illnesses, see page 218. If the rash developed after you were bitten by a tick, see page 71.

Poison ivy and other plant rashes are often red, blistered, and itchy and appear in lines where the leaves brushed against the skin.

When you first get a rash, ask yourself these questions to help determine the cause (also see pages 198 and 218):

- Did a rash that is contained to a specific area (localized) develop after you came in contact with anything new that could have irritated your skin: poison ivy, oak, or sumac; soaps, detergents, shampoos, perfumes, cosmetics, or lotions; jewelry or fabrics; new tools, appliances, latex gloves, or other objects? The location of the rash is often a clue to the cause.

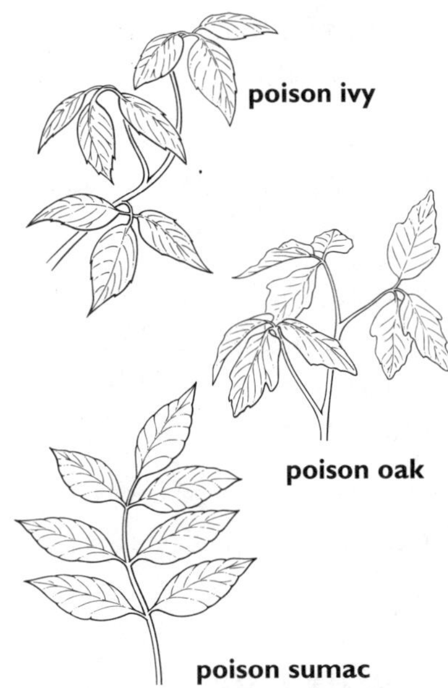

The oil on the leaves of these plants can cause an uncomfortable, itchy, red skin rash with blisters or hives.

- Have you eaten anything new that you may be allergic to?
- Are you taking any new medications, either prescription or nonprescription?
- Have you been unusually stressed or upset recently?
- Is there joint pain or fever with the rash?
- Is the rash spreading?
- Does the rash itch?

Prevention

- If you are exposed to poison ivy, oak, or sumac, wash your skin with dish soap and water within 30 minutes to get the allergy-causing oil off your skin. This may help prevent or reduce the rash. Also wash your clothes, your dog, and anything else that may have come in contact with the plant.

- Avoid products that cause the rash: detergents, cosmetics, lotions, clothing, jewelry, etc.
- Use fragrance- and preservative-free or hypoallergenic detergents, lotions, and cosmetics if you have frequent rashes.
- Rashes on the feet or groin may be due to fungal infections. See page 207.

Home Treatment

- Wash affected areas with water. Soap can be irritating. Pat dry thoroughly.
- Apply cold, wet compresses to reduce itching. Repeat frequently. Also see page 206.
- Leave the rash exposed to the air. Baby powder can help keep it dry. Avoid lotions and ointments until the rash heals. However, calamine lotion is helpful for plant rashes. Use it 3 to 4 times a day.
- Use hydrocortisone cream to provide temporary relief of itching. Use very sparingly on the face and the genital area.

When to Call Kaiser Permanente

- If signs of infection develop:
  - Increased pain, swelling, redness, or tenderness.
  - Heat or red streaks extending from the area.
  - Discharge of pus or honey-colored crust.
  - Fever of 100° or higher with no other cause.
- If you suspect a medication reaction caused the rash.
- If a rash occurs with fever and joint pain.
- If a rash occurs with a sore throat. See scarlet fever on page 168.
- If a rash appears and you aren't sure what is causing it.
- If a rash continues after 2 to 3 weeks of home treatment.

Skin Cancer

Skin cancer is the most common type of cancer. Fortunately, many types of skin cancer are easy to cure.

Most skin cancer is caused by sun damage. Ninety percent of skin cancers occur on the face, neck, and arms, where sun exposure is greatest. Light-skinned, blue-eyed people are more likely to develop skin cancer. Dark-skinned people have less risk.

Most skin cancers are slow-growing, easy to recognize, and easy to treat in a physician's office. A small percentage of skin cancers are more serious.

Skin cancers differ from noncancerous growths in the following ways:

- They tend to bleed more than noncancerous growths do and are often open sores that do not heal.
- They tend to be slow-growing.

Most moles are harmless. However, malignant melanomas (one type of cancerous mole) can be fatal and should be promptly treated.

Prevention

Most skin cancers can be prevented by avoiding excessive exposure to the sun. Most damaging sun exposure has occurred by age 20, so keep your children protected (see page 214). Repeated sun exposure and severe sunburns are major factors in some types of skin cancer.

Home Treatment

Examine your skin with a mirror or another person's help. Look for unusual moles, spots, bumps, or sores that won't heal. Pay special attention to areas that get a lot of sun exposure: hands, arms, chest, neck (especially the back of the neck), face, ears, etc. Report any changes to your physician.

When to Call Kaiser Permanente

Call Kaiser Permanente if you notice any unusual skin changes or growths, especially if they bleed and continue to change.

If your moles do not change over time, there is little cause for concern. If you have a family history of malignant melanoma, let your physician know because you may be at higher risk for malignant melanoma. Call your physician if you notice any of the following "ABCD" changes in a mole:

- **A**symmetrical shape: One half does not match the other half.
- **B**order irregularity: The edges are ragged, notched, or blurred.
- **C**olor not uniform: Watch for shades of red and black, or a red, white, and blue mottled appearance.
- **D**iameter: The mole is larger than a pencil eraser. (Harmless moles are usually smaller than this.)

Asymmetrical shape

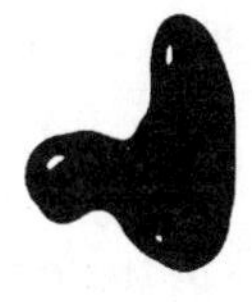

Border irregular

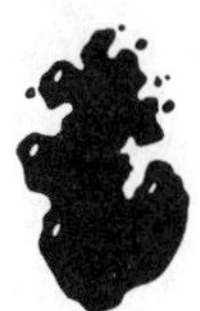

Color varied

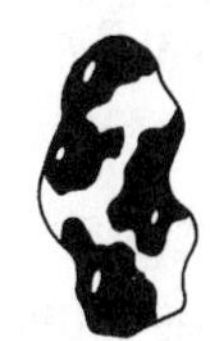

Diameter larger than a pencil eraser

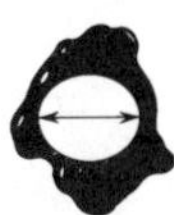

Watch for these "ABCD" mole changes.

- Scaliness, oozing, bleeding, or spreading of pigment into surrounding skin.
- Appearance of a bump or nodule on the mole, or any change in the appearance of the mole.
- Itching, tenderness, or pain.

Sunburn

A sunburn is usually a first-degree burn that involves the outer surface of the skin. Sunburns are uncomfortable but usually are not dangerous unless they are extensive. Severe sunburns can be serious in infants and small children.

Repeated sun exposure and sunburns increase the risk of skin cancer.

Prevention

If you are going to be in the sun for more than 15 minutes, take the following precautions:

- Use a sunscreen that has a sun protection factor (SPF) of 15 or higher. Sunscreens labeled "broad spectrum" can protect the skin from the 2 types of harmful (ultraviolet) rays.
- Apply the sunscreen at least 30 minutes before going in the sun.
- Apply sunscreen to all the skin that will be exposed to the sun, including the nose, ears, neck, scalp, and lips. It needs to be applied evenly over the skin.
- Reapply sunscreen every 2 to 3 hours while in the sun and after swimming or sweating a lot.
- Older adults have sensitive skin and should always use a sunscreen with an SPF of 20 or higher.
- Wear light-colored, loose-fitting, long-sleeved clothes and a broad-brimmed hat to shade your face.
- Drink lots of water. Sweating helps cool the skin.
- Avoid the sun between 10 a.m. and 3 p.m., when the burning rays are strongest.
- Don't forget the kids. Sun exposure may be very hard on their tender skin. Teach your young children safe sun habits—hats and sunscreen—early.

Home Treatment

- Drink plenty of water and watch for signs of dehydration (especially in infants or children). See page 80. Also watch for signs of heat exhaustion. See page 55.
- Cool baths or compresses can be very soothing. Take acetaminophen or aspirin for pain. Don't give aspirin to anyone younger than 20.
- A mild fever and headache can accompany a sunburn. Lie down in a cool, quiet room to relieve headache.
- There is nothing you can do to prevent peeling; it is part of the healing process. Lotion can help relieve itching.

When to Call Kaiser Permanente

- If you develop signs of heat stroke (red, hot, dry skin; confusion). See page 55.
- If symptoms of heat exhaustion (dizziness, nausea, headache) persist after you have cooled off.
- If there is severe blistering (over ½ of the affected body part) with fever or if you feel very ill.
- If you have a fever of 102° or higher.

Warts

Warts are skin growths that are caused by a virus. They can appear anywhere on the body. Warts are not dangerous, but they can be bothersome.

Little is known about warts. Most types are only slightly contagious. They can spread to other areas on the same person but rarely to other people. Genital and anal warts are an exception; they are easily transmitted through sexual contact and may increase a woman's risk for cervical cancer. See page 284.

Plantar warts appear on the soles of the feet. Most of the wart lies under the skin surface and may make you feel like you are walking on a pebble.

Because warts seem to come and go for little reason, it's possible that they are sensitive to slight changes in the immune system. Although there is no scientific explanation for why it works, in some cases you can "think" warts away.

When necessary, your physician can remove warts. Unfortunately, they often come back.

Home Treatment

- Warts appear and disappear spontaneously. They can last a week, a month, or even years. To get rid of your warts, it helps to believe in the treatment. If something works for you, stick with it.
- Try the least expensive method of treating warts first. You may save a trip to your physician.
- If the wart bleeds a little, cover it with a bandage and apply light pressure to stop the bleeding.
- If the wart is in the way, rub it with a pumice stone or a file or apply a nonprescription product containing salicylic acid. (If you have diabetes or peripheral vascular disease, do not irritate the wart or use salicylic acid on it without first discussing these treatments with a health professional.)
- If treatment with salicylic acid causes the area to become tender, taking a 2- to 3-day break from treatment may help relieve pain.
- If you use a pumice stone or file, both the debris from the wart and the area of the pumice stone or file that touched the wart can be infectious. Don't use these items for any other purpose or you may spread

the wart-causing virus. Wash your hands with soap after you touch the debris from the wart or the pumice stone or file.

- For plantar warts, apply a doughnut-shaped pad to cushion the wart and relieve pain. Before you go to bed, apply salicylic acid to the wart, and cover the wart with a bandage (or wear a sock). Wash the medication off in the morning.
- Don't cut or burn off a wart.

When to Call Kaiser Permanente

- If a wart looks infected after being irritated or knocked off.
- If a plantar wart is painful when you walk, and foam pads do not help.
- If you have warts in the anal or genital area. See page 284.
- If a wart develops on your face and is a cosmetic concern.

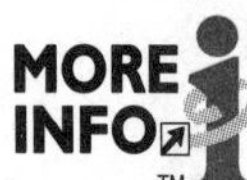

If a wart causes continual discomfort, or if warts are numerous enough to be a problem, they may need to be surgically removed. Talk with your physician about the risks and benefits of surgery to remove warts.

Hair Loss

Many people lose hair as they grow older. Such hair loss is natural and is largely the result of heredity. Balding poses no health risks other than sunburn, which you can prevent by wearing a hat and using sunscreen when outdoors. While men tend to lose hair from the hairline and crown of the head, women's hair becomes thinner all over.

If you are thinking about drug (such as minoxidil) or surgical treatment for hair loss, make sure you understand the risks of treatment, how many treatments you will need, and how long the results will last.

Bald spots are not the same as baldness. Wearing tight braids or habitually tugging or twisting your hair may cause bald spots. Ringworm is a fungal infection that causes scaly bald spots. See page 207. A condition called alopecia areata causes patchy hair loss that may require treatment with steroid medications.

Thinning hair can signal problems such as thyroid disease or lupus. Emotional or physical stress can cause short-term hair loss, as can changes in hormone levels during pregnancy and menopause.

If hair loss is sudden, or if it develops after you start taking a new medication, call your physician.

My mother had a great deal of trouble with me,
but I think she enjoyed it.
Mark Twain

11

Infant and Child Health

When your children get sick or hurt, you are usually the first person to provide care. Your calmness, confidence, and competence in caring for your children's health problems will help them enjoy good health and learn the importance of self-care for their own use as they mature.

Virtually every health problem in this book can affect children. However, a few are almost exclusively childhood concerns. For convenience, we have grouped these problems into this chapter. If the problem you are looking for is not in this chapter, please look for it in the index.

Facts About Infants and Young Children

The following brief notes are of particular concern to parents. This information may help dispel some unnecessary fears and give you some guidance.

Umbilical Cords and Bellybuttons

Clean the bellybutton (navel) 3 to 4 times a day with a bit of cotton moistened with a little rubbing alcohol. Pull the cord up gently but firmly to clean the base (try not to get alcohol on the skin around the navel).

Keep the cord dry and do not give your baby a tub or pan bath until the cord has fallen off and the navel is healed. Fold diapers below and shirts above the cord to promote drying.

The cord will drop off and the navel will heal in 1 to 3 weeks. After the cord comes off, there may be a moist or bloody oozing for a few days. This does not need special treatment.

Call your physician if there is redness or swelling around the navel or a large amount of foul-smelling discharge from the navel.

The appearance of the bellybutton is not affected by the way the cord is tied off. A small lump of tissue sometimes remains after the cord falls off. If it is small, treatment is usually not needed. If it is larger and does not fall off after 2 weeks, call your physician.

Childhood Rashes

Rashes that come with childhood illnesses are hard to tell apart. Review all symptoms before deciding what to do.

Description	Possible Illness
Red, pimple-like spots that turn to blisters; fever	Chickenpox, p. 222.
Rash in diaper area only	Diaper Rash, p. 227.
Red rash on face that looks like slapped cheeks; pink rash that comes and goes on torso; possible fever	Fifth Disease, p. 238.
Red or pink dots on head, neck, shoulders; more common in infants	Prickly Heat, p. 237.
Sudden high fever for 2 to 3 days followed by rose-pink rash on torso, arms, and neck after fever goes down	Roseola, p. 238.
Fine pink rash; starts on face and covers whole body; swollen glands behind ears	Rubella (rare), p. 17.
Fever, runny nose, hacking cough; red eyes 2 to 3 days before spotty red rash covers whole body	Rubeola (measles) (rare), p. 17.
High fever, sore throat, sandpapery rash, and raspberry-textured tongue	Scarlet fever, p. 168.
Blisters on mouth and tongue appearing 1 to 2 days after onset of fever and sore mouth or throat. Painless, blistering rash on fingers, hands, feet.	Hand-Foot-Mouth Disease, p. 234.

Breastfeeding

Breast milk is the ideal food for babies younger than about 6 months. The American Academy of Pediatrics recommends that babies be breastfed for at least the first year of life. However, the length of time that breastfeeding should continue differs for each mother and her child.

Breast milk contains substances that help your baby resist infections and other diseases. Breastfed babies have fewer colds and ear infections, less diarrhea, and less vomiting. Breast milk is easier to digest than formula and, unlike formula, it doesn't cost anything.

Getting some instruction helps ensure that you can breastfeed successfully. If possible, take a breastfeeding class. The La Leche League and the Nursing Mother's Council are other good sources of breastfeeding information, advice, and support.

Nursing mothers need 500 calories more per day than they needed before becoming pregnant. Although you don't need to drink milk to make milk, extra calcium and protein are important, and your physician may recommend a vitamin supplement. Since drugs pass through the breast milk to your baby, avoid drugs, alcohol, and smoking. Limit caffeine to 1 or 2 beverages a day. Do not take any medication while breastfeeding unless it was prescribed by your physician or other health care professional.

Circumcision

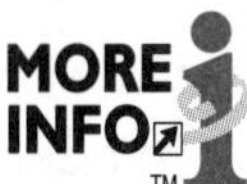

Circumcision is surgery to remove the foreskin of a newborn boy's penis. There are both benefits and risks associated with circumcision. Discuss the risks and benefits with your physician. The decision is entirely up to you.

One major benefit is that circumcision makes it easier to keep the penis clean, which may reduce your baby's risk for urinary tract infections.

The risks of circumcision are slight. Complications of local infection or bleeding occur in about 1 in every 500 cases. Local anesthetic reduces the pain of circumcision. Generally, circumcision is not recommended for sick infants.

If you do have your son circumcised, after the procedure apply petroleum jelly liberally to the head of the penis at each diaper change to prevent the scab from sticking to the diaper. Wash the penis by dripping warm water over it (do not use alcohol or baby wipes). Pat dry with a soft towel. Some redness at the circumcision site is normal. Call your physician if the redness extends down the shaft of the penis.

If you choose not to have your son circumcised, clean the exposed foreskin gently during the first 4 years. Starting around age 4, gently begin to pull back (retract) the foreskin. Do not forcibly retract the foreskin; it may not be fully retractable until puberty. Teach your son to wash his penis well at every bath and to gently retract the foreskin when possible and clean beneath it at least once a week.

Toilet Training

Every child has a unique timetable for becoming toilet-trained. Most children are ready to begin toilet training between 24 and 30 months of age. Look for these signs of readiness in your child:

- Passes stools at about the same time each day.
- Is able to have a dry diaper for at least 2 hours at a time during the day and wakes up dry after a nap.
- Makes certain facial expressions when urinating or passing stools.
- Lets you know when a diaper is dirty and asks to have it changed.
- Seems eager to please and can follow simple instructions.
- Tells you that he or she wants to use the toilet or wear adult underwear.

If you think your child is ready to begin toilet training, the following tips may make it go more smoothly:

- Get your child a potty chair. Let the child get used to using the chair by having him or her sit on it with a diaper on when he or she is passing stools or urinating.
- Let your child watch you or a sibling of the same sex use the toilet. Talk with your child about what you are doing.
- Select clothing for your child that is easy to take off. Clothes with elastic waistbands or easy-to-open fasteners, such as Velcro, work best. Pull-on diapers are also helpful.
- Reward every success with hugs and words of praise. Accidental wetting and soiling are common in the first few weeks, but don't scold or punish your child when they happen. Keep a casual attitude.

Bladder control may take longer than bowel control. If the child is aware of when his or her bladder is full, try putting the child on the potty chair every 30 to 60 minutes. Praise the child for success and give gentle encouragement when the child wets his or her pants.

Sleep Habits

Babies have both deep and light sleep cycles. In each sleep cycle, there are 60 minutes of light sleep, 60 to 90 minutes of deep sleep, and another 30 minutes of light sleep. At the end of this cycle, the baby is semi-alert and can be wakened easily.

Parents can help their baby sleep through the night by helping the baby learn to soothe him- or herself back to sleep during the light sleep cycles.

For babies age 4 to 6 months:

- Put the baby in the crib when he or she is drowsy but awake.
- Make middle-of-the-night feedings short and boring.

- As the baby gets older, delay the middle-of-the-night feeding, and discontinue it sometime after age 6 months.

It is safer for a baby to sleep on his or her back to prevent sudden infant death syndrome (SIDS). Do not force a baby into a sleeping position. Babies are capable of moving themselves.

If You Decide to Bottlefeed

Breastfeeding is the best for your baby, so we encourage you to consider it. Breast milk is your baby's ideal source of nutrition and helps protect your baby from infection. Breastfeeding has benefits for mothers as well. See page 219 for more information about breastfeeding.

However, if you decide you want to exclusively bottlefeed or supplement breastfeeding with some bottlefeeding, you can still use feeding time to bond with your baby. Make this your special time to feel close to your baby by talking, singing, holding, and making eye contact. Remember that it is not safe to prop bottles, so make sure that no one props your baby's bottle.

Choose from 3 types of formula:

- Ready-to-feed: This is the most convenient option because the formula is already prepared for you. This choice is also the most expensive.
- Liquid concentrate: For this option, all you do is add water to the concentrate.
- Powdered: This option is the most economical, but it also requires the most preparation time.

Your baby's health care provider can recommend a specific brand of formula and tell you whether to sterilize or simply wash the bottles and nipples. Many women find that a dishwasher thoroughly cleans both, if they are first scrubbed with a brush.

Always check the expiration date and preparation instructions before you make your baby's formula. Follow the directions exactly.

Bed-Wetting

Bed-wetting (enuresis) in children who have never been dry is common, and most children will outgrow it between the ages of 6 and 10. In almost all cases, bed-wetting is really not a disease, but rather a normal variation in development.

In some cases, a child who has been dry for several months or longer may start to wet the bed again. This can happen without a clear cause, or it may be caused by a urinary tract infection or emotional problems.

Home Treatment

There are a number of ways to deal with bed-wetting. Ask your physician for advice in managing bed-wetting until your child outgrows it.

- Do not punish, embarrass, or blame your child.
- Have your child empty his or her bladder before bed.
- Remind the child to get up during the night to urinate. Providing a bedside potty chair and night light may help.
- Do not force your child to wear diapers at night. Try waterproof, extra-absorbent underwear instead. A thick pad or a vinyl mattress cover will protect the mattress.
- Encourage the child to take responsibility for changing his or her clothes after wetting, for putting a dry towel down on the bed, and for helping wash bed linens.
- Wash underwear and bedding with ½ cup vinegar to eliminate odor.

When to Call Kaiser Permanente

Your physician can rule out or treat any physical causes of bed-wetting and help you and your child manage the problem. Call Kaiser Permanente:

- If bed-wetting occurs with pain or burning during urination or other signs of a urinary tract infection. See page 100.
- If bed-wetting occurs in a child older than 6 years, and home treatment is not successful after 4 to 5 weeks.
- If bed-wetting becomes more frequent or severe despite home treatment.
- If bed-wetting occurs in a child who had previously been dry for several months.
- If a child age 4 or older is having accidental wettings and stool leakage.
- If a child over age 3 has daytime bladder control problems after having been toilet-trained.

Chickenpox

Chickenpox (varicella) is usually a relatively minor illness. For the first couple of days, your child will feel ill, with cold-like symptoms, cough, fever, and abdominal pain. Then a rash of red, pimple-like spots will appear. A child may have as few as 30 spots, or the rash may cover the child's entire body, including the throat, mouth, ears, groin, and scalp.

The spots turn into clear blisters that become cloudy, break open, and crust over. The rash itches a lot. Spots continue to appear for 1 to 5 days and subside over 1 to 2 weeks.

Chickenpox is very contagious. After exposure to the chickenpox virus, symptoms appear in 11 to 20 days. The contagious period starts 1 to 2 days before the rash appears and lasts until all the spots have crusted over. Children can usually return to school or day care after the sixth day of the rash as long as all blisters have crusted over. Encephalitis (see page 160) is a rare complication of chickenpox.

Prevention

The chickenpox vaccine can be given to children age 12 months and older and to teens and adults who have not had the illness. See page 17. It is especially important to immunize teens and adults who have not had chickenpox, because the disease is more severe in adulthood.

Adults who have not been vaccinated and who have not had chickenpox should avoid exposure to children who have it and avoid exposure to people who have shingles (see page 208). Pregnant women who have never had chickenpox and have not been vaccinated should also avoid exposure, since the illness can harm the developing fetus. The vaccine cannot be given during pregnancy.

Home Treatment

- Use acetaminophen to relieve fever. Do not give aspirin to anyone younger than 20 who may have chickenpox because aspirin use is related to Reye syndrome (see page 224).
- Control itching (see page 206). Oral Benadryl and warm baths with baking soda or Aveeno colloidal oatmeal added to the water will help. Avoid Benadryl creams because it is difficult to control the dosage when the medicine is applied to the skin.
- Cut your child's fingernails to prevent scratching. If scabs are scratched off too early, the sores may become infected.

When to Call Kaiser Permanente

- If the child is at risk for complications from chickenpox (is taking steroid medications or receiving cancer chemotherapy, or has a weakened immune system).
- If a child age 3 months to 3 years has a fever of 103° or higher for 12 hours. See Fever on page 231.
- If severe itching cannot be controlled by oral Benadryl and warm baths.
- If bruising appears without injury.
- If sores appear in a child's eyes.
- If you notice signs of encephalitis (see page 160):
  - Fever, severe headache, and stiff neck
  - Unusual sleepiness or lethargy
  - Persistent vomiting

Reye Syndrome

Reye syndrome is a rare, serious disease that can occur at any age, but most often affects people younger than 20. The cause of Reye syndrome is unknown. It usually occurs after aspirin is given to a child who has a viral illness such as chickenpox or flu. Reye syndrome is not contagious.

Reye syndrome causes changes in the body that affect all the organs but are most harmful to the brain and liver.

Symptoms of Reye syndrome include:

- Sudden onset of persistent vomiting that is not related to having flu.
- Drowsiness, lack of energy.
- Rapid, deep breathing (hyperventilation).
- Behavior changes such as extreme irritability, aggressiveness, or confusion.

If Reye syndrome is not treated immediately, it can lead to seizures, coma and, in severe cases, death.

Early treatment of Reye syndrome increases the chance for full recovery. Most people have no long-lasting complications and gradually get better after a few weeks. However, some people may have permanent brain damage.

To prevent Reye syndrome, never give aspirin to anyone younger than 20. Give ibuprofen or acetaminophen instead.

Colic

Colic is not a disease; it is a condition that causes otherwise healthy babies to cry inconsolably, usually in the evening and at night. Physicians aren't sure what causes colic. It is believed to be caused by abdominal pain due to intestinal gas.

All babies cry, so how do you know if your baby has colic? Colic usually follows the "rule of three": Crying starts in the first 3 months after birth and continues more than 3 hours a day, more than 3 days a week.

Fortunately, colic goes away as the baby matures, almost always by the end of the third month—sooner for many babies. Although no single method always works to relieve colicky babies, there are a number of things you can try. Unfortunately, what works one time may not work the next. Be creative and persistent.

Home Treatment

- Most important: Stay calm and try to relax. If you start to lose control, take a minute to calm down. Never shake a baby; it can cause permanent brain damage and even death.
- Make sure your baby is getting enough to eat, but not too much. The problem may be hunger, not colic.
- Make sure your baby isn't swallowing too much air while eating. Feed the baby slowly, holding him or her almost upright. Burp your baby periodically. Prop your baby up for 15 minutes after feeding.

- If your baby is bottlefed, use nipples with holes large enough to drip cold formula at least 1 drop per second. Babies will swallow more air from around the nipple if the hole is too small.
- Heat formula to body temperature. Don't overheat.
- Babies need to suck on something for up to 2 hours a day to be satisfied. If feedings aren't enough, use a pacifier.
- Keep a regular routine for meals, naps, and playtime. Mealtime should be quiet and undisturbed by bright lights and loud noises.
- Make sure your baby's diaper is clean, that he or she isn't too hot or cold, and isn't bored.
- Try rocking or walking your baby. Putting him or her stomach-down over your knee or forearm may be helpful.
- Calm your baby with a car ride or a walk outside. Placing your baby near the hum of a clothes dryer, dishwasher, or bubbling aquarium may have a soothing effect.
- Don't worry about spoiling a baby during the first 3 months; comforting a baby makes both of you feel better.
- Don't leave your baby alone while he or she is crying for more than 5 to 10 minutes. After 10 minutes, try the above suggestions again.

When to Call Kaiser Permanente

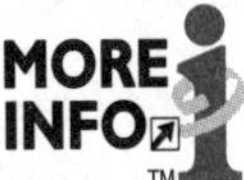

Colic generally does not require professional treatment unless it is accompanied by vomiting, diarrhea, or other signs of a more serious illness. If the baby looks healthy and acts normally between crying episodes, and if your emotions can stand the noise for the first 3 months, you have little cause for worry.

However, if colic lasts more than 4 hours a day, or if you feel like you need help, contact your physician for advice.

In rare cases, colic may be so severe that you and your physician may consider a medication for the baby. Ask about side effects.

Cradle Cap

Cradle cap is an oily, yellow scaling or crusting on an infant's scalp. It is caused by a buildup of normal oils on the skin.

Home Treatment

- Wash your baby's head with baby shampoo once a day. Gently scrub the scalp with a soft-bristled brush (a soft toothbrush works well) for a few minutes to remove the scales. Don't worry about hurting your baby's skull; it is sturdier than you think. Rinse well.

- You can also rub mineral oil on your baby's scalp 1 hour before shampooing to loosen the scales.
- If scrubbing with baby shampoo doesn't work, try using a dandruff shampoo, such as Selsun Blue, Head & Shoulders, or Sebulex. Use these products carefully because they can irritate your baby's eyes.
- If the rash looks irritated and red, applying a mild hydrocortisone cream (such as Cortaid) may help.

Croup

Croup is a respiratory problem that develops most often in children from 2 to 4 years of age. Croup may accompany a viral infection, such as a cold. The main symptom is a harsh cough that sounds like a seal's bark and may cause the child to become very frightened. A fever up to 101° is also common. Croup may last 1 to 7 days. Symptoms usually get worse at night, but they generally improve with each passing night.

Home Treatment

- Do whatever you can to calm your child. Crying can make breathing more difficult.
- Get moisture into the air to make it easier for your child to breathe. Use a cool humidifier (do not use a hot vaporizer). Use only water in the humidifier. Set your child in your lap, and let the cool vapor blow directly into your child's face.
- If your child does not improve after several minutes, take him or her into the bathroom and turn on all of the hot water faucets to create steam. Close the door, and sit with your child while he or she breathes in the moist air for several minutes.
- If your child's breathing still does not improve, bundle him or her up and go outside into the cool night air.

When to Call Kaiser Permanente

- **Call 911 or seek other emergency services immediately** if the child stops breathing or begins to turn blue. Give rescue breathing (see page 36) until help arrives.
- If these signs of respiratory distress appear and persist despite home treatment:
    - Squeaky or raspy sound as the child inhales (stridor).
    - Sucking in or retraction between ribs as the child inhales.
    - Flaring nostrils.
- If the child is so short of breath that he or she can't walk or talk.
- If the child drools or is breathing with the chin jutting out and the mouth open.
- If the child is not calm enough to sleep after being in a room with a humidifier or breathing cold outdoor air for 20 minutes.
- If the child has a fever of 102° or higher, or a fever that does not go away after 48 hours.

- If you or the child becomes hysterical and cannot calm down.
- If this is the first case of croup in your family and you need reassurance.
- If croup lasts longer than 3 nights without improving.
- If your child starts to complain of ear pain.

Diaper Rash

Diaper rash is a skin reaction, usually to the moisture and bacteria in a baby's urine and stools, to the soap used to wash diapers, or to disposable diapers. While it is uncomfortable, diaper rash is usually not dangerous.

Symptoms of the rash are a red bottom and thighs. It will be easier for you to recognize diaper rash after you have seen it the first time.

Prevention

- Change diapers as soon as possible after they have been soiled or wet.
- As often as possible, leave your baby's skin open to the air for 5 to 10 minutes before applying a clean diaper.
- Wash diapers with mild detergent and rinse twice. Do not use bleach.
- If your baby has frequent diaper rash, avoid using plastic pants for a while. They trap moisture against the baby's skin.
- When your baby has diarrhea, protect the diaper area with zinc oxide or another cream.

Home Treatment

- Stop using plastic pants when the rash appears.
- Change diapers frequently. Using a washcloth and water, rinse the skin in the diaper area at every diaper change. Allow the diaper area to air dry if possible. Wash the area with a mild soap once a day.
- Try protecting the skin with Desitin, Diaparene, A & D Ointment, or zinc oxide cream. Apply cream only to dry skin. Discontinue creams if a rash develops or they appear to slow healing.
- Try another brand of disposable diapers. Some babies tolerate one kind better than another.
- Avoid bulky or multilayered diapers.
- Try changing detergents if the rash does not clear.

When to Call Kaiser Permanente

- If the diaper rash becomes very red, raw, or sore-looking, or if it has blisters, pus, peeling areas, or crusty patches.
- If the rash is mainly in the skin creases, because this may indicate a yeast infection.
- If a significant rash lasts longer than 5 days.

Child Safety Seats

Infant and child safety seats save lives. Many states require them for all children under age 4 and those weighing less than 40 pounds. (In California, law now requires them until age 6 or 60 pounds.) Children who are not in child safety seats can be seriously injured or killed during car crashes or even abrupt stops at low speeds. For maximum safety, follow the manufacturer's recommendations for child safety seat use.

All children under age 12 should ride buckled up in the back seat, especially if the car has air bags.

Infants under 20 pounds, regardless of age: Use an infant safety seat that reclines and faces the rear.

Infants younger than 1 year, regardless of weight: Use an infant safety seat that reclines and faces the rear.

Children over 20 pounds and older than 1 year: Use a toddler safety seat that faces the front of the car and has a shield or harness. Some infant safety seats can be converted to toddler safety seats.

Children who have outgrown a safety seat with a harness: Use a booster seat that raises the child so he or she can see out of the window. Use regular lap and shoulder belts. Adjust the shoulder belt to fit across the shoulder, not the neck.

Set a good example for your children by always wearing your own seat belt, and always insist that they buckle up.

Diarrhea and Vomiting

Diarrhea and vomiting may be caused by viral stomach flu or by eating unusual kinds or amounts of food. An infant's developing digestive system sometimes will not tolerate large amounts of juice, fruit, or even milk. Breastfed babies are less likely to develop diarrhea.

Stomach flu often starts with vomiting that is followed in a few hours (sometimes 8 to 12 hours or longer) by diarrhea. Sometimes there is no diarrhea.

Infants and young children, especially those younger than age 1, need special attention when they have diarrhea or are vomiting, because they can quickly become dehydrated. Careful observation of the child's appearance and fluid intake can help prevent problems. For diarrhea in children age 12 and older, see Diarrhea on page 82. For vomiting in children age 4 and older, see Nausea and Vomiting on page 90.

Home Treatment

Diarrhea in babies up to 1 year:

- If your baby is breastfed, continue breastfeeding at more frequent intervals to replace lost fluids.
- If your baby is fed formula, give small feedings at more frequent intervals to make up for lost fluids.

- Supplement feedings with a children's oral electrolyte solution (such as Pedialyte, Ricelyte, or a store brand) only if signs of dehydration develop (see page 80). The amount of electrolyte solution your baby needs depends on his or her weight and degree of dehydration. Call your physician if your baby shows signs of dehydration.
- You can give the oral electrolyte solution a little at a time in a dropper, spoon, or bottle. For children over 6 months of age, you can improve the taste by adding a pinch of NutraSweet or sugar-free Kool-Aid or Jell-O powder.
- Don't use sports drinks, fruit juice, or soda to treat dehydration. These drinks contain too much sugar and not enough of the minerals (electrolytes) that are being lost. Do not give your baby plain water.
- Don't use oral electrolyte solutions as the sole source of fluid for more than 12 to 24 hours.
- Offer your baby easily digestible solid foods (cereal, strained bananas, mashed potatoes) if he or she was eating them before.
- Protect the diaper area with Desitin, Diaparene, A & D Ointment, or zinc oxide cream. Diaper rash is common after diarrhea.

Diarrhea in children 1 year through 11 years:

- Give ½ cup to 1 cup of a children's oral electrolyte solution, half-strength orange juice, or plain water (if the child is eating food) each hour. Add Nutra-Sweet flavorings if needed. Allow your child to drink as much as he or she wants.
- Don't give your child apple juice, chicken broth, sports drinks, soft drinks, or ginger ale. These drinks do not contain the right mixture of minerals and sugar to restore lost fluids and may make the diarrhea worse.
- Give your child frequent small meals of easily digestible foods (cooked cereal, crackers, mashed potatoes, applesauce, bananas). Avoid foods that contain a lot of sugar. Don't use an electrolyte solution as the sole source of fluids and nutrients for more than 24 hours.

As the child gets better, the stools will become smaller and less frequent. Some types of diarrhea may cause watery stools for 4 to 6 days. Watch for signs of dehydration (see page 80). You can treat the illness at home as long as the child is taking in enough fluids and nutrients, is urinating normal amounts, and seems to be improving. For home treatment of diarrhea in children 12 and older, see page 82.

Vomiting in babies up to 6 months:

- Do not feed your baby anything for 30 to 60 minutes after he or she has vomited. Watch your baby closely for signs of dehydration.
- Do not give your baby plain water.

- If your baby is breastfed, offer short but frequent feedings.
- If your baby is fed formula, switch to an oral electrolyte solution (such as Pedialyte or Ricelyte). Offer 1 tablespoon every 10 minutes for the first hour, and double the amount every 20 minutes each hour that your child does not vomit. You can return to regular feedings once 6 hours have passed without your child vomiting.

Vomiting in children 7 months through 3 years:

- After 1 hour has passed since your child last vomited, give 1 ounce of a clear liquid (not plain water) every 20 minutes for 1 hour. Double the amount every 20 minutes each hour that your child does not vomit. Some clear liquids that are safe include children's oral rehydration solution, clear broth, and gelatin dessert.
- Do not use sports drinks (such as Gatorade or Allsport), undiluted fruit juice, or soda. These drinks contain too much sugar. Do not offer plain water or diet soda because they lack the calories and essential minerals your child needs.
- Offer your child regular foods after 6 hours with no vomiting. Avoid high-fiber foods (such as beans) and foods with a lot of sugar, such as candy or ice cream.

For home treatment of vomiting in children 4 and older, see page 90.

When to Call Kaiser Permanente

- If vomiting occurs with severe headache, sleepiness, lethargy, or a stiff neck. See "Encephalitis and Meningitis" on page 160.
- If the diarrhea is bloody, tarry, or dark red.
- If the urine becomes bloody or cola-colored.
- If there is blood in the vomit.
- If signs of severe dehydration appear (also see page 80):
  - Sunken eyes, no tears, dry mouth and tongue.
  - Sunken soft spot (fontanelle) on an infant's head.
  - Little or no urine for 8 hours.
  - Skin that is doughy or doesn't bounce back when pinched.
  - Rapid breathing and heartbeat.
  - Sleepiness, lethargy, listlessness, and extreme irritability.
- If a child with diarrhea or vomiting refuses to drink or cannot take in enough liquid to replace lost fluids.
- If severe vomiting (vomiting most or all clear liquids and feedings) occurs in an infant younger than 3 months of age. In older children, call if severe vomiting continues:
  - Longer than 8 hours in an infant younger than 6 months of age.
  - Longer than 12 hours in a child age 6 months to 4 years.

- If occasional vomiting occurs without other symptoms and the child is able to keep fluids down between vomiting episodes. Call if this continues longer than:
  - 1 to 2 days in an infant under 3 months of age.
  - 2 to 4 days in an infant age 3 to 6 months.
  - 1 to 2 weeks in a child age 7 months to 3 years.
- If severe diarrhea (large loose stools every 1 to 2 hours) continues for longer than:
  - 4 hours in an infant under 3 months of age.
  - 8 hours in an infant age 3 to 6 months.
  - 1 to 2 days in a child age 7 months to 11 years.
- If mild to moderate diarrhea continues without obvious cause or other symptoms for longer than:
  - 24 hours in an infant under 3 months of age.
  - 1 to 2 days in an infant age 3 to 6 months.
  - 4 to 7 days in a child age 7 months to 11 years.
- If vomiting or diarrhea occurs with:
  - A fever of 103° or higher.
  - A low fever for more than 2 days.
- If the child has stomach pain that:
  - Is severe.
  - Is persistent, with frequent vomiting for more than 12 hours but little or no diarrhea.
  - Starts several hours before the vomiting begins and seems like more than just stomach cramps.
  - Is localized to 1 quadrant of the abdomen, especially the lower right quadrant. See illustration on page 77. This may be difficult to determine in a small child.

Fever

Fever is usually defined as a rectal temperature above 100.4°.

For information about taking accurate temperatures in infants and children, see page 342. All temperatures listed in this section are rectal temperatures. Rectal temperatures are the most accurate for checking for fever in a child.

In most but not all cases, fever indicates that an illness is present. By itself, a fever is not harmful; in fact, it may help the body fight infections more effectively.

In children, viral infections, such as colds, flu, and chickenpox, can cause high fevers. Flu (see page 161) can cause a high fever for 5 days or longer. Bacterial infections, such as strep throat and ear infections, also cause fevers. Teething does not cause a fever. If a baby is teething and has a fever, other symptoms may be present that need to be evaluated. Body temperature can also rise above normal when an infant is overdressed or in a room that is too warm.

Children tend to run higher fevers than adults do. Although high fevers are uncomfortable, they do not often cause medical problems. Convulsions from fever (febrile seizures) occur only occasionally. See page 233.

There is no medical evidence that fevers from infection can cause brain damage. The body limits a fever caused by infection from going above 106°. However, heat from an external source (like sunshine on a parked car) can cause the body temperature to go above 107°, and brain damage can occur rapidly.

Home Treatment

It can be hard to know when to call your physician when your child has a fever, especially during the cold and flu season.

The height of a fever may not be related to the seriousness of the illness. The way your child looks and acts is a better guide than the thermometer is.

Most children will be less active when they have a fever. If your child is comfortable and alert, eating well, drinking enough fluids, urinating normal amounts, and seems to be improving, home treatment is all that is needed.

- Encourage the child to drink extra fluids or suck on frozen fruit pops.
- Dress the child lightly, and do not wrap him or her in blankets.

If the fever is higher than 102° and your child is uncomfortable:

- Give acetaminophen or ibuprofen. Do not give aspirin to anyone younger than 20.
- If the fever is 104° or higher, sponge the child with lukewarm water for 20 to 30 minutes. Do not use cold water, ice, or rubbing alcohol. Stop cooling the child if he or she starts to shiver.
- Keep encouraging the child to drink extra fluids, and watch for signs of dehydration (see page 80).

When to Call Kaiser Permanente

- If fever occurs with vomiting, severe headache, sleepiness, lethargy, stiff neck, or a bulging soft spot on an infant's head. See "Encephalitis and Meningitis" on page 160.
- If fever is accompanied by these symptoms:
  - Rapid, difficult breathing.
  - Drooling or inability to swallow.
  - Purple rash that does not lighten when you press on it.
  - Vomiting, diarrhea, and stomach pain (see page 228).
  - Signs of dehydration (see page 80).

- Unexplained skin rash (see page 218 for common childhood illnesses that cause rashes).
- Ear pain (babies often pull at painful ears). See Ear Infections on page 180.
- Pain when urinating (crying when urinating), not caused by painful diaper rash.
- New swelling, pain, redness, or warmth in 1 or more joints.
- Any unusual or severe pain.

- If an infant younger than 3 months of age has a fever of 100.4° or higher.
- If a child age 3 months to 3 years has a fever that:
  - Is 104° or higher.
  - Is 102° to 104° and does not come down after 12 hours.
  - Is 100° to 102° and does not come down after 24 to 48 hours.
- If a child 3 years or older has a fever that:
  - Is 104° or higher and does not come down after 2 hours of home treatment.
  - Is 102° to 104° for 2 days.
  - Is 101° to 102° for 3 days.
  - Is 100° to 101° for 4 days.
- If the child has a fever and seems sicker than you would expect from a viral illness, such as a cold or the flu.
- If the child becomes delirious or has hallucinations.
- If the child's fever began after he or she took a new medication.

Fever Convulsions

Fever convulsions (febrile seizures) are uncontrolled muscle spasms that can happen while a child's temperature is rapidly rising (sometimes the convulsion occurs before you are even aware that the child has a fever). Once a child's fever has reached a high temperature, the risk of a convulsion is probably over.

A child who is having a fever convulsion will lose consciousness. The child's muscles will stiffen, and his or her teeth will clench. Then the child's arms and legs will start to jerk. The child's eyes may roll back, and he or she may stop breathing for a few seconds. The child might also vomit, urinate, or pass stools. Convulsions usually last 1 to 5 minutes.

Although frightening, fever convulsions in children age 6 months to 4 years are seldom serious and do not cause harm. Two to 4 percent of children in this age group are prone to fever convulsions. About 30 percent of children who have a fever convulsion will have another one in the future.

Home Treatment

During a convulsion:

- Try to stay calm, because that will help calm the child.
- Protect the child from injury. Ease the child to the floor, or hold a very small child face down on your lap. Do not restrain the child.
- Turn the child onto his or her side. This will help clear the mouth of any vomit or saliva and will keep the airway open so the child can breathe.
- Do not put anything in the child's mouth to prevent tongue biting, because it may injure the child.
- Time the length of the convulsion, if possible.

After a convulsion:

- If the child is having difficulty breathing, turn his or her head to the side and, using your finger, gently clear the mouth of any vomit or saliva so the child can breathe.
- Check for injuries.
- Reduce the fever with acetaminophen or ibuprofen and lukewarm sponge baths. Do not give aspirin to anyone younger than 20.
- Put the child in a cool room to sleep. Drowsiness is common following a convulsion. Check the child often. The child should return to his or her normal behavior and activity level within 60 minutes of the convulsion.

Hand-Foot-Mouth Disease

Hand-foot-mouth disease is a viral illness that affects many children under 10 as well as young adults. It usually develops during the summer and fall months. Fever, sore throat or mouth, and loss of appetite are early symptoms. Within 2 days, blisters form in the mouth and on the tongue. In children, a painless, blistering rash often develops on the fingers, palms of the hands, and soles of the feet. Infants may also develop a red rash on the buttocks.

There is no treatment for hand-foot-mouth disease other than to give acetaminophen to reduce fever and mouth pain and to make sure the person drinks plenty of fluids. Offer soft, bland foods and cool or warm (not hot) beverages. Frozen fruit pops may help relieve mouth soreness.

The virus that causes hand-foot-mouth disease is easily spread, so a person should not go to day care, school, or work while symptoms are present. All symptoms should go away after about 1 week. The virus is spread through contact with mouth and nasal fluids and stools, so careful hand washing after blowing a runny nose or changing a diaper is important.

When to Call Kaiser Permanente

Call 911 or seek other emergency services immediately:

- If the child stops breathing for longer than 30 to 60 seconds. Begin rescue breathing (see page 36).
- If your child will not become fully awake or looks very sick.
- If your child develops other symptoms, such as vomiting, diarrhea, or difficulty breathing.
- If a convulsion lasts longer than 5 minutes, or if a second convulsion occurs.

Call Kaiser Permanente:

- If the child is younger than 6 months of age, is 6 years old or older, or if the convulsion only affects one side of the body.
- If fever occurs with vomiting, severe headache, sleepiness, lethargy, stiff neck, or a bulging soft spot on an infant's head. See "Encephalitis and Meningitis" on page 160.
- If a convulsion occurs without fever.
- If it is the child's first convulsion, or if you haven't discussed with your physician what to do if there is another one.
- If you are unable to reduce fever to below 102° after a convulsion.

Impetigo

Impetigo is a bacterial infection that is much more common in children than in adults. It often starts when a small cut or scratch becomes infected. Symptoms are oozing, honey-colored, crusty sores that often appear on the face between the upper lip and nose, especially after a cold. Scratching the sores may spread impetigo to other parts of the body.

Prevention

- Wash all scratches and sores with soap and water.
- If your child has a runny nose, keep the area between the child's upper lip and nose clean to prevent infection.
- Keep your child's fingernails short and clean.

Home Treatment

Small areas of impetigo may respond well to prompt home treatment.

- Remove crusts by soaking the area in warm water (use a warm washcloth for the face) for 15 to 20 minutes; then scrub gently with a washcloth and antibacterial soap. Pat dry gently; do not rub. Repeat several times a day.
- Apply an antibiotic ointment. Cover the area with gauze taped well away from the sores. This will help keep the infection from spreading and prevent scratching.

- Adult men with impetigo should shave around the sores, not over them, and use a clean blade daily. Do not use a shaving brush.
- To prevent spreading the infection, do not share towels, washcloths, or bath water.

When to Call Kaiser Permanente

- If impetigo covers a total area larger than 2 inches in diameter.
- If impetigo does not improve after 3 to 4 days of home treatment, or if any new infected areas appear. Your physician may prescribe an antibiotic.
- If there is facial swelling or tenderness, especially near the nose and lips.
- If other signs of infection develop:
  - Pain, swelling, or tenderness.
  - Redness or red streaks extending from the area.
  - Discharge of pus.
  - Fever of 100° or higher with no other cause.

Pinworms

Pinworms are tiny, threadlike worms that infect the digestive tract. Pinworms are most common in 5- to 14-year-olds, although anyone can become infected. The worms live in the upper end of the large intestine, near the appendix, and travel to the outside of the anus to lay their eggs. The egg-laying almost always occurs at night and usually causes the child to scratch the anal area. When the child later sucks a thumb or licks a finger, the eggs are ingested and the cycle begins again. The eggs are very sticky and can survive on clothing and bedding for days, where they can be picked up by other family members.

Anal itching, especially at night, is the most common symptom of pinworm infection. If the infection is severe, there may also be loss of appetite, itching in the genital area, and pain when urinating.

Pinworms are common and affect many families. If you suspect pinworms, it's easy to find out for sure in your own home and at no cost. Go into your child's darkened bedroom 30 minutes after bedtime and shine a flashlight on the child's anus. The light will make the worms move back into the child's anus. If you don't see the worms after checking for 2 or 3 nights, it is unlikely that the child is infected with pinworms.

Prevention

Teach children to wash their hands after using the toilet and before meals.

Home Treatment

- Ask your pharmacist for a nonprescription medication for pinworms. The medication may not be given to children younger than 2 years or used by women who are pregnant.

- Treat every child in the house between the ages of 2 and 10. If infection recurs, consider treating everyone in the family who is older than 2.
- On the first day of treatment, wash all underwear, nightclothes, bedding, and towels in hot water and detergent to get rid of any eggs and prevent reinfection. Sanitize toilet and sleeping areas with a strong disinfectant.
- Trim and keep children's fingernails short.
- Require frequent hand washing, morning showers, and daily changes of pajamas and underwear.

When to Call Kaiser Permanente

- If a person has symptoms of pinworm infection, but you have not seen any worms. If this is the first infection, it is recommended that a health professional confirm the diagnosis.
- If the pinworm medication causes side effects, such as vomiting or pain.
- If you continue to see worms at night despite using a nonprescription medication. Stronger prescription medications are available.
- If a person who has a pinworm infection develops any of the following:
  - Fever or abdominal pain.
  - Redness, tenderness, swelling, or itching in the genital area.
  - Pain when urinating.

Prickly Heat (Sweat Rash)

Prickly heat, also called heat rash, sweat rash, or miliaria, is a rash of red or pink dots that appears on an infant's head, neck, and shoulders. The dots look like tiny pimples.

Prickly heat often develops when parents dress their baby too warmly, but it can develop in any baby when the weather is hot. An infant should be dressed just as lightly as an adult and will be comfortable at the same temperature. It is normal for a baby's hands and feet to feel cold to the touch.

Prevention

Do not overdress your baby. Place your hand between the baby's shoulder blades. If the skin is hot or moist, the baby is too warm.

Home Treatment

- Dress the baby in as few clothes as possible during hot weather.
- Keep the baby's skin cool and dry.
- Keep the baby's sleeping area cool.
- Apply hydrocortisone cream (0.5 percent) to help heal the rash.

When to Call Kaiser Permanente

- If the rash looks infected or lasts longer than 3 days.
- If the infant looks sick.
- If prickly heat is accompanied by a fever of 100.4° in an infant younger than 3 months of age, and the fever doesn't come down after you remove extra clothing from the infant.

Roseola

Roseola (roseola infantum) is a mild viral illness that often starts with a sudden high fever (103° to 105°) and irritability. The fever lasts 2 to 3 days. As the fever drops, a rosy pink rash appears on the torso, neck, and arms. The rash may last 1 to 2 days.

Since the fever is quite high and may come on quickly, fever convulsions may occur (see page 233).

Roseola is most common in children from 6 months to 2 years of age. It is rare after age 4.

Home Treatment

- If the child is uncomfortable, reduce the fever. See page 232.
- Give the child lots of liquids.
- If a fever convulsion occurs, see page 234.

When to Call Kaiser Permanente

See When to Call Kaiser Permanente under Fever on page 232.

Fifth Disease

Another common childhood illness that causes a rash is erythema infectiosum, or "fifth disease." The main symptom is a red rash on the face that looks like slapped cheeks and a lacy, pink rash on the backs of the arms and legs, torso, and buttocks. There may be a low fever. The rash may come and go for several weeks in response to changes in temperature and sunlight.

A child with fifth disease is most contagious the week before the rash appears. Once the rash has developed, the child is no longer contagious.

Home treatment for fifth disease is simply to keep the child comfortable and watch for signs that a more serious illness is present (fever over 102°; child seems very sick).

Fifth disease is harmless in children, but it poses a slight risk to developing fetuses. Pregnant women should avoid exposure if possible. If you are pregnant and are exposed to a child with fifth disease, or if you develop a fifth disease-like rash, contact your obstetrician.

If you want to get well, take the initiative.
Filipino proverb

12

Chronic Conditions

Most of the conditions described in this book are acute illnesses, which means that they get better after a short while. Chronic conditions, on the other hand, last long periods of time or come and go, often for the rest of your life. Having a chronic disease does not mean you can no longer enjoy the good things in life: chronic diseases may not be curable, but they can often be controlled.

Kaiser Permanente offers many classes and programs to help members manage chronic conditions. Ask your health professional for more information, or contact your local Health Education Department.

Some conditions that can be chronic are covered in other places in this book.

- Allergies, see page 141.
- Arthritis, see page 117.
- Asthma, see page 146.
- Back problems, see page 103.
- Bronchitis (chronic obstructive pulmonary disease, or COPD), see page 150.
- Depression, see page 313.
- Fibromyalgia, see page 129.
- Headaches, see page 189.
- Irritable bowel syndrome, see page 87.
- Neck problems, see page 113.
- Osteoporosis, see page 129.
- Skin conditions such as acne and psoriasis, see pages 197 and 199.

Diabetes

During digestion the starches and sugars in the food you eat are converted to glucose, a sugar that your body uses for energy. Insulin is a hormone produced by the pancreas that helps control the amount of glucose in blood. Without insulin, your body cannot use or store glucose, so too much sugar stays in your blood.

Over a long period of time, high blood sugar levels may damage blood vessels and nerves, increasing your risk for problems that can affect the eyes, heart, kidneys, legs, and feet.

Type 1 diabetes occurs when the pancreas makes little or no insulin. Type 1 diabetes usually develops in childhood or adolescence but can develop at any age. People with type 1 diabetes must give themselves insulin shots every day.

Type 2 diabetes occurs when the pancreas cannot make enough insulin to meet the body's needs or when the body does not use insulin properly. Type 2 diabetes often develops in adults, especially those who are overweight and over age 40. Many people with type 2 diabetes are able to control their blood sugar through regular physical activity, healthful eating, frequent self-testing of blood sugar, and maintaining a healthful weight. Some may need insulin shots or oral medications to lower their blood sugar.

Risk factors for type 2 diabetes include:

- Having a family history of type 2 diabetes.
- Being age 40 or over.
- Being overweight (20 percent more than ideal weight).
- Having an inactive lifestyle.
- Being of African-American, Hispanic, Pacific Island, or Native American descent.
- Having a history of diabetes during pregnancy (gestational diabetes) or delivery of a baby over 9 pounds.
- Being a woman with polycystic ovarian syndrome (PCOS).
- If your blood glucose has ever been higher than normal though not in the diabetes range (what we now call prediabetes).
- Having hypertension.
- Having an HDL cholesterol level lower than or equal to 35 mg/dl (milligrams per deciliter) or triglycerides higher than 250 mg/dl.

The symptoms of diabetes vary from person to person. A person may believe that his or her symptoms are due to an illness or to aging, not diabetes. Symptoms include:

- Dry mouth and increased thirst.
- Frequent urination (especially at night).
- Increased appetite.
- Unexplained weight loss.
- Feeling weak, tired, and dizzy.
- Frequent skin infections and slow-healing wounds.
- Recurrent vaginal infections.
- Blurry vision.
- Tingling or numbness in the hands or feet.

Your physician needs to do a blood test to accurately diagnose diabetes.

Prevention

At this time, there is no known way to prevent type 1 diabetes.

The risk for developing type 2 diabetes runs in families. However, even if you have a history of type 2 diabetes in your family, you may be able to delay or prevent its onset by maintaining a healthful body weight and exercising regularly.

Home Treatment

- If insulin or other medications are prescribed to control your blood sugar, take them as directed. If you improve your diet and get regular physical activity, you may need less medicine. Check with your physician before making any changes in your medication.
- Eat a healthful diet to help keep your blood sugar in control and maintain a healthy weight. Pay special attention to eating low-fat foods and to the other diet recommendations in Chapter 17.
- Get regular physical activity to help control your blood sugar level, reduce your risk for heart disease, and control your weight. Work closely with your physician to determine how your activity level affects your blood glucose levels and medication needs.
- It may help you to keep your blood sugar level within good control if you track the following daily:
    - The time and content of each meal you eat.
    - The kind and amount of exercise you get.
    - How tired or energetic you feel.
    - If you have a home glucose monitor, check and record your blood sugar level as often as directed by your physician. This record will help you understand how your body reacts to different foods and exercise, so you can keep your blood sugar level in good control.
- Learn to recognize the symptoms of low blood sugar. Talk with your physician about how to treat extremely low blood sugar. Symptoms of low blood sugar are:
    - Sweating
    - Fatigue, weakness, nausea
    - Extreme hunger
    - Blurry vision
    - Dizziness, headache
    - Rapid heartbeat, anxiousness
    - Confusion, irritability, slurred speech
- Take good care of your feet. Diabetes may damage nerves and reduce blood flow to your feet, increasing your risk for infection. Take care to avoid cuts and sores, and promptly treat any injuries to your feet.
- Get regular eye exams. Eye changes caused by diabetes often have no symptoms until they are quite advanced. Diabetic retinopathy is one form of diabetic eye

disease that can cause blindness. Early detection and treatment of diabetic retinopathy may slow its progress and save your sight.

- Have regular medical checkups. Talk to your physician about how often you need them.

Believe that you can control diabetes. Controlling diabetes requires making significant, long-term lifestyle changes that may seem overwhelming at first. However, if you adopt a "take charge" attitude about your health and focus on making one change at a time, you are more likely to be successful.

The National Diabetes Information Clearinghouse (1 Information Way, Bethesda, MD 20892-3560, (301) 654-3327, www.niddk.nih.gov) is a good resource for more information about diabetes.

When to Call Kaiser Permanente

Call 911 or seek other emergency services immediately if a person with diabetes is losing consciousness or becomes unconscious and you cannot tell if the person's blood sugar is too low or too high.

Call Kaiser Permanente:

- If signs of unusually high blood sugar develop in a person who has diabetes:
  - Fast, shallow breathing
  - Fruity-smelling breath
- If your blood sugar levels are higher or lower than usual and you cannot explain them.
- If you have been diagnosed with diabetes and are sick and need advice.
- To get a blood sugar test if you suspect that you have diabetes but have not yet been diagnosed.

High Cholesterol

Cholesterol is a fat-like substance that is produced by your body and is also found in foods that come from animal sources (meat and dairy products, poultry, and fish). Your body's cells need cholesterol to function properly. However, it is common for excess cholesterol in the blood to build up inside your arteries (atherosclerosis), causing them to narrow. Atherosclerosis is the starting point for most heart and circulation problems.

Good and Bad Cholesterol

Cholesterol travels through your bloodstream attached to protein, in a combination called a lipoprotein. Two lipoproteins are the main carriers of cholesterol: low-density lipoprotein (LDL) and high-density lipoprotein (HDL).

- LDL ("bad cholesterol") carries cholesterol from the liver to other parts of the body. Under certain conditions, LDL cholesterol can build up on the walls of the arteries. Having a high LDL cholesterol level increases your risk for coronary artery disease (CAD), heart attack, and stroke.

- HDL ("good cholesterol") helps clear LDL cholesterol from the body by picking up cholesterol from the bloodstream and taking it back to the liver for disposal. Increasing your HDL cholesterol level may reduce your risk for heart disease.

Triglycerides are another type of fat that can be found in the bloodstream. A high triglyceride level may also increase your risk of developing coronary artery disease and having a stroke.

Cholesterol Screening

Experts don't agree on the best schedule for cholesterol testing. You and your physician can determine the schedule that is best for you based on your risk factors for coronary artery disease. Most adults age 20 and older should have their cholesterol tested every 5 years. High-risk adults should have it tested more often.

If your total cholesterol is greater than 200 mg/dl (milligrams per deciliter), or if you have any of the following risk factors for coronary artery disease, you may want to have your cholesterol checked more often:

- Having a family history of early heart attack (before age 55 in father or brother; before age 65 in mother or sister).
- Being a cigarette smoker.
- Having high blood pressure (over 140/90) or taking high blood pressure medication.
- Having diabetes.
- Having an HDL level below 40.
- Having a triglyceride level over 200.

If your total cholesterol is over 200 mg/dl, and you don't know what your HDL and LDL levels are, more extensive testing can help you better estimate your actual risk.

How to Reduce Your Cholesterol

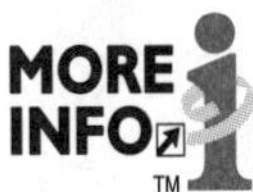

For many people, a low-fat diet and physical activity are all that are needed to lower cholesterol. People who have very high cholesterol, diabetes, or who already have coronary artery disease (or who are at very high risk for CAD) may need medication as well as exercise and a low-fat diet to lower their cholesterol.

- Eat less total fat, especially saturated fat. Follow the guidelines for eating less fat on page 302.
- Attend a nutrition workshop or consult a registered dietitian to learn ways to lower your saturated fat intake to 7 percent or less of total calories and your dietary cholesterol to less than 200 mg per day. Your total fat intake can be up to 35 percent of total calories, as long as most of it is unsaturated fat.

- Eat 2 to 3 servings (3 to 4 ounces) of baked or broiled fish per week. The safety and value of fish oil supplements is not yet known.
- Eat more soluble fiber (fruit, dry beans and peas, oats, and soy foods). See page 299.
- Exercise more. Exercise increases your HDL cholesterol level.
- If you smoke or use other tobacco products, consider getting help to quit. See page 26 for tips on quitting. Smoking increases the risk of heart attack and stroke, even in people with low cholesterol.
- Lose weight. Losing even 5 to 10 pounds can lower LDL and triglyceride levels and raise HDL levels.

What Do the Numbers Mean?

There are guidelines doctors rely on to evaluate your cholesterol numbers and assess your risk for heart disease. The importance of the numbers varies from person to person, depending on whether a person has diabetes, additional risk factors for heart disease, or actually has heart disease. The following ranges apply to people who are at average risk for heart disease.*

Total cholesterol

Desirable: Less than 200

Borderline high: 200 to 239

High: 240 and above

HDL cholesterol

High (desirable): Above 60

Acceptable: 40 to 60

Low (not desirable): Less than 40

LDL cholesterol

Optimal: Less than 100

Near optimal: 100 to 129

Borderline high: 130 to 159

High: 160 to 189

Very high: 190 and above

Triglycerides

Normal: Less than 150

Borderline high: 150 to 199

High: 200 to 499

Very high: 500 and above

**Figures provided by the National Cholesterol Education Program (NCEP), Adult Treatment Panel III, National Institutes of Health (NIH).*

High Blood Pressure

Blood pressure is a measurement of the force of blood against the walls of the arteries. Blood pressure readings include 2 numbers, for example, 130/80. The first number in the reading is called the systolic pressure. It is the force that blood exerts on the artery walls as the heart contracts. The second number in the reading is the diastolic pressure. It is the force that blood exerts on the artery walls between heartbeats, when the heart is at rest.

When you have high blood pressure, also called "hypertension," the force of blood against your artery walls is too strong. Hypertension is called the "silent killer" because it does not cause symptoms even if it is severely high.

The National Institutes of Health recently released revised guidelines for "normal" blood pressure, "prehypertension," and hypertension.

- Normal blood pressure is 119/79 or below.
- Prehypertension is 120/80 to 139/89.
- Stage 1 (moderate) hypertension is 140/90 to 159/99.
- Stage 2 (severe) hypertension is 160/100 or higher.

Despite what a lot of people think, high blood pressure usually does not cause headaches, dizziness, or lightheadedness. It usually has no symptoms. However, high blood pressure increases your risk for heart attack, stroke, and kidney or eye damage. Your risk of developing these problems increases as your blood pressure rises.

Risk factors for high blood pressure include:

- Smoking
- Being overweight.
- Having a family history of high blood pressure.
- Being of African-American descent.
- Having an inactive lifestyle.
- Drinking too much alcohol.
- Having too much salt or not enough potassium in the diet.
- Using certain medications, including birth control pills, steroids, decongestants, and anti-inflammatory drugs.

Prevention

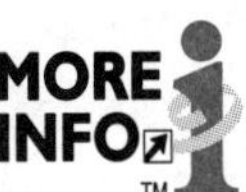

Changes in your lifestyle may help you prevent high blood pressure or help you lower your blood pressure if it's too high.

- Maintain a healthful weight. This is especially important if you tend to put on weight around the waist rather than in the hips and thighs. Losing even 10 pounds can help you lower your blood pressure.

- Be physically active at least 30 minutes on most days of the week. This will help you lower your blood pressure (and may also help you lose weight).
- Drink alcohol only in moderation:
  - For men, have no more than two 12-ounce beers, two 4- to 5-ounce glasses of wine, or two 1-ounce shots of hard alcohol per day.
  - For women, have no more than one 12-ounce beer, one 4- to 5-ounce glass of wine, or one 1-ounce shot of hard alcohol per day.
- Use salt moderately. Too much salt in the diet can be a problem for some people who have high blood pressure and are also salt-sensitive.
- Make sure you get enough potassium, calcium, and magnesium in your diet. Eating plenty of fruits (such as bananas and oranges), vegetables, legumes, and low-fat dairy products will ensure that you get enough of these minerals.
- Reduce the saturated fat in your diet. Saturated fat is found in animal products (milk, cheese, and meat). Limiting these foods will help you lose weight, lower cholesterol, and reduce your risk for coronary artery disease. See page 301.
- If you smoke or use other tobacco products, consider getting help to quit. See page 26 for tips on quitting. Tobacco use increases your risk for heart attack and stroke.
- Learn how to check your blood pressure at home. See page 355.

Home Treatment

- Follow the prevention tips above even more closely if you already have high blood pressure.
- Take any prescribed blood pressure medications exactly as directed, and see your physician at least once a year.
- If you are taking blood pressure medication, talk to your physician before taking decongestants or anti-inflammatory drugs, because they can raise your blood pressure.

When to Call Kaiser Permanente

- Call immediately if you have high blood pressure and:
  - You have pain in the upper abdomen with chest pain that is crushing or squeezing, feels like a heavy weight on your chest, or occurs with any other symptoms of a heart attack (see page 54).
  - You are experiencing symptoms of a stroke (see page 70).
  - Your blood pressure rises suddenly.
  - You have a sudden, severe headache that is worse than any headache you've had before.

Reversing Coronary Artery Disease

There is some evidence that coronary artery disease can be reversed by making major lifestyle changes, including eating a strict low-fat diet. Other studies indicate that moderate restriction of dietary fat is probably as good as a strict low-fat diet.

The Lifestyle Heart Trial found that people who followed a low-fat vegetarian diet, quit smoking, began exercising, and practiced relaxation techniques daily actually showed some decrease in the amount of fat and calcium build-up in their arteries. Although this was a very small study, other studies have shown similar improvements with less severe diet restrictions.

In the past, cholesterol-lowering drugs were only given to people with high cholesterol. Newer studies show that such drugs may also help people with normal or borderline high cholesterol levels who have signs of or risk factors for heart disease. In these people, cholesterol-lowering drugs may help prevent atherosclerosis from developing or getting worse. They also appear to lower the risk of heart attack and stroke.

- Call if your blood pressure is higher than 140/90 on 2 or more occasions (taken at home or in a community screening program). If 1 blood pressure reading is high, have another taken by a health professional to verify the first reading.
- Call if you develop uncomfortable or disturbing side effects from any medication taken for high blood pressure.

Behind every successful woman is herself.
New American Proverb

13 Women's Health

This chapter focuses on health problems that are unique to women. If you are looking for general guidelines for making healthful lifestyle choices to prevent illness and injury, see Chapter 2, Living a Healthy Life. Specific tips for developing a fitness plan, eating a healthful diet, maintaining a healthful body weight, managing stress, and preventing sexually transmitted diseases are included in other chapters. Use the index to find the information you need.

Breast Health

Breast cancer is the leading cause of cancer deaths in women who are 40 to 55 years old. The good news is that breast cancer can often be highly treatable if it is detected early. There are 3 methods of early detection: mammography, clinical breast exam, and breast self-exam.

One of the most important risk factors for breast cancer is age. The risk goes up significantly after age 50. Women younger than 50 are at relatively low risk for breast cancer. However, if your mother or a sister had breast cancer before menopause, talk with your physician about starting mammography and other screenings before age 40.

Mammography

A mammogram is a breast X-ray that can reveal breast tumors that are too small to be detected by breast self-exam or a clinical breast exam.

Studies have shown that mammograms save lives. In women over 50, mammograms reduce breast cancer death rates by up to 1/3. The outcomes of studies for women younger than 50 are less clear.

Your physician may tell you how often he or she would like you to get a mammogram. The following is a schedule that a physician may recommend for a woman who is not at high risk for breast cancer:

- Younger than 40: mammograms not usually done.

- Age 40 to 50: offer mammograms every 1 to 2 years depending on a schedule agreed upon by the woman and her physician.
- Over 50: mammograms every 1 to 2 years.

Yearly mammograms are recommended for any woman who has had cancer in one breast. If you have a female relative (mother, sister) who had breast cancer before menopause, talk to your physician about when to start and how often to have mammograms.

Getting all the facts and thinking about your own needs and values will help you make a wise decision about mammography.

Preparing for a Mammogram

- Arrange to have your mammogram 1 to 2 weeks after your period ends.
- Do not wear deodorant, perfume, powder, or lotion, because they can affect the quality of the X-ray.
- Wear clothing that allows you to easily undress from the waist up.

Clinical Breast Exam

During a clinical breast exam, a physician or nurse looks at your breasts and gently feels them for lumps or other unusual changes. During the exam, the physician or nurse can also teach you how to examine your breasts yourself.

A clinical breast exam is recommended with gynecological exams every 1 to 2 years after age 40. A clinical breast exam is also done whenever a woman has symptoms indicating that there may be a problem with her breasts.

Breast Pain

Breast pain is common and, fortunately, is rarely a serious problem. Many women's breasts become achy, heavy, or sore a week or so before their menstrual periods start. This is called cyclic pain. It is caused by hormonal changes that occur during the menstrual cycle. The symptoms usually go away at the end of a woman's period. Cyclic breast pain usually ends after a woman completes menopause.

Noncyclic breast pain, which is not associated with a woman's periods, is usually described as sharp or burning. This pain usually occurs on one side only; it may go up towards the armpit; and it may come and go. Pain in one spot that does not go away should be checked by a health professional.

Stress, caffeine use, estrogen therapy, and the use of tranquilizers and other medications can make breast pain worse. Sore breasts can also be a sign of pregnancy.

If pain or any other changes in your breasts concern you, talk to your health professional. If you are over 40 or have a family history of breast cancer, discuss breast cancer screening with your physician.

Breast Self-Exam

Most women's breast tissue has some lumps or thickening. When in doubt about a particular lump, check the other breast. If you find a similar lump in the same area on the other breast, both breasts are probably normal. Be on the lookout for a lump that feels much harder than the rest of the breast. Have any areas of concern checked by your health professional.

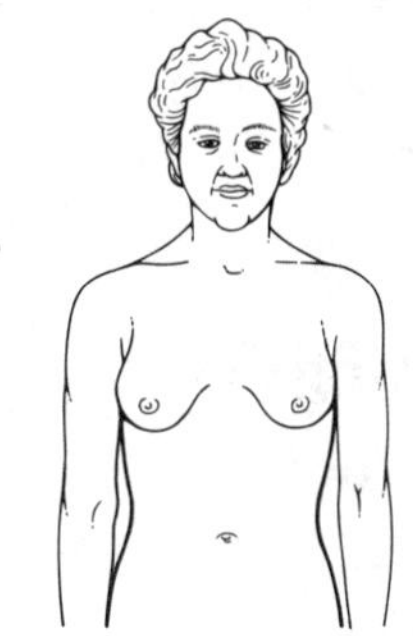

Look at your breasts in a mirror.

The breast self-exam is a simple technique to help you learn what is normal for you and how to recognize any changes.

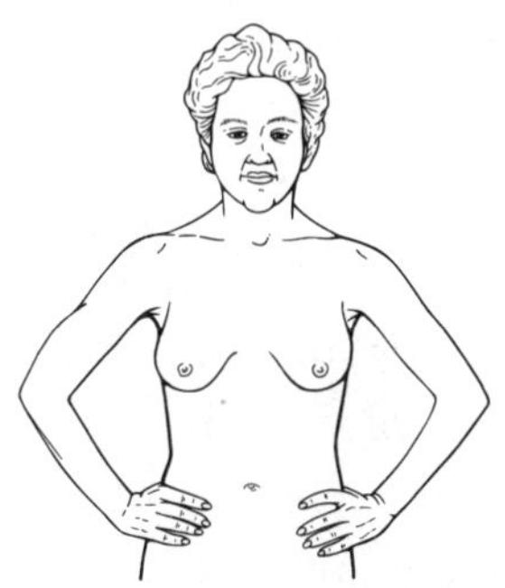

Put your hands on your hips.

Establish a regular time to examine your breasts. A few days after your period when your breasts are not swollen or tender is a good time. Women who do not menstruate (after menopause and hysterectomies) can examine their breasts anytime.

The breast self-exam takes place in 2 stages.

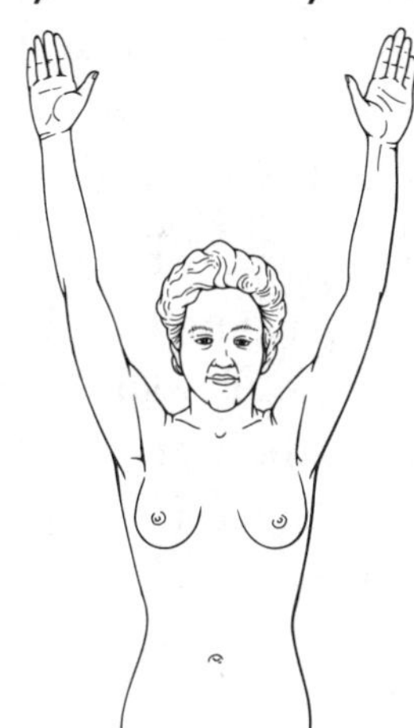

Raise your arms.

Stage 1: In front of the mirror

Examine your breasts visually in a mirror. Few women have breasts that match exactly. It is normal for one breast to be slightly larger than the other. Learn what is normal for you.

Stand and look at your breasts in 4 positions:

- With your arms at your sides
- With your arms on your hips
- With your arms raised overhead
- While bending forward

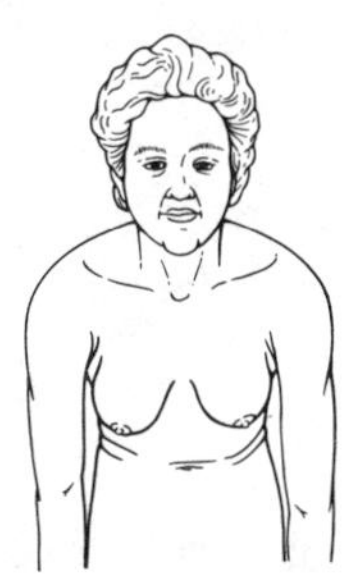

Bend forward, still looking in the mirror.

In each position, look for changes in the contour and shape of your breasts, the color and texture of the skin and nipples, and any discharge from the nipples.

Stage 2: Lying down

To examine your right breast, place a pillow or folded towel under your right shoulder. If your breasts are large, lie on your left side and turn your right shoulder back flat to spread the breast tissue more evenly over your chest wall.

Use the pads of 3 middle fingers of your left hand to examine your right breast. Move your fingers in small, dime-sized circles. Use light to medium pressure in each spot to feel the full thickness of the breast tissue. Don't lift your fingers away from the skin. You are feeling for lumps, thickening, or changes of any kind.

Examine your entire breast using a vertical strip pattern (see illustration). Examine all tissue from the collarbone to the armpit and from just under the breast (the bra line) to the breastbone. Start in the armpit and work down to the underside of the breast (bottom of the bra line). Move 1 finger-width toward the middle and work up to the collarbone. Repeat until you have covered all the breast tissue.

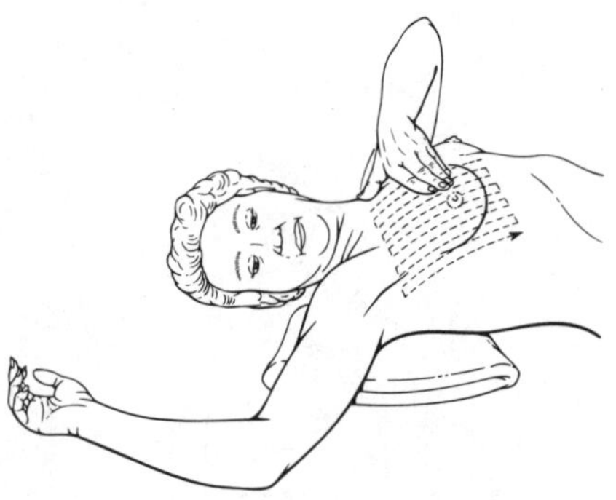

Vertical strip pattern: move your fingers up and down across the breast.

If you discover any unusual lumps, thickening, or changes of any kind, or if there is a discharge from the nipple when you are not squeezing it, report them to your physician immediately. Most lumps are not malignant (cancer), but your physician needs to make a diagnosis.

If you examine your breasts monthly, you will learn what is normal for you and quickly recognize if something changes. The breast self-exam takes some practice. Ask your physician or health care professional for help in learning the technique.

Prevention and Early Detection of Breast Cancer

We do not know for sure how to prevent breast cancer. However, the following suggestions may help.

- Limit alcohol to 1 drink per day. Moderate to heavy drinking increases your risk for breast cancer.
- Eat a low-fat diet. Fat in the diet is linked to an increased risk for breast cancer.
- Eat foods that contain vitamins A and C, such as dark green and orange vegetables and fruits. Eat more cruciferous vegetables

(broccoli, cabbage, kale). There is some evidence that a diet that includes these foods may reduce your risk for breast cancer.

Early Detection of Breast Cancer

- Have a clinical breast exam every 1 to 2 years after age 40 or according to a schedule that you and your physician agree upon.
- Have a mammogram every 1 to 2 years after age 50.
- Do a breast self-exam every month (see page 251).

When to Call Kaiser Permanente

- If you find a lump that concerns you, particularly if it is hard and unlike any other tissue in your breasts.
- Any time you find a breast lump if you are past menopause and are not taking hormones.
- If you have a bloody or greenish discharge from a nipple, or a watery or milky discharge that occurs without pressing on the nipple or breast.
- If one of your breasts changes shape, or if it seems to pucker or "pull" when you raise your arms.
- If the skin of one breast becomes dimpled ("orange peel skin").
- If you notice a change in the color or feel of the skin of a breast or the darker area (areola) around a nipple.
- If you have any signs of infection in a breast, which include:
  - Pain, swelling, redness, heat, or tenderness in or around the breast.
  - Pus draining from the nipple or a sore or wound on the breast.
  - Fever of 100° or higher without another cause.
  - Swollen, tender glands (lymph nodes) under the arm.

Gynecological Health

Regular pelvic exams and Pap tests are vital components of women's health. These exams can give you early indications of any abnormalities in your reproductive organs. It is better to catch any disease in its early stages, when it may be easier to treat.

Self-Exam

Self-exams will help you better understand your own body and what is normal for you. Periodically examine your entire genital area for any sores, warts, red swollen areas, or unusual discharge. A normal vaginal discharge may be white to yellowish white and smell slightly like vinegar. It can be either thick or thin and present in large or small amounts; every woman is different. During ovulation (the midpoint between periods), there is often a large amount of clear, slippery mucus. If your discharge seems unusual in amount, smell, or texture, see Vaginitis on page 266.

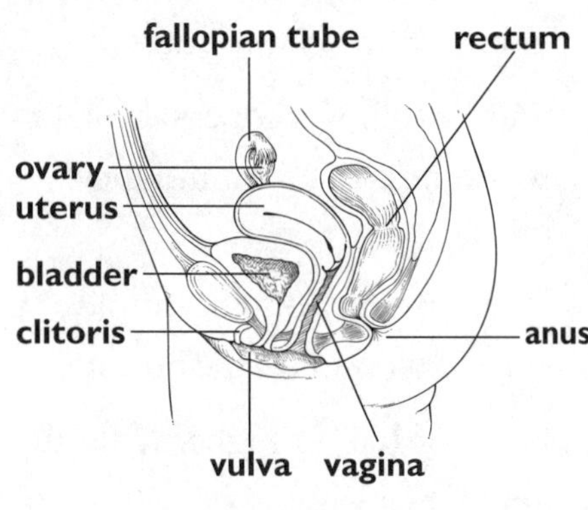

Female pelvic organs

There should be no pain or straining when you urinate, and the urine should come out in a fairly steady stream. The urine should be pale yellow, and it should not have a strong ammonia smell. If you experience pain or burning when you urinate, see Urinary Tract Infections on page 100 or Vaginitis on page 266. If you have problems with bladder control, see Urinary Incontinence on page 98.

Pelvic Exam and Pap Test

A pelvic exam given by a health professional will generally consist of an external genital exam, a Pap test, and a manual exam.

The Pap test is the screening exam for cancer of the cervix (the lower part of the uterus). The Pap test detects 90 to 95 percent of cervical cancers, making it a reliable and important test. To do the test, your health professional will insert an instrument (speculum) into your vagina to spread apart the vaginal walls. Then, using a cotton swab, small brush, or wooden spatula, your health professional will gather several samples of cells from your cervix. The cells are put on a slide and sent to a lab for classification. Your health professional should let you know the results of your Pap test when they return from the lab. Ask for an explanation of your results if you don't understand them.

If your Pap test results are abnormal, you will be asked to return for more testing. You may have another Pap test, or your physician may try to find the area in your cervix that contains abnormal cells using a special magnifying device (colposcopy).

To do a manual exam, your health professional will insert 2 gloved and lubricated fingers into your vagina and press on your lower abdomen with his or her other hand to feel for any abnormalities in the shape or size of your ovaries and uterus.

Scheduling a Pelvic Exam

It is recommended that you have your first Pap test when you become sexually active or at age 21, whichever comes first. After that, Pap tests are recommended every 2 years, depending on your risk factors.

If you have risk factors for cervical cancer or a history of abnormal Pap tests, it is recommended that you have a Pap test each year. Discuss the best schedule for Pap tests for you with your physician.

Arrange to have the test 1 to 2 weeks after your period ends. Do not douche, have sexual intercourse, or use feminine hygiene products for at least 24 hours before a Pap test, because doing any of these things can alter the test results.

Morning Sickness

Many women experience nausea and vomiting during the first few months of pregnancy. Morning sickness, which can occur at any time of day, is a normal result of the body's adjustment to the hormones of pregnancy. The following home treatment can help.

- Eat 5 or 6 small meals a day to avoid having an empty stomach. Include some protein in each of the meals.
- Eat crackers or dry toast as soon as you get up in the morning.
- Increase your intake of vitamin B_6 by eating more whole grains and cereals, wheat germ, nuts, seeds, and legumes. Talk with your health professional before taking vitamin supplements during early pregnancy. They may cause nausea.
- Avoid foods (or food smells) that make you nauseous.
- Get plenty of rest.

Call your health professional if your symptoms are so severe that you cannot hold down food or liquids, if you are vomiting more than 3 times a day, or if you are losing weight.

Pregnancy: How to Make a Healthy Baby

You can increase the chances that your baby will be healthy. The following guidelines will help.

Before Conception

Your health, both before conception and during the first weeks after, is particularly important for your baby's health. Start helping your baby even before you become pregnant.

- Get a thorough physical checkup. If any problems or needs are found, deal with them early. Have a blood test to check your rubella immunity. If you test negative, you will need an immunization. It is recommended that you wait at least 3 months after being vaccinated before you get pregnant. Exposure to rubella during early pregnancy can harm your baby.
- Testing for genetic problems is important for some couples. If you have reasons to worry, genetic testing will help you make decisions about your pregnancy. Testing may include questions about family history of Down syndrome, sickle cell disease, Tay-Sachs disease, spina bifida, hemophilia, muscular dystrophy, and other conditions. Couples may want to get genetic testing if:
    - They have had a child with a genetic disease or abnormality.
    - Either partner has a family history of hereditary diseases.

    - The woman has had 3 or more abortions.
    - The woman will be 35 years old by the time she delivers the baby.
- If you have diabetes, high blood pressure, seizure disorders, or any inherited diseases, talk with your physician before getting pregnant. Your physician may want to modify your treatment and may be able to prescribe medicine that is safer for the developing baby.
- See your dentist and, if possible, have any necessary fillings or other work done before you get pregnant.
- If you have symptoms of a sexually transmitted disease or are unsure of your partner's sexual history, read pages 283 to 285 and arrange for an examination and testing.
- Eat well. Make sure your diet includes plenty of green, leafy vegetables and legumes, and take a multivitamin supplement that contains 0.4 mg of folate (folic acid). Folic acid helps prevent certain birth defects such as spina bifida. Other good sources of folic acid include fortified cereal and whole-wheat bread.
- Get physical activity and control your weight as advised by your physician.
- If you smoke or use other tobacco products, consider getting help to quit. See page 26 for tips on quitting.
- Cut down on caffeinated drinks, such as coffee, tea, and cola drinks.
- Stop drinking alcoholic beverages, such as beer, wine, and hard liquor.
- Stop all illegal drug use and eliminate any medications that are not absolutely essential.
- If you are anxious or depressed, get help. See pages 312 and 313.
- Buy a good book on pregnancy and start reading.

Early Pregnancy (Weeks 1 to 14)

- Continue to avoid smoking, alcohol, and drugs.
- Make the first visit to your caregiver in the first 10 to 12 weeks of your pregnancy.
- Get tested for HIV infection.
- Continue to improve your nutrition. Call your local WIC (Women, Infants, and Children) agency to learn whether you are eligible for this program. WIC provides vouchers for nutritious food, nutrition education, and breastfeeding support to pregnant women, women with new babies, and children younger than 5.
- Continue taking a multivitamin supplement containing 0.4 mg of folate.
- Avoid touching cat feces and litter boxes. Also, wash your hands after handling raw meat and cook all meat well before you eat it. Cat feces and raw or undercooked

meat can carry toxoplasmosis, an infection that can cause a miscarriage or brain damage in the fetus.

- Avoid all chemical vapors, paint fumes, and poisons.
- If you drink coffee or soda with caffeine, cut back to 2 cups per day.

Middle Pregnancy (Weeks 15 to 28)

- Continue with the guidelines described above.
- Reduce your risk for injury and falls:
    - Wear sensible shoes.
    - Continue moderate levels of your regular exercises, but do not become exhausted or significantly short of breath.
    - Avoid sports with a high risk for falls or impact, such as skiing or horseback riding.
- Increase your calcium intake by drinking more milk (1 quart of skim or low-fat milk per day) or through other sources of calcium. See page 304.

Late Pregnancy (Weeks 29 to 40)

- Follow all of the guidelines listed above.
- Get plenty of rest.
- Take childbirth classes with your partner or designated coach.
- Educate yourself about early signs of labor.
- Have your other children take a class to help them adjust to the new baby.
- Practice relaxation exercises (see page 328). They will be helpful during labor.
- Develop a written birth plan with your health professional that outlines your wishes and expectations throughout the labor and delivery.
- Maintain a good sense of humor.

Cesarean Deliveries

Most babies are delivered vaginally, just as nature intended. However, when the health of the baby or mother is at risk, physicians can deliver the baby through an incision in the mother's abdomen. This is called a Cesarean delivery.

There are 3 main concerns with Cesarean deliveries:

- More risk. Many mothers who have Cesarean deliveries develop infections or bleeding that requires additional medications or treatment. Although more women die as the result of having a Cesarean delivery than do women who have vaginal deliveries, the death rate for both types of delivery is very low.
- Longer recovery. You can usually go home within 1 day after a vaginal delivery. The hospital stay after a Cesarean delivery may be 2 to 3 days. After a Cesarean delivery,

you must limit your activity over the next 4 to 6 weeks to allow the incision to heal.

- Less involvement. The mother and other family members can be more involved with a vaginal delivery. Cesarean delivery is a surgery, which limits family involvement.

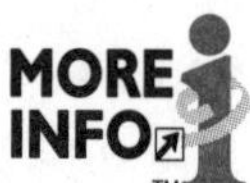

Cesarean deliveries are a good idea when either the baby or the mother is in danger. A Cesarean delivery should not be done just because it is easier to schedule. If you previously had a Cesarean delivery, you can probably have a vaginal delivery with your next pregnancy. Ask your caregiver what you can do to help avoid the need for a Cesarean delivery.

Breastfeeding

Breast milk is the ideal food for your new baby. Consider taking a breastfeeding class before your baby is born. See page 219.

A nursing mother needs to consume 500 more calories per day than she did before becoming pregnant. Although you don't need to drink milk to make milk, extra calcium and protein are important, and your physician may prescribe a vitamin supplement. Avoid smoking and drinking alcoholic or caffeinated beverages. Do not take any medication while breastfeeding unless it is prescribed by a health professional.

Bleeding Between Periods

Many women experience bleeding or spotting between periods. It does not necessarily mean a serious condition is present. Use of an intrauterine device (IUD) may increase your chances of spotting. Some minor bleeding is common during ovulation and during the first few months of using birth control pills. Other hormonal birth control methods, such as Norplant implants and Depo-Provera injections, can cause bleeding between periods. Women who are breastfeeding often have irregular vaginal bleeding or spotting. Stress and hormonal imbalances are other common causes of irregular bleeding. In all of these situations, if the bleeding is not heavy and occurs only occasionally, there is probably no cause for concern. Avoid aspirin, which may prolong the bleeding.

There are other, less common causes of bleeding between periods that may be more serious:

- A woman who is pregnant may continue to have 1 or 2 periods at her usual time. Any bleeding that occurs between those periods is abnormal and may indicate a problem with the pregnancy.
- A woman who is having a miscarriage usually will have cramping, lower abdominal pain, and vaginal bleeding.

- Ectopic pregnancy (when a fertilized egg attaches somewhere other than the uterus, also called tubal pregnancy) usually causes lower abdominal pain, and there may be vaginal bleeding.
- Noncancerous uterine growths (uterine fibroids) can cause spotting or bleeding between periods in some women.
- A pelvic infection also may cause bleeding between periods. Fever, cramping pain, painful sexual intercourse, and a bad-smelling vaginal discharge are other symptoms.
- If the opening of the uterus (cervix) is inflamed, there may be bleeding, especially after sexual intercourse or douching.
- A woman who has gone through menopause should no longer have vaginal bleeding if she is not on hormone replacement therapy (HRT). If she does, she may have an abnormal growth in her uterus and should see a health professional.

When to Call Kaiser Permanente

Call 911 or seek other emergency services immediately if you have severe vaginal bleeding (soaking more than 8 pads or super tampons in 8 hours) and signs of shock (see page 67).

Call Kaiser Permanente:

- If you are pregnant and have any vaginal bleeding.
- If you have new lower abdominal pain with unexpected vaginal bleeding.
- If the bleeding is severe, but you do not have signs of shock.
- If you have irregular vaginal bleeding and a fever of 100° or higher.
- If bleeding between periods lasts longer than 1 week or occurs 3 months in a row.
- If bleeding occurs after sexual intercourse or douching.
- If you are over 35 and have any bleeding between periods or prolonged bleeding with periods.
- If you are using a hormonal method of birth control and your periods are different from what your physician told you to expect.
- If bleeding recurs after you have gone through menopause.

Menopause

For most women, menopause occurs between the ages of 45 and 55, when the production of female hormones (estrogen and progesterone) begins to decline. You may have changes in your menstrual periods before they stop altogether. Every woman is unique and will experience menopause differently.

Osteoporosis is linked to the decrease in estrogen that comes with menopause. See pages 129 and 261.

Women can expect to live 1/3 of their lives after menopause, so it is important to manage any problems related to menopause.

Irregular periods may mean that a woman's menstrual flows are lighter or heavier than usual; that the intervals between periods are shorter or longer; or that there is spotting between periods. Some women have regular periods until their periods stop suddenly, and others have irregular periods for a long time until menopause.

Although you are less fertile during the years before the onset of menopause, you may continue to release eggs (ovulate), so you could become pregnant. If you do not wish to become pregnant, continue to use birth control until your physician confirms that you have reached menopause or until you have not had a menstrual period for 12 months.

Hot flashes are sudden periods of intense heat, sweating, and flushing. A hot flash usually begins in the chest and spreads out to the neck, face, and arms. Seventy-five to 80 percent of women going through menopause will have hot flashes. Hot flashes may occur as frequently as once an hour and last as long as 3 to 4 minutes. If they occur at night, they may disrupt your sleep patterns. Disrupted sleep can lead to insomnia, fatigue, irritability, or inability to concentrate.

Hot flashes usually stop within 1 or 2 years but may persist for several years.

Vaginal dryness, the loss of lubrication and moisture in the vagina, may lead to soreness during and after sexual intercourse. These vaginal changes may also increase your risk for vaginal infections and urinary incontinence. See Vaginitis on page 266 and Urinary Incontinence on page 98.

Mood changes are caused by the hormonal and physical changes of menopause. Symptoms such as nervousness, lack of energy, insomnia, moodiness, or depression are common.

Many women think that menopause means emotional upset and the loss of sexuality. On the other hand, many women look forward to the freedom that menopause brings, particularly freedom from menstrual cycle discomfort and the need for birth control. Understanding what is happening to you and using home care techniques to relieve any discomfort will help you through menopause.

Home Treatment

Irregular periods

Keep a written record of your periods in case you need to discuss them with a health professional.

Hot flashes

Hot flashes usually improve after 1 to 2 years. In the meantime:

- Keep your home and workplace cool.
- Wear layers of loose clothing that can be easily removed.
- Drink lots of water. Drink cold beverages rather than hot ones.
- Eat smaller, more frequent meals to avoid the heat generated by digesting large amounts of food.
- Try the relaxation tips on page 328.

Hormone Therapy

During and after menopause, a woman's body produces much less of the hormone estrogen. Hormone therapy is often prescribed to treat symptoms of menopause and to reduce a woman's risk for osteoporosis. There are 2 types of hormone therapy:

- Estrogen therapy (ET) is estrogen alone. Because ET may increase the risk of cancer in the lining of the uterus (endometrial cancer), it is usually prescribed only for women who have had a hysterectomy. Estrogen is available as tablets or skin patches.
- Hormone therapy (previously called HRT, now called HT or EPT for estrogen progesterone therapy) combines estrogen with progestin, another female hormone. Progestin reduces the effect of estrogen on the uterine lining and protects against cancer of the uterus. Progestins are available as tablets.

Hormone therapy reduces the discomfort of menopausal symptoms such as hot flashes and vaginal dryness. However, hormone therapy can have unpleasant side effects, including bloating, cramping, nausea, breast tenderness, and irregular vaginal bleeding. Estrogen can also be used as a vaginal cream or in a vaginal ring to relieve dryness. With this approach very little hormone is absorbed into the bloodstream; therefore, side effects are unusual and risks are very low.

Hormone therapy is not recommended for women who have had breast cancer, heart disease, stroke, trouble with blood clots, liver disease, or undiagnosed uterine bleeding. According to recent studies, it slightly increases your risk for breast cancer, heart disease, stroke, blood clots, and dementia.

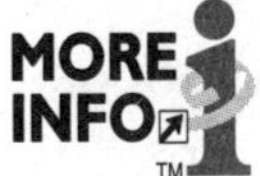

Hormone therapy is no longer recommended for improving general health or even for osteoporosis. It is suggested that HT be used only for a short time to manage severe menopausal symptoms. Talk to your physician or nurse practitioner before deciding whether hormone therapy is a good idea for you.

Vaginal dryness

Use a water-soluble vaginal lubricant, such as Astroglide or Replens, to ease discomfort during sexual-intercourse. Vegetable oil will also work. Do not use Vaseline or other petroleum-based products.

Mood changes

The best thing you can do for yourself is realize that you are not alone. Discuss your symptoms with other women. Give yourself, and ask others for, abundant amounts of love, caring, and understanding. Try to develop a relaxed attitude about menopause. Tension and anxiety may make your symptoms worse.

Hormone therapy may improve hot flashes, vaginal dryness, and mood changes. If these symptoms are very bothersome, talk to your physician about hormone therapy. See page 261.

When to Call Kaiser Permanente

- If your menstrual periods are unusually heavy, irregular, or prolonged (1½ to 2 times longer than normal).
- If bleeding occurs between periods when your periods have been regular.
- If bleeding recurs after periods have stopped for 6 months.
- If your symptoms are interfering with your life and home treatment does not help (see Home Treatment on page 260).
- If you are considering hormone therapy.
- If you have unexplained bleeding (different from what your health professional told you to expect) while you are taking hormones.

Menstrual Cramps

Many women suffer from painful menstrual cramps (dysmenorrhea). Symptoms include mild to severe cramping in the lower abdomen, back, or thighs; headaches; diarrhea or constipation; nausea; dizziness; and fainting. During the menstrual cycle, the lining of the uterus produces a hormone called prostaglandin. This hormone causes the uterus to contract, often painfully. Women who get severe cramps may produce higher-than-normal amounts of prostaglandin or may be more sensitive to its effects.

An intrauterine device (IUD) can cause increased cramping during your period for the first few months of use. If menstrual cramping persists or gets worse, you may need to consider having the IUD removed and choosing another birth control method. Pain caused by endometriosis (a condition in which cells from the lining of the uterus become implanted on other pelvic organs) usually occurs 1 to 2 days before menstrual bleeding begins and continues through the period. Pelvic infections may cause pain at any time, but the pain often occurs after menstrual bleeding has begun. Some women who have noncancerous uterine growths (uterine fibroids) have menstrual cramps.

Home Treatment

- Exercise. Regular workouts decrease the severity of cramps. See Chapter 16.
- Ibuprofen and naproxen sodium generally help ease cramps better than aspirin and acetaminophen do. Take either ibuprofen or naproxen sodium the day before your period starts, or at the first sign of pain. Take these products with milk or food. Otherwise, they may upset your stomach.
- Use heat (hot water bottles, heating pads, or hot baths) to relax tense muscles and relieve cramping.
- Herbal teas (such as chamomile, mint, raspberry, and blackberry) may help soothe tense muscles and anxious moods.
- Try using sanitary pads instead of tampons.
- If symptoms other than cramping (such as weight gain, headache, and tension) occur before your period begins, see Premenstrual Syndrome on page 264.

When to Call Kaiser Permanente

- If sudden, severe pelvic pain occurs, with or without menstrual bleeding.
- If your menstrual cramps have become worse.
- If pelvic pain seems unrelated to your menstrual cycle.
- If you have cramps and a fever of 100° or higher.
- If cramps begin 5 to 7 days before your period starts or continue after your period stops.
- If cramps do not respond to home treatment for 3 cycles, or if they interfere with your normal activities.
- If you suspect that your intrauterine device (IUD) is causing cramps, and the pain is more than you can stand or is worse than what your physician told you to expect.

Missed or Irregular Periods

Missed or irregular periods have a variety of causes. Pregnancy is usually the first cause to be considered, but other common causes include:

- Stress; weight loss or weight gain; increased exercise (missed periods are common in endurance athletes); and travel.
- Use of hormonal birth control methods, such as birth control pills, Depo-Provera injections, and Norplant implants, all of which may cause lighter, less frequent, or skipped periods.

- Menopause or menarche (the start of menstrual periods). For the first few years of menstruation, periods may be irregular.
- Medications, including steroids, tranquilizers, and diet pills.
- Hormonal imbalance or problems in the pelvic organs.
- Breastfeeding.
- Other medical conditions.

If you've skipped a period, try to relax. Restoring your life to emotional and physical balance may help. Many women miss periods now and then. Unless you are pregnant, chances are your cycle will return to normal next month. If you could be pregnant, treat yourself as if you are until you know for sure.

Home Treatment

- If you had sex during the previous month, do a home pregnancy test.
- Avoid fad diets that greatly restrict calories and food variety, and avoid rapid weight loss. To maintain a healthful weight, focus on eating a variety of low-fat foods. See Chapter 17.
- Increase exercise gradually. If you are an endurance athlete, cut back on training or talk with a physician about hormone and calcium supplements to protect against bone loss.
- Learn and practice relaxation techniques to reduce and cope with stress. See page 328.
- If you are age 45 or older, you may be starting menopause. See page 259.

When to Call Kaiser Permanente

- Call immediately if it is possible that you may be pregnant and you are having lower abdominal pain.
- If it is possible that you may be pregnant, make an appointment to confirm your home pregnancy test and begin pregnancy counseling and/or prenatal care.
- If you have missed 2 regular periods, and there is no obvious cause such as those listed previously.
- If you are an endurance athlete who is unable to cut back on training. You may need to take hormones or calcium supplements.
- If you miss 2 or 3 periods while taking birth control pills, and you have not skipped any pills.
- If you have not started having menstrual periods by age 16.

Premenstrual Syndrome

Many women have mild symptoms related to menstruation, such as cramps and mild breast tenderness. These symptoms are considered a normal part of the menstrual cycle. A diagnosis of premenstrual syndrome (PMS) is reserved for symptoms that occur during the

2 weeks before a woman's period begins and that are severe enough to disrupt her life.

About 40 percent of women are affected by PMS at some time in their lives. PMS occurs most often in women in their 20s and 30s and is rare in teenagers.

Many physical and psychological symptoms have been attributed to PMS. Symptoms vary greatly from woman to woman. They can include physical changes such as breast swelling, water retention, bloating, weight gain, and acne; mood and behavior changes such as irritability, depression, difficulty concentrating, decreased sex drive, and aggression; painful symptoms such as headaches, breast tenderness, and muscle aches; and other symptoms such as food cravings, lack of energy, and sleep disturbances.

If you suspect that you have PMS, keep a menstrual diary in which you record:

- Your symptoms and how severe they are.
- Dates when symptoms occur.
- Days when you have your period.

If symptoms consistently occur before your period and end shortly after your period, you may want to follow the home treatment recommendations. Many women find that making small changes in their lives significantly improves their PMS symptoms.

Hysterectomy Guidelines

Hysterectomy is the surgical removal of the uterus. It is generally done to treat disease. However, there are times when other treatments may work as well with fewer risks.

Hysterectomy may be recommended for the following conditions:

- Uterine or cervical cancer.
- Severe uterine bleeding that cannot be controlled by other treatments.
- Ovarian cancer.
- Large, noncancerous tumors (fibroids) that cause severe bleeding and pain or press on the bladder.
- Severe uterine prolapse (uterus falls into the opening of the vagina).

Other treatments may work better for:

- Cervical cancer that develops before menopause and has not spread.
- Abnormal uterine bleeding that responds to drug and other treatments.
- Fibroids that cause mild symptoms.
- Uterine prolapse that responds to nonsurgical treatments.
- Pelvic inflammatory disease that responds to drug and other treatments.

Getting all the facts and thinking about your own needs and values will help you make the best decision about hysterectomy.

Home Treatment

- Eat small meals every 3 to 4 hours that include plenty of whole grains, fruit, and vegetables. Limit fats and sweets, and reduce salt to help limit bloating.
- Eliminate tobacco, alcohol, and caffeine. This may help relieve some symptoms. If you smoke or use other tobacco products, consider getting help to quit. See page 26 for tips on quitting.
- Exercise regularly to help minimize PMS symptoms.
- Try a nonprescription PMS medication such as Midol or Pamprin. Many products contain a combination of drugs to help relieve symptoms of cramps, bloating, and headache.
- Be good to yourself. Reduce your stress level as much as possible. Try relaxation techniques such as yoga and deep breathing. See Chapter 18.
- Talk with others. Your PMS also affects those with whom you live and work. Join a PMS self-help group.
- Take a calcium supplement (600 mg, twice a day). A recent study showed a reduction in PMS symptoms for ½ of women who took a calcium supplement. Taking 400 to 500 mg of magnesium per day can also help reduce PMS symptoms.

When to Call Kaiser Permanente

- If PMS symptoms regularly disrupt your life and keep you from doing your regular activities.
- If you feel out of control because of PMS symptoms.
- If PMS symptoms do not end within a few days after your menstrual bleeding starts.

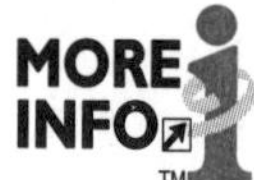

If irritability or mood changes caused by PMS are severely disrupting your life, make an appointment with your physician. He or she may prescribe medication to reduce these symptoms.

Vaginitis

Vaginitis is any vaginal infection, inflammation, or irritation that causes a change in normal vaginal discharge. General symptoms include a change in the amount, color, odor, or texture of vaginal discharge; itching; painful urination; and pain during sexual intercourse. Common types of vaginitis include yeast infection (see page 268), bacterial vaginosis, and trichomoniasis, which is caused by a parasite spread through sexual contact (see page 285). Some other sexually spread diseases can cause unusual vaginal discharge or vaginal irritation. See page 283. In addition, irritation caused by douching frequently, wearing tight clothing, or using strong soaps, perfumed feminine hygiene products, or spermicides may contribute to vaginal irritation or infection.

If you have burning and pain when you urinate and feel the need to urinate often, see Urinary Tract Infections on page 100.

Symptoms of bacterial vaginosis often include a thin, grayish white, fishy-smelling vaginal discharge. The odor is often worse after sex. Bacterial vaginosis is commonly associated with having multiple sex partners, using an intrauterine device (IUD) or diaphragm, exposure to a sexually transmitted disease (STD), or frequent douching, but it may occur in women who don't have these risk factors.

Symptoms of trichomoniasis may include a large amount of frothy, foamy, white, yellow, green, or gray vaginal discharge; vaginal redness, irritation, and swelling; and vaginal odor.

Prevention

- Limit the number of your sex partners and use condoms during sexual intercourse. Having multiple sex partners may increase your risk for vaginitis by changing the normal environment of your vagina.
- If you think frequent vaginal infections may be related to use of a diaphragm or IUD, spermicidal foams or jellies, or condoms, discuss other birth control options with your health professional.
- Wipe from front to back after using the toilet. This will help you avoid spreading bacteria from your anus to your vagina.
- Wash your vaginal area once a day with plain water or a mild, nonperfumed soap. Rinse well and dry thoroughly. Avoid douching unless your health professional instructs you to do so.
- Avoid the use of feminine deodorant sprays and other perfumed products. They irritate and dry tender skin.
- During your period, change tampons at least 3 times a day, or alternate tampons with pads. Remember to remove the last tampon used during your period.
- Antibiotic medications can kill the healthy bacteria that grow in your vagina. If you are taking an antibiotic, drink acidophilus milk or eat yogurt that contains live *Lactobacillus* cultures to help prevent vaginitis.
- Avoid panty hose and tight nylon underwear, which limit air circulation to your vaginal area.

Home Treatment

A vaginal infection may clear up without treatment in 3 or 4 days. If your symptoms do not improve, call Kaiser Permanente.

- Avoid sexual intercourse to give irritated vaginal tissues time to heal.
- Do not scratch. Relieve itching with a cold water compress or cool baths.
- Make sure the cause of vaginitis is not a forgotten tampon or another foreign object.
- Do not douche unless your health professional instructs you to do so.
- Wear loose-fitting, cotton clothing; avoid nylon and synthetics.
- If you think you may be pregnant, do a home pregnancy test.
- If itching is the most bothersome symptom, try a nonprescription vaginal cream or suppositories for yeast infections. See Yeast Infections on page 268.

When to Call Kaiser Permanente

- If you have pelvic or lower abdominal pain, fever, and unusual vaginal discharge.
- If you have pain or bleeding after sexual intercourse (and the pain is not eased by using a vaginal lubricant such as Astroglide).
- If you have an unusual or foul-smelling vaginal discharge.
- If you have vaginal itching that does not go away after you use a nonprescription medication for yeast infections.
- If you think you've been exposed to a sexually transmitted disease (see page 283). Your sex partner may need to be treated too.
- If you plan to see a health professional, do not douche, use vaginal creams, or have sexual intercourse for 48 hours before your appointment. Doing these things may make your problem more difficult to diagnose.

Yeast Infections

A vaginal yeast infection (candidiasis) is caused by an excess growth of yeast organisms in the vagina. Yeast infections are common in women of childbearing age. They can cause severe discomfort but rarely cause serious problems.

Common symptoms of yeast infection include vaginal itching (often severe); white, curdy, usually odorless vaginal discharge; and pain when urinating and during sexual intercourse. The skin around the vagina (labia) may be red and irritated. If you have burning and pain when urinating and feel the need to urinate often, see Urinary Tract Infections on page 100.

Yeast infections are not spread by sexual contact. However, some physicians feel that treating your sex partner with antifungal medications may help prevent recurrent yeast infections.

Yeast infections are commonly associated with antibiotic or steroid use, pregnancy, diabetes, and illnesses that weaken the immune system. In addition, douching frequently, wearing tight clothing, or using strong soaps or perfumed feminine hygiene products may contribute to vaginal irritation or infection.

Prevention

- Drink acidophilus milk or eat yogurt that contains live *Lactobacillus* organisms. Yogurt has been shown to prevent vaginal yeast infections.
- Wear cotton or cotton-lined underwear. Avoid tight-fitting pants and undergarments. They increase heat and moisture in the vaginal area, which may allow yeast to grow more easily in your vagina.
- Avoid feminine sprays, talcs, or perfumes in your vaginal area, because they may affect the balance among the microorganisms in your vagina. Do not douche unless your health professional instructs you to do so.
- Wipe your vaginal area from front to back after using the toilet and when bathing.
- If you have diabetes, limiting your sugar intake and controlling your diabetes will help prevent yeast infections.

Home Treatment

Left untreated, vaginal yeast infections often clear up on their own, usually when your period begins. Be sure you have a yeast infection before you try self-treatment.

- Use a nonprescription antifungal medication for yeast infections (such as Gyne-Lotrimin, Monistat 7, or a store brand) as directed.
- Drink acidophilus milk or regularly eat yogurt that contains live *Lactobacillus* cultures.
- Douche with yogurt that contains live *Lactobacillus* cultures. Talk with your physician before using a yogurt douche.
- Avoid excessive cleaning of your vaginal area. Wash once a day with plain water or a mild, nonperfumed soap.
- Don't use tampons while using a topical treatment (cream or vaginal suppositories) for a vaginal yeast infection. The tampons can absorb the medication. Use sanitary pads instead.
- If sexual intercourse causes discomfort, avoid it until your symptoms go away.

When to Call Kaiser Permanente

- If you develop lower abdominal pain or a fever greater than 101° along with symptoms of a vaginal yeast infection.
- If you think this is the first time you've had a yeast infection, or if you aren't sure whether your symptoms are being caused by a yeast infection.
- If home treatment with a nonprescription antifungal product fails to clear up a yeast infection within 3 or 4 days, or if you are using antifungal creams repeatedly.
- If you have symptoms of a urinary tract infection. See page 100.
- If you are or may be pregnant.
- If symptoms of a yeast infection return within 2 months and you have not been taking antibiotics.

If you plan to see a health professional, do not douche, use vaginal creams, or have sexual intercourse for 48 hours before your appointment. Doing these things may make your problem more difficult to diagnose.

The man who says it cannot be done should not interrupt the man doing it.
Old Chinese Proverb

14

Men's Health

This chapter focuses on health problems that are unique to men. If you are looking for general guidelines for making healthful lifestyle choices to prevent illness and injury, see Chapter 2, Living a Healthy Life. Specific tips for developing a fitness plan, eating a healthful diet, maintaining a healthful body weight, managing stress, and preventing sexually transmitted diseases are included in other chapters. Use the index to find the information you need.

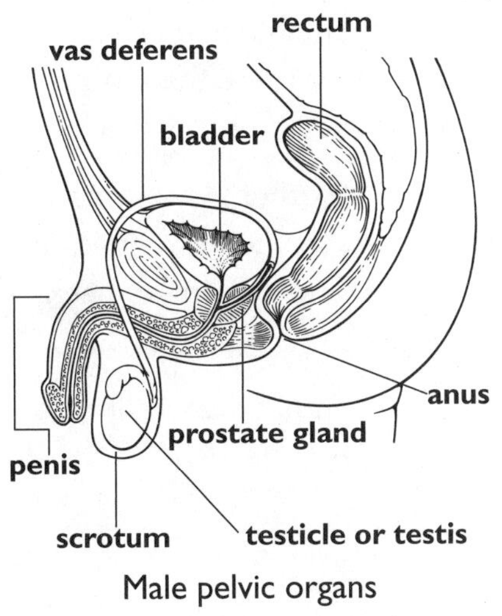

Male pelvic organs

Genital Health

Daily cleansing of the penis, particularly under the foreskin of an uncircumcised penis, can prevent bacterial infection. Daily washing also reduces the already low risk of penile cancer. Boys should be taught by age 3 or 4 to start to gently pull back (retract) the foreskin. The foreskin may not be fully retractable until puberty. Wash the penis, and replace the foreskin over the head of the penis after cleansing. Do not forcibly retract a child's foreskin if it is painful or difficult to do so.

Erection Problems

Erection problems are common and can often be solved with self-care. By definition, an erection problem is difficulty in raising or maintaining an erection capable of intercourse.

Erection problems are often caused by stress at work, tension in relationships, depression, fatigue, lack of privacy, physical injury, alcohol, or side effects of medications. These causes are generally temporary and will usually resolve with home treatment. Other, less reversible causes include diabetes, a long history of smoking, nerve damage, and vascular disease.

The ease of gaining and sustaining erections generally decreases with age. However, with the right foreplay and environment, there is no age limit to the ability of healthy men to have erections.

Prevention

Most erection problems can be prevented or resolved by taking a more relaxed approach to lovemaking and watching for possible side effects from medications or illnesses.

Home Treatment

- Rule out medications first. Many drugs, especially blood pressure medicines, water pills (diuretics), and mood-altering drugs, have side effects that can cause erection problems. Ask your physician or pharmacist to check your medications for possible effects on sexual function, or look it up yourself.
- Avoid alcohol and smoking, which make erection problems worse. If you smoke or use other tobacco products, consider getting help to quit. See page 26 for tips on quitting.
- Cope with stress (see Chapter 18). Tension in your life can distract you and make getting erections difficult. Regular physical activity and other stress-relieving activities may help ease tension.
- Take time for more foreplay. Let your partner know that you would enjoy some stroking. Slow down; then slow down some more.
- Make sure you're ready. If you have recently experienced a loss or change in a relationship, you may not yet be emotionally ready for erections. Generally, your stress will subside and your erection problem will disappear over time. Do what you can to relax.
- Find out if you can have erections at other times. If you can have an erection during masturbation or on awakening, the problem is probably stress-related or may be caused by an emotional problem.

When to Call Kaiser Permanente

- If you think that a medication may be causing the problem. Your physician may prescribe a different medication.
- If you are unable to have an erection at all, or think that your problem may be a physical one.
- If you have other symptoms such as urinary problems, pain in the lower abdomen or lower back, or fever.
- If your symptoms are related to a recent injury.

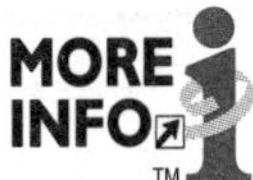

If you have tried home treatment for a few months but your symptoms have not improved, you may wish to talk with your physician about erection-producing medications or injections, a vacuum device, or a penile implant. Getting all the facts and thinking about your own and your partner's needs and values will help you make a wise decision about treatment for erection problems.

Prostate Infection (Prostatitis)

The prostate is a doughnut-shaped gland that lies under the bladder, about halfway between the rectum and the base of the penis. It encircles the urethra, the tube that carries urine from the bladder out through the penis. This walnut-sized gland produces some of the fluid that transports sperm during ejaculation.

There are 4 types of prostatitis. They include nonbacterial prostatitis, which has no known cause; acute and chronic bacterial prostatitis; and prostatodynia, which is often related to stress or anxiety. Symptoms are similar for all forms of prostatitis. With the exception of acute bacterial prostatitis (in which the symptoms are severe, come on suddenly, and may include fever and chills), it is difficult to determine the exact kind of prostatitis a man has based on symptoms alone.

Symptoms may include:

- Frequent urge to urinate, but passing only small amounts of urine.
- Burning sensation when urinating; inability to empty the bladder completely.
- Difficulty starting urination; interrupted or weaker-than-normal urine flow; and dribbling after urinating.
- Urinating excessively at night.
- Pain or discomfort in the lower back; the scrotum; the area between the scrotum and the anus; the lower abdomen; the upper thighs; or above the pubic area.
- Prostate pain or vague discomfort during ejaculation.
- Pain during ejaculation and blood in the semen.
- Difficulty achieving or maintaining an erection.

Bacterial prostate infections usually respond well to self-care and antibiotics. If the infection recurs, long-term antibiotic treatment may be needed. Prostate infections that are not caused by bacteria usually respond to home treatment.

Prevention

There is no reliable way to prevent prostatitis. Taking the full amount of the antibiotic prescribed by your physician for acute or chronic bacterial prostatitis can reduce the possibility of having another infection in the future.

Home Treatment

- Avoid alcohol, caffeine, and spicy foods, especially if they make your symptoms worse.
- Take hot baths to help soothe pain and reduce stress.
- Eat plenty of high-fiber foods, and drink enough water to avoid constipation. Straining to pass stools can be very painful when your prostate is inflamed.
- Taking aspirin or ibuprofen may help ease painful prostate symptoms.

When to Call Kaiser Permanente

- If urinary symptoms occur with fever, chills, vomiting, or pain in the back or abdomen.
- If your urine is red or pink and there is no dietary reason for this (see page 102). Always call your physician if you have blood in your urine.
- If symptoms continue for 5 days despite home treatment.
- If your symptoms suddenly change or get worse.
- If you have pain during urination or ejaculation. If there is also an unusual discharge from your penis, see pages 283 to 285.
- If you have urinary symptoms, such as trouble starting to urinate, inability to empty your bladder completely, or frequent urination (especially at night), that are not related to drinking more fluids.

Prostate Enlargement

As men age, the prostate may enlarge (benign prostatic hyperplasia). This seems to be a natural process and is not really a disease. However, as the gland gets bigger, it tends to squeeze the urethra and cause urinary problems, such as:

- Difficulty getting the urine stream started and completely stopped (dribbling).
- Frequent urge to urinate, or being awakened by the urge to urinate.
- Decreased force of the urine stream.
- Having the sense that the bladder is not completely empty after urinating.

An enlarged prostate gland is not a serious problem unless urination becomes extremely difficult or backed-up urine causes bladder infections or kidney damage. Some dribbling after urination is very common and not necessarily a sign of prostate problems.

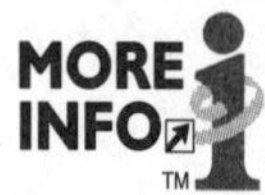

Surgery is usually not necessary for an enlarged prostate. Although surgery used to be a common treatment, recent research shows that most cases of prostate enlargement do not get worse over time. Many men find that their symptoms are stable, and sometimes symptoms even clear up on their own. In these cases, the best treatment may be no treatment at all. Drugs are available that may help improve symptoms in many men. Your physician can advise you about the various treatment options.

Prevention

Since the prostate produces seminal fluid, there is a long-standing belief that ejaculating regularly (2 to 3 times per week) will help prevent an enlarged prostate. There is no scientific proof of this, but it is risk-free.

Home Treatment

- Avoid antihistamines and decongestants, which can make urinary problems worse.
- If you are bothered by a frequent urge to urinate at night, cut down on beverages before bedtime, especially alcohol and caffeine. Continue to drink at least 8 glasses of water and other fluids during the day.
- Don't postpone urinating, and take plenty of time. Try sitting on the toilet instead of standing.
- If dribbling after urinating is a problem, wash your penis once a day to prevent skin infections.
- Also see Urinary Incontinence on page 98.

When to Call Kaiser Permanente

- If you are unable to urinate, or if you feel as if you cannot empty your bladder completely.
- If you develop fever, back or abdominal pain, or chills.
- If there is blood or pus in your urine.
- Water pills (diuretics), tranquilizers, antihistamines, decongestants, and antidepressants can aggravate urinary problems. If you take any of these drugs, ask your physician if there are other medications you could use that do not cause these urinary side effects.
- If the symptoms of an enlarged prostate come on quickly, are bothersome enough that you want help, or last longer than 2 months.

Prostate Cancer

Prostate cancer is the second leading cause of cancer deaths in men. When detected early, before it has spread to other organs, prostate cancer may be curable. A man's risk for prostate cancer increases with age, and most cases develop in men over 65. Since it tends to develop late in life and usually grows slowly, prostate cancer does not usually shorten a man's life. However, the younger you are and the larger or more advanced the cancer is, the more serious the disease may be.

There are no specific symptoms of prostate cancer. Most men have no symptoms at all. In a few cases, it can cause urinary symptoms very similar to those of prostate enlargement (see page 274). In advanced cases, other symptoms, such as pain, may develop if the cancer spreads to other organs or to the bones.

Prostate cancer sometimes runs in families, is more common in African-American men, and tends to be more common in men who eat a high-fat diet.

Prevention

Eating a low-fat diet that includes plenty of fruits and vegetables is the only known way to reduce your risk for prostate cancer. There is some evidence that eating more foods that contain cooked tomatoes (7 to 10 servings per week) may decrease your risk for prostate cancer.

There is controversy about the value of using digital rectal exams and the prostate-specific antigen (PSA) blood test to screen all men for prostate cancer. Using these tests to detect early prostate cancer may not improve quality of life or prolong life, especially in men who are older or have other serious health problems. Therefore, many experts are uncertain whether routine digital rectal exams or PSA tests are appropriate for all men. Talk with your physician for more information about prostate cancer screening.

Home Treatment

Prostate cancer treatment is tailored to each individual. Work with your physician to be sure that you will receive the long-term benefits from the treatment you choose.

Learn all you can about the available treatment options, which may include watchful waiting, so that you and your physician can select the one best suited for you. Your age, overall health, other medical conditions, and the characteristics of the cancer are all important factors to consider when you make treatment decisions.

When to Call Kaiser Permanente

- If any urinary symptoms (see Prostate Enlargement on page 274) come on quickly, are bothersome enough that you want help, or last longer than 2 months.
- If you want to discuss screening for prostate cancer, especially if you have a relative who developed prostate cancer.

Testicular Problems

The testicles produce sperm and male hormones. Males usually have 2 testicles, located behind the penis inside a sac of skin called the scrotum. It is normal for one testicle to be slightly larger than the other.

Each testicle is suspended at the end of a spermatic cord, a network of blood vessels that carry blood to and from the testicle. Sperm cells leave the testicle through the epididymis (a coiled tube located at the top of the testicle). Then they move through a tube called the vas deferens and are deposited in the seminal vesicles, which are near the prostate gland.

Sperm mix with fluids produced by the seminal vesicles and the prostate to create semen, which exits the body through the penis during sexual activity.

The location of the testicles makes them prone to injury, especially during contact sports. Wearing a protective athletic "cup" can prevent injuries. Pain caused by a testicular injury usually goes away within an hour or so. However, if pain persists, or if a testicle becomes swollen or bruised, see a health professional.

Testicular torsion occurs when one of the testicles rotates, twisting the spermatic cord and cutting off blood flow to the testicle. Testicular torsion can occur at any age, but it is most common in young boys. It may occur after strenuous physical activity or after an injury, but it often has no specific cause and may occur while a boy is sleeping.

Symptoms of testicular torsion include sudden, severe pain in one testicle that may radiate to the lower abdomen; swelling high in the scrotum; nausea and vomiting; and fever.

Testicular torsion is a medical emergency. Surgery is often needed to restore blood flow to the testicle. If the procedure is not done within a few hours after the onset of symptoms, the testicle can be permanently damaged and may have to be removed.

Epididymitis is inflammation of the epididymis. It can be caused by a bacterial infection (including chlamydia, which is spread through sexual contact, see page 283). Irritation resulting from a bladder infection or injury is another cause of epididymitis. Epididymitis causes pain and swelling in the scrotum that develops gradually, over hours or days, and can become severe. The scrotum may feel hot and be tender to the touch, and the person may have a fever. Bacterial epididymitis is usually treated with antibiotics.

Orchitis is inflammation of the testicle. It may be caused by a bacterial infection or by a virus such as the mumps virus. Orchitis can also occur with epididymitis or a prostate infection (prostatitis). Symptoms include scrotal pain; swelling (usually on one side of the scrotum); and a feeling of heaviness in the scrotum. If it is not treated, orchitis can cause infertility.

Testicular cancer is rare and most often affects males between the ages of 15 and 34. Those at highest risk include males whose testicles have not descended or did not descend until after age 6, and males with a family history of testicular cancer. Testicular cancer usually affects only one testicle and responds well to treatment if detected early. Symptoms of testicular cancer may include a painless lump or swelling or a feeling of heaviness in one testicle.

Prevention

- Prevent testicular injury by wearing a protective athletic "cup" when you play sports.

- Prevent bacterial infections that are spread through sexual contact by following the safer sex guidelines on pages 285 and 287.
- Make sure your child has completed the measles, mumps, and rubella (MMR) vaccination series. See page 17.
- Teenage boys and men who are at increased risk for testicular cancer should do a testicular self-exam once a month. After taking a warm bath or shower:
    - Stand and place your right leg on an elevated surface such as the side of the bathtub or the toilet seat.
    - Examine the surface of your right testicle by gently rolling it between the thumb and fingers of both hands. Feel for any hard lumps or nodules. The testicle should feel round and smooth.
    - Feel for any enlargement of the testicle or a change in its consistency. It is normal for one testicle to be slightly larger than the other. Report any major size differences to a health professional.
    - Repeat the exam on your left testicle.

Home Treatment

- Elevating the scrotum with a pillow and applying ice may help relieve pain caused by an injury.
- Wearing a jock strap daily may relieve scrotal pain.

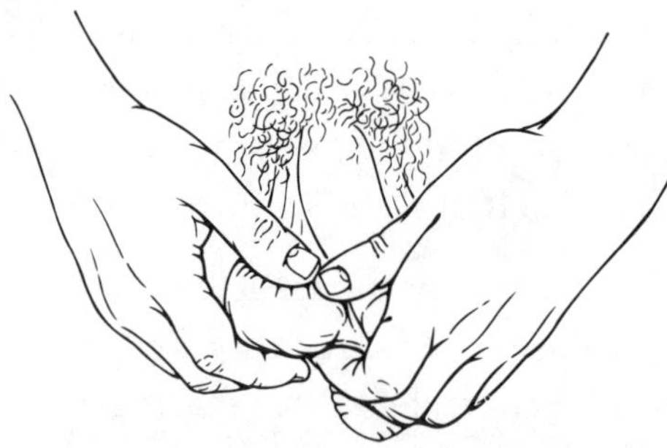

Gently feel each testicle for hard lumps or a change in size.

- Take aspirin or acetaminophen to relieve pain caused by orchitis. Do not give aspirin to anyone younger than 20. Warm baths may also help relieve pain.

When to Call Kaiser Permanente

- If you find a lump in a testicle.
- If you notice any enlargement in a testicle or a change in its consistency.
- If pain in a testicle or the scrotum comes on suddenly and is severe.
- If pain and/or swelling in a testicle or the scrotum worsens over a period of several hours or days.
- If pain and/or swelling in a testicle or the scrotum is accompanied by fever.
- If pain and/or swelling in the scrotum develops after exposure to the mumps virus.
- If pain resulting from an injury does not go away or if swelling does not lessen after a few days.
- If you have a feeling of heaviness in one testicle.

I wasn't kissing her, I was whispering in her mouth.
Groucho Marx

15 Sexual Health

This chapter covers some issues of concern to people who are sexually active, including birth control and sexually transmitted diseases (STDs). Infection with the human immunodeficiency virus (HIV), which causes AIDS, is also included.

Birth Control

Birth control can help prevent unplanned pregnancies. However, no birth control method (except abstinence) is 100 percent effective and without risks. The text that follows and the chart on page 280 briefly describe the most common birth control methods.

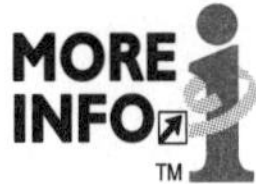

Review each of the birth control methods presented in this chapter with your partner before deciding which one meets your needs. Your health professional can help you better understand the effectiveness and risks of each method.

Use all birth control methods exactly as your physician or the package instructions recommend. Proper use helps ensure effectiveness.

If you have sexual intercourse without using a birth control method and are concerned about a possible pregnancy, call your physician or advice nurse as soon as possible for information about emergency contraception. Emergency contraceptive pills can prevent pregnancy AFTER you have had sex without using birth control. These pills can be taken anytime within 72 hours (3 days) after having unprotected sex. The sooner you take them after having sex, the more effective they are in preventing pregnancy. See "Emergency Contraception" on page 281.

Hormonal methods of birth control for women either prevent the ovaries from releasing an egg each month (ovulation) or thicken the mucus at the opening of the uterus so sperm can't get to the uterus to fertilize an

Birth Control

Method	Pregnancies*	Comments
Sterilization Tubal ligation (women) Vasectomy (men)	Fewer than 1	Consider it permanent.
Hormonal Methods		
Oral contraceptives (the Pill)	5	Decreases risk of uterine and ovarian cancer. Increased risk of circulatory disorders and high blood pressure in women who smoke.
Emergency contraception pill	1	Use within 72 hours after having unprotected sex.
Depo-Provera (shot) Lunelle (shot)	Fewer than 1	Depo-Provera may cause irregular menstrual bleeding. Monthly period with Lunelle.
Intrauterine Device (IUD)	Fewer than 1	Effective for 5 to 10 years, depending on type. May be expelled without being noticed. May cause bleeding and cramping. Levonorgestrel IUD decreases bleeding and cramping.
Barrier Methods		
Condom (male)	14	For maximum protection against STDs, use latex or polyurethane condoms every time you have sex.
Condom (female)	21	
Diaphragm (with spermicide)	20	
Cervical cap (with spermicide)	20 to 40	
Spermicides		
Jelly, cream, foam, suppositories	26	Use with a condom for best protection.
Used with condom	6	
Periodic Abstinence (natural family planning: basal body temperature, mucus, or rhythm/calendar method)	25	
Withdrawal	19	
No method (chance)	85	

*Typical number of accidental pregnancies per 100 women in 1 year. When birth control methods are used exactly as directed, pregnancy rates are lower. Adapted from: R. Hatcher et al., *Contraceptive Technology, 1998.*

egg. All hormonal birth control methods require a physician's prescription. Hormonal methods of birth control do not protect against STDs.

Oral contraceptives (the Pill) are taken daily. Depo-Provera is a hormone injection given by a health professional once every 3 months. Lunelle is a monthly hormone injection.

The intrauterine device (IUD) is a plastic device that is inserted into the uterus by a physician, nurse practitioner, or certified nurse midwife. Some IUDs, such as the levonorgestrel intrauterine system (Mirena), release a hormone to prevent conception. Other IUDs release copper, which appears to kill sperm. IUDs do not provide any protection against STDs. IUDs are ideal for women who want a reversible form of birth control and are in a mutually monogamous relationship.

Barrier methods of birth control kill sperm and/or keep sperm from entering the uterus and reaching the egg. Barrier methods work best when 2 methods are combined; for example, male condoms used with spermicidal foam.

Emergency Contraception

Emergency contraception either prevents the release of an egg from a woman's ovaries (ovulation) or prevents a fertilized egg from implanting in the uterus. It can be very effective for preventing unintended pregnancy if you use it soon after you have unprotected sex.

Sometimes called the "morning-after pill," emergency contraceptive pills (usually a high-dose form of regular birth control pills) can be taken anytime within 72 hours after you have unprotected sex. Inserting a copper-bearing intrauterine device (IUD) within 5 to 7 days after intercourse is another method of emergency contraception.

Regardless of method, the sooner you use emergency contraception, the more effective it is in preventing pregnancy.

If you have sexual intercourse and are concerned about a possible pregnancy because you did not use birth control or because your birth control may have failed (for instance, if a condom or diaphragm tore or you skipped a birth control pill), call your health professional immediately for information about emergency contraception.

The male condom is a thin, flexible tube of latex rubber or animal skin that is placed over the man's erect penis before sexual intercourse to catch ejaculated semen. There are also condoms for women that fit inside the vagina to protect against STDs and unplanned pregnancy. Latex or polyurethane condoms provide the most reliable, but not total, protection against STDs, including HIV. Lambskin condoms are not effective in preventing STDs. Condoms are available without a physician's prescription. Many condoms are lubricated with a spermicide. Condoms can be used with other birth control methods for added protection against STDs.

Spermicides are foams, jellies, and suppositories that contain chemicals which kill sperm. Spermicides are available without a physician's prescription. Most spermicides contain nonoxynol-9. Some people are allergic to nonoxynol-9 and may develop sores in the vagina or on the penis after coming in contact with it. Sometimes the allergic reaction is triggered by other chemicals in the spermicide, and switching to a different product solves the problem.

The diaphragm and cervical cap are small rubber caps that are filled with spermicide and inserted into the vagina to cover the opening to the uterus (cervix) before sexual intercourse begins. They are left in place for 6 hours or longer after sexual intercourse. Both the diaphragm and the cervical cap require a physician's prescription. When used alone, these barrier methods provide minimal protection against STDs.

Surgical methods of contraception include vasectomy (men) and tubal ligation (women). During a vasectomy, the tubes (vas deferens) that carry a man's sperm from his testes are clamped or cut off, thus preventing sperm from being ejaculated in semen. Tubal ligation procedures close off or cut the tubes (fallopian tubes) that carry a woman's eggs from her ovaries to her uterus. This prevents eggs from being fertilized or implanting in the uterus. Both vasectomy and tubal ligation should be considered permanent, but in some cases they can be successfully reversed with surgery. Surgical methods of birth control do not protect you against STDs.

Natural family planning (fertility awareness) methods help a couple estimate when the woman is most likely to become pregnant (during ovulation) so they can avoid sexual intercourse during that time. To estimate when ovulation occurs, a woman records her temperature, examines her vaginal mucus discharge, and tracks her menstrual periods. Natural family planning is the least effective method of birth control. It does not provide protection against STDs.

Sexually Transmitted Diseases

Sexually transmitted diseases (STDs) or venereal diseases (VD) are infections passed from person to person through sexual intercourse (vaginal or anal), genital contact, or contact with fluids such as semen, vaginal fluids, and blood (including menstrual blood). Many of these diseases can also be spread by sharing needles and other items that may be contaminated with infected blood or body fluids. Chlamydia, trichomoniasis, genital herpes, genital warts, gonorrhea, hepatitis B, and syphilis are among the most common STDs. HIV infection, which causes AIDS (acquired immune deficiency syndrome), is also an STD and is discussed on page 286.

Chlamydia, gonorrhea, hepatitis B, herpes simplex virus, HIV, and syphilis can be spread from an infected mother to her unborn baby or infant. At this time, the hepatitis B vaccine is the only immunization available to prevent the spread of disease from mother to child. If you are infected with any of these diseases, talk to your physician about how you can protect your baby before and after it is born.

Chlamydia is a bacterial infection that affects millions of men and women. It may be difficult to detect chlamydia; about 75 percent of women and 20 percent of men with the disease have no symptoms, but they can still infect their sex partners. If symptoms do show up, they occur 1 to 3 weeks after exposure to the bacteria. In women, symptoms may include vaginal discharge or irregular menstrual bleeding, pain when urinating, or lower abdominal pain. In men, there may be a discharge from the penis and pain when urinating.

All sexually active females between the ages of 15 and 25 should get tested for chlamydia every year.

Chlamydia is easily treated with antibiotics. If undetected and untreated, chlamydia can cause pelvic inflammatory disease (infection in the ovaries and fallopian tubes), which may lead to sterility (inability to conceive a child).

Genital herpes is caused by the herpes simplex virus, which also causes cold sores (see page 204). Genital herpes is easily spread from one partner to another or from one part of the body to another through direct contact with a herpes sore. Oral sex (mouth on genitals) can pass herpes from the mouth to the genitals or from the genitals to the mouth.

Symptoms of the first genital herpes outbreak occur 2 to 7 days after contact with an infected person. It is also possible to be infected with genital herpes and have no symptoms.

The first case of genital herpes may be quite severe, with many painful sores or blisters. Fever, swollen glands, and headache or muscle aches may also occur. If the sores develop inside the urethra (the tube that carries urine out of the body) or the vagina, there may be pain when urinating or vaginal discharge. The sores crust over and disappear in 2 to 3 weeks.

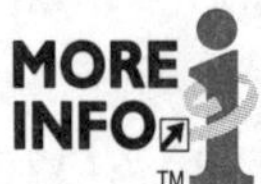

There is no known cure for genital herpes. Most people with genital herpes have recurrent outbreaks. Having 4 outbreaks per year is typical. Outbreaks tend to become less frequent and less severe over time. Itching, burning, or tingling may occur at the place where the sores will later appear. Medication may be helpful if you have very frequent and severe outbreaks.

Genital warts are caused by the human papillomavirus (HPV), which is spread through sexual contact. The warts generally look like small, fleshy bumps or flat, white patches on the lips around the vagina (labia), inside the vagina, on the penis or scrotum, or around the anus. A person infected with HPV may never develop genital warts, or the warts may be too small to be seen. Certain types of HPV seem to increase the risk of cervical cancer in women. A Pap test can occasionally detect the virus.

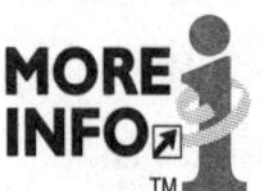

If genital warts are bothersome or develop on the cervix, they can be removed by a health professional. However, wart removal does not cure HPV infection, and the warts may recur. There does not appear to be an effective cure for HPV infection at this time. However, in many people the infection goes away by itself and does not cause further problems.

Gonorrhea is a bacterial infection that is spread through sexual contact. Symptoms, which appear 2 days to 2 weeks after infection, may include painful or frequent urination, vaginal discharge, irregular menstrual bleeding, or a thick discharge from the penis. Many people who are infected have no symptoms.

Untreated gonorrhea can lead to pelvic inflammatory disease and sterility in women; it can lead to prostate infection (see page 273) in men. Gonorrhea sometimes spreads to a person's joints, causing arthritis. Antibiotic treatment cures the infection. Both sex partners need to be treated to keep from passing the infection back and forth.

Hepatitis B is a viral infection that is spread through contact with infected blood, semen, or vaginal fluid (see page 97). The hepatitis B virus (HBV) is very contagious and may be spread to household contacts (other than sex partners) by sharing such things as razors and toothbrushes. Most people with hepatitis B recover completely after 4 to 8 weeks, but a small percentage of adults remain infected for months or years. Chronic infection can lead to life-threatening liver damage. Drug treatment for chronic HBV infection is not very effective.

People at risk for HBV infection (those with more than 1 sex partner; men who have sex with men; people who use intravenous drugs; and health care workers) should receive the hepatitis B vaccine. The vaccine is also recommended for all infants. See page 18.

Syphilis is a bacterial infection spread through sexual contact and through sharing needles contaminated with an infected person's blood. When syphilis is spread through sexual contact, symptoms appear about 3 weeks after infection occurs. The first symptom is a red sore that appears on the genitals, rectal area, or mouth. The sore is usually painless and may go unnoticed. Swollen lymph nodes near the sore are another possible symptom.

If syphilis is not treated early, it can proceed to a second phase after about 2 months. Symptoms of the second phase include a rash, patchy hair loss, fever, swollen lymph nodes, and flu-like symptoms that are easily confused with other illnesses. Syphilis can be treated with antibiotics. If untreated, syphilis may cause serious problems and premature death.

Trichomoniasis is a bacterial infection that is spread through sexual contact. In women, the bacteria usually infect the vagina or urethra. In men, infections can develop in the urethra or under the foreskin of the penis.

Up to ½ of women who have trichomoniasis have no symptoms, and symptoms in infected men are rare. If symptoms do appear, they do so 4 to 28 days after infection occurs. Symptoms in women may include vaginal discharge, itching, and irritation and pain during sexual intercourse and when urinating. In men there may be a discharge from the penis and pain when urinating.

Trichomoniasis usually does not lead to serious illness. However, the infected person and his or her sex partner need to be treated with antibiotics to keep from passing the infection back and forth. Condoms should be used until treatment is completed.

Prevention

Preventing a sexually transmitted disease is easier than treating an infection once it occurs. Only monogamy (you and your partner have sex only with each other) between uninfected partners or sexual abstinence completely eliminates the risk.

- Avoid sexual contact while you or your partner is being treated for a sexually transmitted disease.
- If you or your partner has herpes, avoid sexual contact when a blister or any open sore is present. Use condoms unless you are in a stable, monogamous relationship and you have considered the risks associated with having unprotected sex with a person who has genital herpes.

- The same behaviors that reduce your risk for HIV infection also reduce your risk of getting other STDs. See page 287 for additional prevention guidelines, including condom use.

When to Call Kaiser Permanente

Call if you notice any unusual discharge from the vagina or penis; sores, redness, or growths on the genitals; or if you suspect that you have been exposed to an STD.

STDs need to be diagnosed and treated by a health professional. Your physician or a clinician at your local health department can diagnose and treat STDs. Your sex partner may also need to be treated, even if he or she has no symptoms. Otherwise, your partner may reinfect you or develop serious complications.

HIV Infection and AIDS

Human immunodeficiency virus (HIV) is spread when blood, semen, or vaginal fluids from an infected person enter someone else's body. Once a person becomes infected, the virus attacks and gradually weakens his or her immune system. AIDS is the last phase in HIV disease, when the body is no longer able to fight infection or disease. Without treatment, AIDS develops in most people 12 to 13 years after they first become infected with HIV. With treatment, AIDS may be delayed for many more years.

A person is said to be HIV-positive if antibodies to the virus are detected in his or her blood. It may take up to 6 months after infection for the antibodies to appear. However, the virus can be spread to others before antibodies or symptoms are apparent.

The specific behaviors that spread HIV include:

- Sharing injection needles, syringes, or drug-use equipment with someone who is HIV-positive.
- Unprotected (without a condom) rectal entry intercourse (anal sex) with someone who is HIV-positive. Anal sex often tears the rectal blood vessels, allowing the virus to enter the body.
- Vaginal intercourse without a condom or oral sexual activity with someone who is HIV-positive.

Babies born to or breastfed by women who are HIV-positive are also at high risk for becoming infected with the virus. Anti-HIV viral medications taken during pregnancy and labor greatly reduce the chances of passing the virus from mother to child.

Because all donated blood has been tested for HIV since 1985, the risk of getting the virus from transfused blood or blood products is extremely low.

HIV is not spread by mosquitoes; toilet seats; being coughed on by an infected person; casual contact with someone who is HIV-positive or who has AIDS; or by donating blood. Being touched, hugged, or lightly kissed by someone who is HIV-positive will not transfer the virus to you.

A simple, confidential blood test, available from your physician or a health department, can determine if you are HIV-positive. All pregnant women and any individual who is at high risk should have this test. Although new tests may detect HIV as early as 3 weeks after infection, it may take up to 6 months for HIV antibodies to develop. The virus can be transmitted even before antibodies have developed. Even after antibodies develop, some people remain free of symptoms for well over 10 years but can still transmit the virus to others.

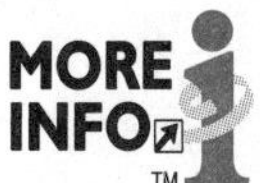

People who educate themselves about HIV infection learn how to make wise health decisions about preventing the spread of the virus and seek treatments that may improve their chances for staying healthy longer.

Symptoms of HIV Infection

Early symptoms of HIV infection may mimic flu and can also include a rash and swollen glands. Common symptoms of later-stage HIV infection include:

- Rapid, unexplained weight loss.
- Unexplained fever and night sweats.
- Severe fatigue.
- Diarrhea or other bowel changes.
- Shortness of breath and a persistent dry cough.
- Mouth sores.
- Swollen lymph nodes in the neck, armpits, or groin.

These symptoms can be caused by many illnesses other than HIV infection. However, if any symptom develops or persists without a good explanation, especially if your behavior puts you at risk for HIV infection, call your physician.

Researchers believe that most people who are HIV-positive will eventually develop AIDS. Although there is still no cure for HIV infection or AIDS, new treatments have dramatically improved the lives and health of people with HIV. Early diagnosis by testing is the key. If you find out that you have been infected, there are many resources available to help you.

Prevention

Only monogamy (you and your partner have sex only with each other) between uninfected partners or sexual abstinence completely eliminates the risk of HIV infection and other sexually transmitted diseases. The following **safer sex guidelines** will help you reduce your risk.

- If you are beginning a new sexual relationship:
  - Take time before having sex to talk about HIV and other STDs. Find out if your partner has ever been exposed to or infected with an STD or if your partner's behavior puts him or her at risk for HIV infection. Tell your partner if you've ever engaged in high-risk behavior. Remember that it is possible to be infected with an STD without knowing it.
  - Use latex condoms every time you have sex (vaginal, anal, or oral) until you are certain that neither you nor your partner has any STDs and that neither of you will have unprotected sexual contact with anyone else while your relationship lasts.
  - If you plan to use HIV testing to decide whether it is safe to have unprotected sex, have the test done 6 months after the last time you engaged in high-risk behavior. In the meantime, use condoms every time you have sexual contact.
- Avoid unprotected sexual contact with anyone who has symptoms of or who has been exposed to an STD, or whose behavior puts him or her at risk for HIV infection. Keep in mind that a person may still be able to transmit STDs even if no symptoms are present.
- Avoid unprotected vaginal, anal, or oral sex with anyone whose sexual history may not be risk-free. Use latex condoms from the beginning to the end of sexual contact. "Natural" or lambskin condoms do not protect against HIV infection or other STDs.
- Do not rely on spermicides or a diaphragm to protect against STDs. Latex condoms provide the best protection against STDs, including HIV.
- Female condoms also are effective. These are similar to a polyurethane condom with a diaphragm on one end and a plastic ring on the other. A woman can insert the condom before having sex.

In addition to the guidelines above, taking the following precautions will reduce your risk of getting HIV and hepatitis B:

- Avoid activities that may spread HIV (see page 285). Safer activities include closed-mouth kissing, hugging, massage, and other pleasurable touching.
- Never share needles, syringes, or other personal items that could be contaminated with blood.

If your job or behavior puts you at risk for HIV infection, or if you come in contact with HIV-infected blood (for example, an accidental needle stick), contact a health professional immediately. In some cases, medications may prevent HIV infection if they are started within a few hours after you are exposed to the virus. Have a blood test 6 months after any activity or accident that puts you at risk for HIV infection.

For more information, call the National AIDS Hotline at 1-800-342-AIDS.

When to Call Kaiser Permanente

- If your behavior puts you at risk for exposure to HIV, or if your sex partner has high-risk behavior or is HIV-positive.
- If you are pregnant and have reason to believe that you may have been exposed to HIV or another STD.
- If you have symptoms, including fatigue, weight loss, fever, diarrhea, cough, or swollen glands, that do not go away after a short period of time and do not seem to be related to another illness.
- If you are HIV-positive and you develop any of the following:
  - Fever higher than 103°.
  - Fever higher than 101° that lasts 3 days or longer.
  - Increased outbreaks of cold sores or any unusual skin or mouth sores.
  - Severe numbness or pain in the hands and feet.
  - Rapid, unexplained weight loss.
  - Unexplained fever and night sweats.
  - Severe fatigue.
  - Diarrhea or other bowel changes.
  - Shortness of breath and a persistent dry cough.
  - Swollen lymph nodes in the neck, armpits, or groin.
  - Personality changes, difficulty concentrating, confusion, or severe headache.

If exercise could be packed into a pill, it would be the single most widely prescribed, and beneficial, medicine in the nation.
Robert Butler, MD

16

Fitness and Physical Activity

Staying fit is not only good for your health, it is good for you. If you want to enjoy life more, the tips in this chapter can help.

The Benefits of Exercise

No amount of exercise can guarantee a long life. However, even moderate amounts of physical activity can improve the likelihood of a healthy life. Along with a positive attitude and a healthful diet, your fitness level plays a major role in how well you feel, what illnesses you avoid, and how much you enjoy life.

Consider the benefits of fitness presented here and find one or more reasons to commit to your own fitness program.

Are You Ready to Get Started?

- Any activity is better than no activity . . . and you never have to run a marathon. You can start with a 5-minute walk **today**, and presto! You're started!
- Then, you can look for ways to liven up every day with a few minutes of walking, gardening, bicycling, dancing, swimming, taking the stairs, basketball, hiking, skating, playing games, etc.
- Some people like to write down all of their activity on their calendar. Then they can step back and say, "I did it!"

Benefits of Exercise

- Relieves tension and stress
- Provides enjoyment and fun
- Stimulates the mind
- Helps maintain stable weight
- Controls appetite
- Boosts self-image
- Improves muscle tone and strength
- Improves flexibility
- Lowers blood pressure
- Relieves insomnia
- Increases "good" (HDL) cholesterol
- Reduces risk of diabetes
- Increases energy and helps decrease fatigue
- Reduces anxiety and depression
- Improves balance and coordination
- Helps prevent constipation

Your Personal Fitness Plan

No one can prescribe the perfect fitness plan for you. You have to figure it out based on what you enjoy doing and what you will continue to do. The next few pages can be a big help.

Consistency is the most important, the most basic, and the most often neglected part of fitness. Consistency in regular exercise or moderate activity delivers all of the fitness benefits.

A good fitness plan has 3 parts: aerobic fitness, muscle strengthening, and flexibility. Read the section on each part. Then see Setting Your Fitness Goals on page 294.

Aerobic Fitness

Aerobic conditioning strengthens your heart and lungs. Good aerobic exercises include brisk walking, running, stair climbing, biking, swimming, aerobic dance, or anything else that raises your heart rate and keeps it up for a while.

How Hard Should I Exercise?

Nice and easy does it. Exercise does not have to be intense to be of value. In fact, if you exercise too hard, you get less benefit than if you go at a moderate pace.

Above all, listen to your body. If the exercise feels too hard, slow down. You will reduce your risk of injury and enjoy the exercise much more.

Try the "talk-sing test" to determine your ideal exercise pace:

- If you can't talk and exercise at the same time, you are going too fast.
- If you can talk while you exercise, you are doing fine.
- If you can sing while you exercise, it would be safe to exercise a little faster.

Your exercise is most effective when you can talk, but not sing, while doing it.

Target Heart Rate

Another way to see how hard you are exercising is to check your heart rate. You gain the most aerobic benefits when your exercise heart rate is 60 percent to 80 percent of your maximum heart rate. This is your target heart rate. After exercising for about 10 minutes, stop and take your pulse for 10 seconds (see page 57). Compare the number to the chart on page 293. Adjust the intensity of your exercise so that your heart rate stays between the two numbers. However, the target heart rate is only a guide. Each individual is different, so pay attention to how you feel.

Target Heart Rate

Age	10-second heart rate
20	20–27
25	20–26
30	19–25
35	19–25
40	18–24
45	18–23
50	17–23
55	17–23
60	16–22
65	16–21
70	15–20

Target heart rate is 60 percent to 80 percent of maximum heart rate (maximum heart rate = 220 minus your age).

How Often and How Long Should I Exercise?

Most studies show that exercising for 30 minutes on most days each week is what it takes to improve fitness. However, sometimes it's easier to make exercise a habit if you do it every day.

With aerobic exercise, harder is not better, but longer is. Although you can get good fitness benefits from as little as 10 minutes of aerobic exercise per day, extending your exercise time will increase your rewards. This is true for up to 1 hour of exercise per day. Beyond that, there may be diminishing health returns and increasing risk of injuries.

Warm Up and Cool Down

For the first 5 minutes of your exercise routine, start out slowly and easily so your muscles have a chance to warm up.

End your exercise with a little cool-down period. If you've been running or walking quickly, gradually slow your pace, then do a few light stretches to improve flexibility. See page 295.

Drink some extra water before and after exercising.

Muscle Strengthening

Strengthening your muscles improves your work and athletic performance and prevents fatigue. Muscle-strengthening exercises will also improve your posture and help you feel more energetic.

Resistance training, with free weights, weight-training equipment, or inexpensive rubber tubing, can quickly increase your muscle strength.

Other simple, safe, and effective strengthening exercises include bent-knee curl-ups, chin-ups, push-ups, side leg-lifts, and other calisthenics to improve abdominal, neck, arm, shoulder, and leg strength.

Flexibility

Stretching can increase your range of motion and reduce stiffness and pain. Stretching is particularly important during the cool-down phase after exercising when your muscles are warm. See the stretches on page 295.

- Stretch slowly and gradually. Don't bounce. Maintain a continuous tension on the muscle.
- Relax and hold each stretch for a count of 20.
- Exhale as you stretch, to further relax your muscles. If stretching hurts, you have gone too far or you are doing something incorrectly.

Try to stretch a little every day. Take a stretch break instead of a coffee break.

Overcome Barriers to Exercise

There are 6 barriers to exercise that are all easy to overcome.

1. No time? Try shorter periods of activity spread throughout the day, such as three 10-minute walks.

2. Too tired? It's often lack of exercise that makes you tired. Exercise gives you energy. Try it.

3. Embarrassed? Many people are, especially at first. Be proud that you're taking care of your body.

4. No partner? Yes, it's more fun to exercise with a friend. If your regular exercise partner quits, find another one. You could also join a fitness club, take a class, or exercise to a video.

5. Bad weather? Too hot, too cold, too wet, too windy—it never seems right for exercise. Lots of people exercise come rain or shine. Try a variety of indoor and outdoor activities.

6. Too costly? You had to let the fitness club membership expire. You can't afford a mountain bike. You panic at the price of running shoes. It all costs money. But can you afford not to exercise? Try a low-cost option, such as walking instead of driving.

Setting Your Fitness Goals

Are you as strong, flexible, and physically fit as you would like to be? If you are, good for you. We hope this chapter has helped you reaffirm the exercises you are already doing. However, if you want to make some improvements, here's one piece of advice: Try to improve a little bit at a time.

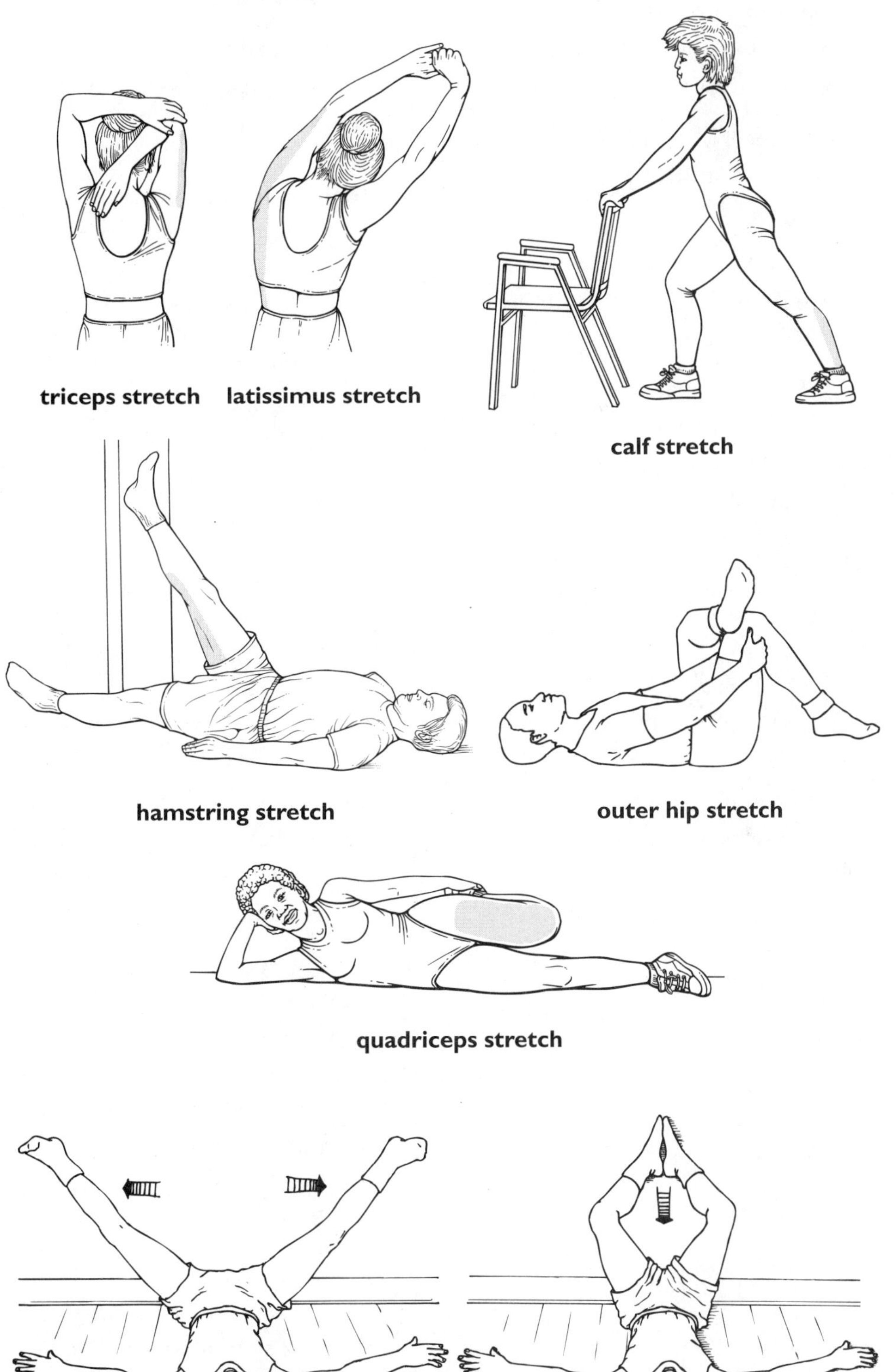

Stretching exercises

The only way to walk a mile is to take 1 step at a time. The only way to improve your fitness level is to take it 1 step at a time.

- Pick 1 aspect of fitness (aerobic, strength, flexibility) you want to improve first.
- Pick an activity that you enjoy. You're more likely to keep doing something you like.
- Set a 1-month goal that you think you can reach. For example, plan to walk for 10 minutes at lunch 3 days a week, or stretch for 5 minutes each morning.
- Start today. Keep a record of what you do.
- When you reach your first goal, reward yourself! Then set a new one.

Consistency brings success. Each success may be a small one, but small successes can quickly add up to physical fitness that will make a big difference in your life.

Exercise Cautions

Moderate exercise is safe for most people. To be safe, start slowly and gradually increase the intensity of your exercise. However, if you can answer "yes" to any of the following questions, talk with your physician before beginning an exercise program.

- Do you have heart trouble?
- Do you have undiagnosed chest pains?
- Do you have high blood pressure?
- Do you often feel faint or dizzy?
- Do you have arthritis or other bone or joint problems that might be aggravated by improper exercise?
- Do you have diabetes? You may want to talk with your physician about how increased exercise affects your insulin needs.

Men over age 40 who have been inactive or who have 2 or more risk factors for heart disease* and who plan to start a vigorous exercise program (running or fast bicycling or swimming) may wish to talk with their physicians about any possible risks.

**Cholesterol over 200 mg/dl, blood pressure over 140/90, smoking, diabetes, or family history of heart disease before age 45.*

Never eat more than you can lift.
Miss Piggy

17

Nutrition

This chapter gives some guidelines for good eating and some hints on how to help your children establish healthful eating habits. Children learn best by example, so practice good eating habits along with them.

10 Simple Guidelines for Eating Well

The Dietary Guidelines for Americans are aimed at improving health and reducing the risk of disease, especially high blood pressure, heart disease, stroke, type 2 diabetes, and cancer.

1. Aim for a healthful weight. Healthy bodies come in a variety of shapes and sizes. Work toward achieving and maintaining a weight that is best for you by choosing a variety of healthful foods and getting regular physical activity. If you would like to lose weight, Kaiser Permanente can help. Talk to your physician or call your local health education department for more information.

2. Be physically active every day. Regular physical activity that is vigorous enough to raise your heart rate has many benefits. When combined with a balanced diet, being physically active is the best way to maintain a healthful body weight.

3. Let the Pyramid guide your food choices. The Food Guide Pyramid on page 300 is a simple, flexible guide designed to help you create a balanced diet. It encourages eating a variety of foods in balance with one another so that you get the nutrients your body needs each day. The Food Guide Pyramid can help you get the most out of your food choices.

4. Choose a variety of grains daily, especially whole grains. Foods made from grains, such as wheat, rice, and oats, are the foundations of good nutrition. They provide vitamins, minerals, starches, and fiber and are often low in fat. Whole grains may also help protect against heart disease and high blood pressure.

5. Choose a variety of fruits and vegetables daily. Fruits and vegetables are key parts of your daily diet, but most people eat fewer than the 5 servings that are recommended. They taste great, are easy to prepare, and may protect you from some types of cancer.

6. Keep food safe to eat. Prevent food poisoning by keeping hot foods hot and cold foods cold. Bacteria can grow rapidly when food is not stored or handled properly. See Stomach Flu and Food Poisoning on page 93 for more information on keeping food safe.

7. Choose a diet that is low in saturated fat and cholesterol, and moderate in total fat. Watching your fat intake can reduce your risk for heart disease, cancer, and high blood pressure. Choosing more grains, fruits, and vegetables can help you reduce the amount of total fat in your diet.

8. Choose beverages and foods that limit your intake of sugars. Added sugars have no other nutrients and, when consumed in excess, they crowd healthier foods out of your diet.

9. Choose and prepare foods with less salt. You can reduce your chances of developing high blood pressure by consuming less salt. Reducing your salt intake can also help you lower your blood pressure if it's currently high.

10. If you drink alcoholic beverages, do so in moderation. Alcohol supplies calories but few or no nutrients. Drinking alcohol is the cause of many health problems and accidents, and it can lead to addiction. Moderate alcohol consumption is defined as no more than 2 drinks a day for men and no more than 1 drink a day for women. Women who are pregnant or trying to become pregnant should avoid alcoholic beverages altogether.

Eating Well: A Basic Plan

Eat a variety of foods from the Food Guide Pyramid on page 300 each day. Most people who follow the diet outlined by the Pyramid will get all the vitamins, minerals, and other nutrients their bodies need and will have little trouble controlling their weight.

Grain Products

Whole grains, such as wheat, oats, brown rice, and potatoes, contain large amounts of vitamins, minerals, fiber, and water. Contrary to popular belief, foods made from whole grains are not fattening. They are primarily carbohydrates, which have less than ½ as many calories per gram as fats do.

Whole-grain foods become fattening only when you or the companies who make them add fat (or if you eat too much of them). Try substituting nonfat yogurt or salsa for butter and sour cream on a baked potato.

Use fresh vegetable and tomato sauces instead of rich cream sauces on pasta.

Fruits and Vegetables

Fruits and vegetables provide vitamins, minerals, and fiber and are naturally low in fat. Choose any form of fruits and vegetables: fresh, frozen, canned, or dried.

Many fruits and vegetables contain compounds that appear to protect against some cancers, such as the antioxidant vitamins A (carotenoids) and C and beta carotene. Carotenoids are found in deep orange and dark green vegetables and fruits, such as carrots, sweet potatoes, pumpkin, spinach, and in collard and turnip greens. Vitamin C is found in citrus fruits and citrus fruit juices, such as oranges and orange juice, and in cantaloupe, strawberries, peppers, broccoli, and tomatoes.

Vegetables in the cabbage family, including broccoli, cauliflower, and Brussels sprouts, contain other compounds that appear to protect against several types of cancer.

A diet that contains a variety of fruits and vegetables protects against heart disease and high blood pressure too.

Aim to eat at least 2 servings of fruits and at least 3 servings of vegetables each day.

Fiber

Fiber is the indigestible part of plants. It is not absorbed into the bloodstream like other nutrients are. However, it plays an important role in keeping your digestive tract healthy by providing "bulk." A high-fiber diet may protect you against colon cancer.

There are 2 types of fiber found in foods: insoluble fiber and soluble fiber.

Insoluble fiber, which can be found in whole-grain products, such as whole-wheat flour, provides bulk for your diet. Together with fluids, insoluble fiber stimulates your colon to keep waste moving out of your bowels. Without fiber, waste moves too slowly, increasing your risk for constipation, diverticulosis, and probably colon cancer.

Soluble fiber, which is found in fruit, legumes (dry beans and peas), and oats, helps lower blood cholesterol, reducing your risk for heart disease. Soluble fiber, especially the fiber in legumes, can also help regulate your blood glucose level.

Do you need more fiber in your diet? If your stools are soft and easy to pass, you probably get plenty of fiber. If they are hard and difficult to pass, more fiber and water may help. See page 78 for more information about constipation.

To increase fiber in your diet:

- Eat at least 5 servings of fruits or vegetables a day (see the Food Guide Pyramid on page 300). Eat fruits with edible skins and seeds: kiwi fruit, figs, blueberries, apples, and raspberries. Eat more raw or lightly cooked vegetables.

Guide to Eating Well

Grains (breads, cereals, rice, pasta) form the foundation of a healthful diet. Serving sizes: 1 slice of bread, 1 oz. of cereal, ½ bagel, ½ cup of pasta or rice.

Eat plenty of fruits and vegetables. Serving sizes: ¾ cup fruit or vegetable juice; ½ cup raw, canned, or cooked fruits or vegetables; 1 medium apple or banana; 1 cup raw leafy vegetables.

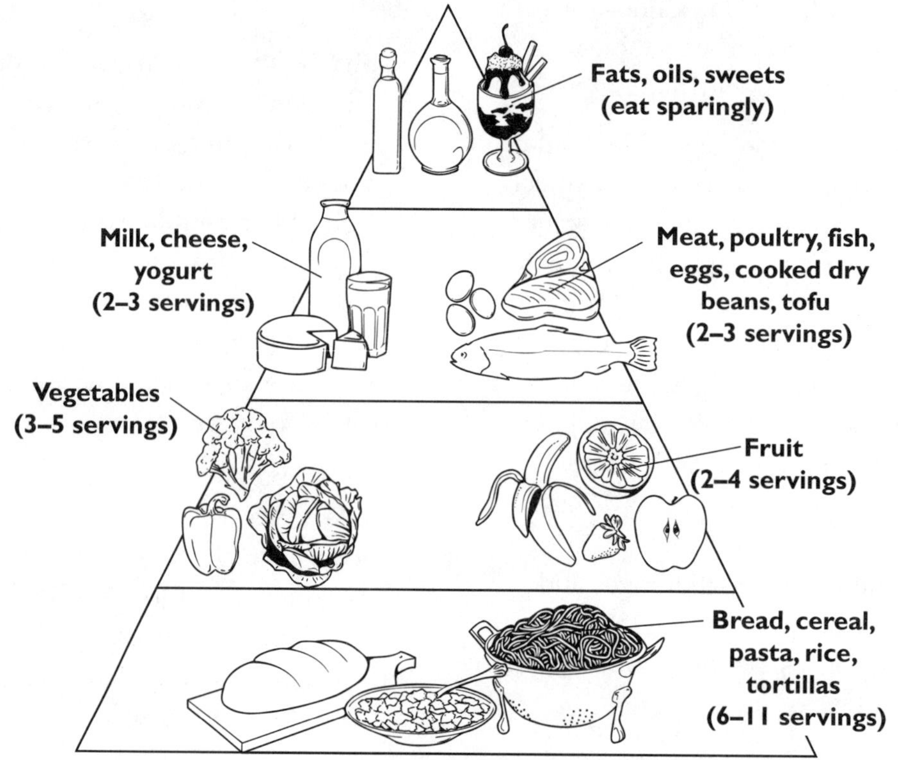
Fats, oils, sweets
(eat sparingly)
Milk, cheese, yogurt
(2–3 servings)
Meat, poultry, fish, eggs, cooked dry beans, tofu
(2–3 servings)
Vegetables
(3–5 servings)
Fruit
(2–4 servings)
Bread, cereal, pasta, rice, tortillas
(6–11 servings)

The Food Guide Pyramid (USDA)

Choose lean meats, fish, or poultry and cooked dry beans to reduce fat. Serving sizes: 2–3 oz. cooked lean meat, poultry, or fish; ½ cup cooked dry beans; 1 egg; 2 tbsp. peanut butter.

Choose nonfat or low-fat dairy products. Serving sizes: 1 cup milk or yogurt, 1½–2 oz. low-fat cheese, ½ cup cottage cheese.

Eat foods from the top of the Pyramid only in moderation. Examples: cooking oil, butter or margarine, high-fat salty snacks, alcohol, candy.

- Switch to whole-grain and whole-wheat breads, pasta, tortillas, and cereals. The first ingredient listed should be whole-wheat flour.
- Eat more cooked dry beans, dry peas, and lentils. These high-fiber, high-protein foods can replace some of the high-fat, no-fiber meats in your diet.
- Popcorn is a good high-fiber snack. However, avoid added oil, butter, and salt. Use an air or microwave popcorn popper to eliminate oil, and add flavor with salt substitute or herb mixtures.

Water

One easy way to improve your diet is to drink more water. Active people need 2 quarts of water a day, and people who exercise regularly need even more. Start your day by drinking a big glass of water when you first get up; then drink 6 to 8 more glasses (8 ounces each) throughout the day. If you drink other fluids, you can get by with less water, but plain water is best. (Milk is another good choice, with the added bonus of a boost of calcium.)

Sugar

In moderation, sugar does little harm. However, if too many of your calories come from sugar, you will gain weight and/or not get enough of the other nutrients you need. Sugar also contributes to dental cavities.

To reduce sugar in your diet:

- Be aware that all sugars are basically alike. Honey and brown or raw sugar have no advantage over other sugars. Corn syrup is another commonly used form of sugar.
- Processed foods and drinks can be full of sugar. Flavored yogurt, breakfast cereals, canned fruits, and desserts often have sugar added. Look for breakfast cereals that have 6 grams or less of added sugar per serving.
- Limit foods and drinks that list sugar among the first few ingredients.
- You can reduce the amount of sugar added to homemade baked goods by up to ½ without affecting the texture. Try using more sweet spices, such as cinnamon and nutmeg, in your recipes.
- Make it a habit to eat a sweet piece of fruit instead of a sugary dessert most of the time.
- Drink water instead of soft drinks or fruit drinks.

Fats in Foods

The Dietary Guidelines for Americans recommend that less than 30 percent of your total calorie intake come from fat. Reducing dietary fat to 30 percent will slow the development of heart disease, reduce your cancer risk, and improve your overall diet. No more than 10 percent of total calories should come from saturated fats.

The 80-20 Rule

If you are generally healthy, you don't need to worry about maintaining a perfect diet. If you make healthful eating choices 80 percent of the time, occasionally eating high-fat or high-calorie foods the remaining 20 percent of the time won't be a problem.

However, some scientists think that getting 30 percent of your total calories from fat is still too much for a healthy heart. A diet that consists of 20 percent fat (no more than 7 percent saturated fat) may further reduce your risk for heart disease and can also help less active people stay closer to a healthful weight.

If you need help reducing fat in your diet, a registered dietitian can create a menu plan that will help you meet your goal.

Simple Ways to Reduce Saturated Fat

When eating meat:

- Reduce serving sizes to 2 or 3 ounces (about the size of a deck of cards), and don't eat second helpings. If you eat red meat, choose the leanest cuts, such as tenderloin, sirloin, or top and bottom round. Cut off any visible fat.
- Eat more fish and poultry (without skin). They contain less saturated fat than red meat does.
- Bake or broil red meats, poultry, and fish instead of frying them in butter or fat.
- Occasionally serve tofu, other soy products, or a combination of legumes (dried beans, peas, lentils) and grains in place of a meat entree.

When using dairy products:

- Use fat-free or low-fat milk.
- Choose cheeses made with fat-free or low-fat milk, or look for cheeses that have no more than 5 grams of fat per ounce (read the label).
- Try fat-free or low-fat cottage cheese or yogurt in place of cream and sour cream; or use fat-free sour cream and fat-free cream cheese.

When cooking:

- Steam vegetables. If you choose to sauté them, use 1 tablespoon of oil (or less), or try using other liquids such as wine or defatted broth.
- Use nonstick pans, or add a small amount of oil to a preheated pan (less oil goes farther this way).
- Season vegetables with herbs and spices instead of butter and sauces; or try a butter substitute such as Butter Buds or Molly McButter. Dress salads with lemon juice, fat-free mayonnaise, or fat-free dressing.
- Use a cooking oil that is liquid at room temperature (such as canola, olive, or corn oil) and use it sparingly (1 teaspoon at a time).

- Experiment with using less oil than is called for in recipes. You may need to increase other liquids. Use applesauce, prune puree, or mashed bananas to replace some or all of the fat in baked goods.

Dietary Cholesterol

For many people, foods high in cholesterol raise the amount of cholesterol in the blood. These foods include liver, other organ meats, egg yolks, and dairy fats. Limit how much you eat of these foods.

Protein

Protein is important for maintaining healthy muscles, tendons, bones, skin, hair, blood, and internal organs. Most adult Americans get all the protein they need in their diets. If you eat animal products (milk, cheese, eggs, fish, meat), your diet will contain plenty of protein. However, if you eat little meat, poultry, or fish and use no dairy products, your diet will require careful planning in order for you to get all the protein and other nutrients you need.

Vitamins

Vitamins are tiny elements of food that have no calories, yet are essential to good health. Vitamins A, D, E, and K are fat-soluble and can be stored in the liver or in fat tissue for a relatively long time. Other vitamins, including all the B vitamins and vitamin C, are water-soluble, and your body can only retain them for a short time, so it is important that you consume them often.

Most people who eat a variety of foods from the Food Guide Pyramid (page 300) get all the necessary vitamins. However, if you typically eat fewer than 1,500 calories per day, you may want to consider taking a vitamin-mineral supplement. Choose a balanced, multivitamin-mineral supplement rather than a specific vitamin or mineral, unless your physician prescribes a specific supplement. Avoid taking much more than 100 percent of the recommended daily allowance of any vitamin or mineral unless it is prescribed by a physician.

Certain vitamins found in foods have been shown to prevent some diseases. However, researchers are still trying to determine whether those vitamins have the same preventive effects when taken as supplements. If possible, add more variety and balance to your diet rather than trying to make up for a poor diet by taking supplements.

Minerals

Minerals have many important roles in the structure and function of your body. You need minerals to build and maintain healthy teeth and bones; to carry nerve signals to and from your brain; to carry oxygen to your cells; to regulate blood sugar levels; and to maintain a healthy immune system.

A total of 60 minerals have been discovered in the body, and 22 are essential to health. Eating a variety of foods is the best way to get all the minerals you need.

Lactose Intolerance

People whose bodies produce too little of the enzyme lactase have trouble digesting the lactose (sugar) in milk. Symptoms of lactose intolerance include gas, bloating, cramps, and diarrhea after drinking milk or eating milk products.

If you have mild to moderate lactose intolerance:

- Eat small amounts of milk products at any one time.
- Try eating cheese. Most of the lactose in cheese is removed during processing.
- Eat yogurts made with active cultures, which provide their own enzymes that digest the lactose in milk.
- Drink pretreated milk (such as Lactaid), or try enzyme tablets (such as Lactaid or Dairy Ease), which will help you digest lactose.
- You may be able to tolerate milk if you drink it with snacks or meals.

If you have severe lactose intolerance:

- Read labels to avoid any form of lactose in foods.
- Be sure to include non-dairy sources of calcium in your diet. See page 304. You may need calcium supplements to get enough calcium. Ask your physician or a dietitian.
- Find ways to get enough of the nutrients supplied by the milk group from the rest of your diet.

Calcium

Calcium is the primary mineral needed for building and maintaining strong bones. Calcium is especially important for growing children and for women, especially in the peak bone-building years between the teens and early 30s. Calcium also helps women prevent osteoporosis, which can occur after menopause. See page 129.

Children from 1 to 3 years of age need 500 mg of calcium per day; those from 4 to 8 years of age need 800 mg per day; and those from 9 to 18 years of age need 1,300 mg per day. Adults between 19 and 50 years of age need 1,000 mg per day. Adults age 51 and older need 1,200 mg per day.

Fat-free or low-fat dairy products are the best source of dietary calcium. One cup of fat-free milk contains about 313 mg of calcium. Fat-free and low-fat yogurt have 442 mg per cup. Milk products provide other nutrients in addition to calcium, such as protein. Other foods, such as tofu, fortified soy milk, broccoli, greens, and calcium-fortified orange juice, provide calcium in varying amounts.

While dietary calcium is preferred, low-dose calcium supplements (calcium citrate) can also help keep bones strong.

Salt

Most people get far more salt (sodium) than they need. For some people, excess salt causes high blood pressure. See page 245.

In general, processed foods contain the most salt, while unprocessed foods, such as fresh fruits and vegetables, have the least. If you want to cut back on the salt in your diet:

- Read the Nutrition Facts labels on foods for sodium content. Choose foods that contain less sodium.
- Limit ready-mixed sauces and seasonings, frozen dinners, and canned or dehydrated soups. These foods are usually packed with salt. Products labeled "low sodium" contain less than 140 mg of sodium per serving.
- Eat lots of fresh or frozen fruits and vegetables. These foods contain very little sodium.
- Don't put the salt shaker on the table, or get a salt shaker that allows very little salt to come out. Use salt substitute or "lite salt" sparingly.
- Always measure the salt in recipes, and use ½ of what is called for.
- Avoid fast foods, which are usually very high in salt. In a restaurant, ask the chef not to salt food during cooking.

Iron

Your body needs small amounts of iron to make hemoglobin, which carries oxygen in your blood. Adult men need 10 mg of iron per day; adult women need 15 mg per day. People who have increased blood loss caused by ulcers or heavy menstrual periods, or who lose blood from taking blood thinners (anticoagulants) or arthritis medications (such as aspirin), are at high risk for iron deficiency anemia. Symptoms of iron deficiency anemia include paleness and fatigue. A blood test is needed to confirm the diagnosis, and further testing may be needed to determine the cause of the blood loss.

To get more iron in your blood:

- Increase the amount of vitamin C in your diet. Vitamin C helps you absorb more iron from food. To get the most iron from a bowl of iron-enriched cereal, drink a glass of orange or other citrus juice when you eat the cereal. High-iron cereals have at least 25 percent of the Daily Value (DV) of iron.
- Eat meat and vegetables or grains together. The iron in animal tissues (heme iron) improves absorption of the iron in other foods.
- Avoid caffeinated tea with meals. It interferes with iron absorption.

Iron Supplements

Women who menstruate and who eat fewer than 1,500 calories per day may wish to consider taking a multivitamin-mineral supplement that contains iron. (Men are much less likely to need iron supplements.) A low-dose ferrous-form iron supplement containing no more than 20 mg is safe for most women to take daily. However, too much iron can cause a number of serious medical problems or mask the development of others. Do not take more than 20 mg of iron per day without consulting your physician first. Take iron supplements between meals, at bedtime, or on an empty stomach. Keep iron supplements away from children.

Non-Nutrients in Foods

In addition to the essential nutrients, foods also contain non-nutrient compounds that act on your body in some way. These include phytochemicals (found in plants), many of which protect against cancer.

Some foods contain compounds that have medicinal effects, such as the compound found in cranberries that may flush bacteria from the urinary tract and prevent urinary tract infections.

The non-nutrients in foods are of great interest today, and many of them are just being discovered. Foods are made of hundreds of chemicals that cannot be duplicated in a supplement. Taking a supplement cannot provide "insurance" against a poor or inadequate diet. If you think that your diet is poor, then the best advice is to improve it.

Nutrition for Children

Your whole family can follow the diet outlined in the Food Guide Pyramid (page 300). Offer nutritious foods as well-planned, pleasant meals and snacks. Then sit back and let your child decide how much to eat (or even if he or she wants to eat at all). This is a good division of responsibility that allows children to tune in to their own appetite and takes the pressure off the parents.

Child-Sized Environment

Imagine yourself eating at a giant's table. That's how a child can feel eating at an adult-sized table in an adult-sized chair.

- Provide a booster seat and child-sized utensils. However, fingers are fine until a child can hold utensils easily.
- Give children smaller plates and smaller servings (1 tablespoon per year of age is a good serving size guide). If the child is hungry for seconds, he or she will ask for them.

Healthful Snacks

Young children have small stomachs and high energy needs, so they need frequent snacks to supplement meals. Plan between-meal snacks as part of the day's total food intake. Snacks should provide good nutrition, not just empty calories.

- Fruits and fruit juices are good snacks. Other good choices are raw vegetable sticks with fat-free dressing, cereal, yogurt, cheese, or soup.
- Serve meals and snacks on a regular schedule. Do not serve snacks so close to a meal that they interfere with the child's appetite.
- Choose desserts that are low in fat and high in nutrients. Fruit, yogurt, and other foods found in the Food Guide Pyramid are good choices.

He who laughs, lasts.
Mary Pettibone Poole

18

Mental Health Problems and Mind-Body Wellness

This chapter is organized in 2 sections. The first section covers some common mental and emotional health problems and describes what you can do to treat them at home and when you should seek professional help. The second section describes the relationship between your mental health and your physical health.

This chapter does not address all mental health problems. If you have symptoms of a mental health problem that are not described here, contact a health professional.

> **Medical Emergencies**
>
> **If you think you have an emergency medical condition, call 911 or go to the nearest hospital.**
>
> An emergency medical condition is a medical or psychiatric condition that manifests itself by acute symptoms of sufficient severity (including severe pain) such that you could reasonably expect the absence of immediate medical attention to result in serious jeopardy to your health, serious impairment to your bodily functions, or serious dysfunction of any bodily organ or part.

Mental Health Problems

Mental health problems are similar to other health problems: some can be prevented; others will go away on their own with home treatment; and some need professional attention. Many mental health problems begin when physical stress (such as an illness or injury) or emotional stress (such as the loss of a loved one) triggers chemical changes in your brain. The goal of treatment for mental health problems—including self-care and professional treatment—is to reduce stress and restore the normal chemical processes in your brain.

In general, it is a good idea to seek professional help for a mental health problem when:

- A symptom becomes severe or disruptive.
- A symptom becomes a continuous or permanent pattern of behavior and does not respond to self-care.
- Symptoms become numerous, affect all areas of your life, and do not respond to self-care or communication efforts.
- You are thinking about suicide.

Alcohol and Drug Problems

The overuse or abuse of alcohol or other drugs is called substance abuse. It is common, costly, and associated with many medical problems.

Alcohol Problems

A person has an alcohol use problem if he or she continues to drink even though alcohol is interfering with his or her health or daily living. Alcoholism is defined as a physical or psychological dependence on alcohol.

Alcohol abuse patterns vary. Some people get drunk every day. Some drink large amounts of alcohol at specific times, such as weekends. Others may be sober for long periods and then go on drinking binges that last for weeks or months.

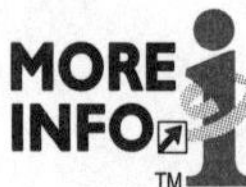

Long-term heavy drinking causes liver, nerve, heart, and brain damage; high blood pressure; stomach problems; sexual problems; and cancer. Alcohol abuse can also lead to violence, accidents, social isolation, and difficulties at work, at home, or with the law.

Signs that a person's body is dependent on alcohol include personality changes, blackouts, drinking more and more for the same "high," and denial of the problem. A person with alcoholism may gulp or sneak drinks, drink alone or early in the morning, and suffer from the shakes. He or she may also have family or work problems or get in trouble with the law due to drinking.

A person whose body is dependent on alcohol may suffer serious withdrawal symptoms (such as trembling, delusions, hallucinations, sweating, and seizures) if he or she stops drinking suddenly. Once alcohol dependency develops, it is very difficult for a person to stop drinking without outside help. Medical detoxification may be needed.

Drug Problems

Drug abuse includes the use of marijuana, cocaine, heroin, or other "street drugs," and the abuse of legal prescription drugs. Some people turn to drugs as a way to get a "high" or to deal with stress or emotional problems.

Are You a Problem User?

Answer the following questions honestly. They refer to your use of alcohol and drugs, including prescribed and illegal drugs.

- Have you ever felt that you ought to cut down on your drinking or drug use?
- Do you get annoyed at criticism of your drinking or drug use?
- Do you ever feel guilty about your drinking or drug use?
- Do you ever take an early morning drink or use drugs first thing in the morning to get the day started or to eliminate the "shakes?"

A person who answers "yes," "sometimes," or "often" to 2 or more of these questions may have a problem with alcohol or drugs. Call a health professional to arrange for other tests to diagnose alcohol or drug dependence.

Tranquilizers, sedatives, painkillers, and amphetamines are misused most often, sometimes unintentionally.

Drug dependence (addiction) occurs when a person develops a physical or psychological need for a drug. A person may not be aware that he or she has become dependent on a drug until he or she tries to suddenly stop taking it. Withdrawing from the drug can cause uncomfortable symptoms such as muscle aches, diarrhea, or depression. The usual treatment for drug dependence is to reduce the dose of the drug gradually until it can be stopped completely.

Prevention

- Look for signs of mental stress. Try to understand and resolve sources of depression, anxiety, or loneliness. Don't use alcohol or drugs to deal with these problems.
- Educate your children about the effects of alcohol. Children are less likely to use alcohol or other drugs if their parents teach them early (during the elementary school years) about the effects of alcohol.
- If you drink, do so in moderation: not more than 2 drinks a day for men and not more than 1 drink a day for women. One drink is 12 ounces of beer, 5 ounces of wine, or 1 ounce of hard liquor.
- Don't drink alcohol or use drugs if you are pregnant.
- Ask your pharmacist or physician if any of your current medications could potentially lead to overuse or dependence. Be especially cautious of painkillers, tranquilizers, sedatives, and sleeping pills. Follow the instructions carefully, and do not exceed the recommended dose.
- Do not suddenly stop taking any medication without your physician's supervision.
- Avoid alcohol when you are taking medications. Alcohol can react with many drugs and cause serious complications.

Signs of Drug Use

- Chronic red eyes, sore throat, dry cough, and fatigue (in the absence of allergies).
- Major changes in sleeping or eating habits.
- Moodiness, hostility, or abusive behavior.
- Work or school problems, absenteeism.
- Loss of interest in favorite activities.
- Social withdrawal or changes in friends.
- Stealing, lying, and poor family relationships.

Home Treatment

- Recognize early signs that alcohol or drug use is becoming a problem. See "Are You a Problem User?" on page 309.
- Attend an Alcoholics Anonymous meeting (a self-help group devoted to helping members get sober and stay sober).

If you are concerned about another person's alcohol or drug use:

- Never ignore the problem. Discuss it as a medical problem.
- Build up the person's self-esteem and reaffirm his or her value as a person. Help the person see that he or she can be successful without alcohol or drugs. Let the person know you will support his or her efforts to change.
- Ask if the person will accept help. Don't give up if you get a negative response; keep asking periodically. If the person eventually agrees, act that very day to arrange for help. Call a health professional or Alcoholics Anonymous for an immediate appointment.
- Attend a few meetings of Al-Anon, a support group for family members and friends of alcoholics. Read some 12-step program information.

When to Call Kaiser Permanente

- If a person loses consciousness after drinking alcohol or taking drugs.
- If a person who has been drinking alcohol or using drugs threatens to commit suicide.
- If a person who suddenly stops using alcohol has withdrawal symptoms (trembling, hallucinations, seizures).
- If you answer "yes," "sometimes," or "often" to 2 or more of the questions under "Are You a Problem User?" on page 309.
- If you recognize an alcohol or drug problem in yourself and are ready to accept help. Both outpatient and inpatient treatment programs are available.

Anger and Hostility

Anger signals your body to prepare for a fight. When you get angry, adrenalin and other hormones are released into your bloodstream. Your blood pressure, pulse, and respiration rate all go up.

Anger is a normal response to daily events. It is the appropriate response to any situation that poses a threat. Anger can be directed to become a positive, driving force behind your actions.

Hostility is being ready for a fight all the time. Continual hostility keeps your blood pressure high and may increase your risk for heart attack and other illnesses. Being hostile also isolates you from other people.

Home Treatment

- When confronted with a situation that might trigger an angry response, ask yourself:
  - Is this really important enough to get angry about?
  - Am I justified in getting angry?
  - Will getting angry really make a difference?
- Try to understand the real reason why you are angry. Is it the current situation that is making you angry or something that happened at some earlier time?
- Notice when you start to become angry, and take steps to deal with your anger in a positive way. Don't ignore your anger until you "blow up." Express your anger in healthy ways:
  - Count to 10 or practice some other form of mental relaxation (see page 328). When you have calmed down, you will be better able to discuss the conflict rationally.
  - Try screaming or yelling in a private place, not at other people.
  - Go for a short walk or jog.
  - Talk about your anger with a friend.
  - Draw or paint to release the anger, or write about it in a journal.
- Use "I" statements, not "you" statements, to discuss your anger. Say "I feel angry when my needs are not being met," instead of "You make me mad when you are so inconsiderate."
- If you are angry with someone, listen to what the other person has to say. Try to understand his or her point of view.
- Forgive and forget. Forgiving helps lower blood pressure and ease muscle tension so you can feel more relaxed.
- Read books about anger and how to handle it. See page 321 for additional information about anger and violent behavior.

When to Call Kaiser Permanente

- If anger has led or could lead to violence or harm to you or someone else.
- If anger or hostility interferes with your work, family life, or friendships.

Anxiety

Feeling worried, anxious, and nervous is a normal part of everyday life. Everyone frets or feels anxious from time to time. However, when anxiety becomes overwhelming and interferes with your daily life, it is not normal.

Anxiety can cause both physical and emotional symptoms. A specific situation or fear can cause some or all of these symptoms for a short time. When the situation passes, the symptoms go away.

Physical Symptoms

- Trembling, twitching, or shaking
- Lightheadedness or dizziness
- Feeling of fullness in the throat or chest
- Muscle tension, aches, or soreness
- Restlessness
- Fatigue
- Insomnia
- Breathlessness or rapid heartbeat
- Sweating or cold, clammy hands

Emotional Symptoms

- Feeling keyed up and on edge
- Excessive worrying
- Fearing that something bad is going to happen
- Poor concentration
- Irritability or agitation
- Constant sadness

Many people, including children and teens, develop anxiety disorders in which many of these symptoms occur when there is no identifiable cause.

Phobias and panic disorder are two common anxiety-related disorders. Phobias are irrational, involuntary fears of common places, objects, or situations. Panic disorders occur when a person has periods of intense fear and anxiety when there is no clear cause or danger. Physical symptoms that may occur during a panic attack include chest pain, feelings of choking or suffocation, nausea, shaking, sweating, pounding heart, and dizziness or faintness.

Self-care, often combined with professional treatment, can be effective in managing anxiety.

Home Treatment

The following home treatment tips can relieve simple anxiety and also help in combination with medical care.

- Recognize and accept your anxiety about specific fears or situations. Then say to yourself, "This is not an emergency. I feel uncomfortable, but I am not in danger. I can keep going even if I feel anxious."

- Be kind to your body:
  - Relieve tension with vigorous exercise or massage.
  - Practice relaxation techniques. See page 328.
  - Get enough rest. If you have trouble sleeping, see Sleep Problems on page 317.
  - Avoid alcohol, caffeine, chocolate, and nicotine. They increase your anxiety level.
- Schedule worry time. Set aside a specific time each day (15 to 60 minutes) to do all your worrying. Write down all your fears. When worries come to mind during other parts of the day, save them as a list for your next scheduled worry time.
- Engage your mind:
  - Get out and do something you enjoy, such as going to a funny movie or taking a walk or a hike.
  - Plan your day. Having too much or too little to do can make you more anxious.
- Keep a record of your symptoms. Discuss your fears with a good friend. Confiding with others sometimes relieves stress.
- Get involved in social groups or volunteer to help others.

When to Call Kaiser Permanente

- If you are seriously considering harming yourself or someone else.
- If anxiety interferes with your daily activities.
- If you have sudden, severe attacks of fear or anxiety with intense physical symptoms (shaking, sweating) when there is no apparent reason to be afraid.
- If intense, irrational fears of common places, objects, or situations interfere with your daily life.
- If symptoms of anxiety are still severe after 1 week of home treatment.
- If you suffer from nightmares or flashbacks to traumatic events.
- If you are unable to feel certain about things (e.g., whether you unplugged the iron) no matter how many times you check, or if repetitive actions that you cannot control interfere with your daily activities.

Depression

Most people experience some form of depression at some point in their lives. Depression can range from a minor problem to a major life-threatening illness. Fortunately, effective treatments are available for most people who suffer from depression.

Sadness or Depression?

If you have experienced 5 or more of the following symptoms nearly every day for more than 2 weeks, you may be suffering from depression:

- Feelings of sadness, anxiety, or hopelessness.
- Lack of interest or pleasure in usual activities or pastimes.
- Increase or decrease in appetite or unexplained gain or loss of weight.
- Frequent backaches, headaches, stomach problems, or other aches that don't respond to treatment.
- Insomnia or excessive sleepiness.
- Low energy, fatigue.
- Feeling restless or irritable.
- Feeling worthless or guilty.
- Inability to concentrate, remember, or make decisions.
- Frequent thoughts of suicide or death.

Home treatment may be all that is needed for mild depression. However, if you are feeling suicidal or if home treatment doesn't help lift your mood within 2 weeks, contact a health professional. With counseling, medication, and continued home treatment, you can overcome most cases of depression.

Depression is probably caused by a combination of factors, including the genetic traits that a person inherits from his or her parents. Most major depressions involve problems with the chemical messengers (neurotransmitters) in the brain. The amount of stress in a person's life and the way a person copes with stress also contribute to depression.

Ongoing depression affects a person's body, mind, and social behavior.

Many things can trigger depression, including:

- Drinking alcohol or using illegal drugs.
- Having a major illness or injury.
- Grieving the death of a loved one.
- Going through major life changes (loss of a job, divorce, children leaving home, retirement).
- Being under long-term stress, such as having a family member with a chronic illness.
- Taking certain medications or having certain health conditions.
- Having recently had a baby (postpartum depression).

Reduced daylight during the winter seems to cause a form of depression called seasonal affective disorder in some people. See page 315.

Everyone gets sad. Gauging how deep and pervasive your sad feelings are can help you decide what to do. See "Sadness or Depression?" on page 314 to help determine if you are depressed.

Seasonal Affective Disorder

Seasonal affective disorder (SAD), sometimes called the winter blues, is a mental health problem that usually occurs in the months when there is less sunlight. There is no known cure, but it can be controlled, and it improves in the spring when there are more hours of daylight. The main symptoms include depressed mood, decreased energy, and food cravings. If you notice such a pattern developing during the winter, consider trying the following:

- Go out into the sun as often as possible. Protect your skin—it's your eyes' exposure to the sun that will help.
- Take a vacation to a sunny place.
- Get regular exercise, either outdoors or indoors near a window that lets in sunlight.

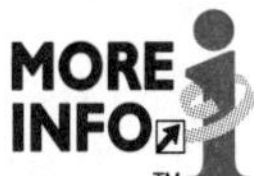
Light therapy (phototherapy) is sometimes successful in treating SAD. It involves sitting, working, or reading in front of high-intensity lights for up to several hours a day.

Medication can also be helpful, either alone or in combination with light therapy.

Because many things can contribute to depression, combining self-care and professional treatment is often most effective. The most common form of treatment combines counseling (psychotherapy) with medication. Inpatient treatment is sometimes needed in severe cases.

Home Treatment

For many people, self-care alone can improve symptoms of mild depression. For more serious depression, self-care can add to the benefits of professional treatment.

- Consider what might be causing or adding to your depression:
  - Are medications causing it? Review your prescription and nonprescription medications with a pharmacist or physician.
  - If it's wintertime or you haven't been out in the sun for a while, read the information about seasonal affective disorder on page 315.
- Pace yourself according to your energy level. Choose what is most important to get done and do those things first.
- Do not make major life decisions when you are depressed. If you must make a major decision, ask someone you trust to help you.
- Do not drink alcohol or use medications that have not been prescribed by your health professional.

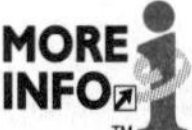

- Spend time with other people. Do things you usually enjoy, even if you don't feel like doing them.
- Get enough sleep. If you are having difficulty sleeping, see Sleep Problems on page 317.
- Eat a healthful diet (see Chapter 17). If you don't feel like eating, eat small snacks rather than large meals.
- Exercise regularly. Getting 20 to 30 minutes of exercise each day is good for your body and your mind. Go for a walk. Take the stairs instead of the elevator. Dance.
- Believe that this mood will pass. Then look for signs that it is ending.
- Give yourself time to heal. Do not expect too much from yourself too soon.

When to Call Kaiser Permanente

- If you are feeling suicidal or are planning to hurt someone else.
- If you hear voices that tell you to hurt or kill yourself or someone else.
- If you have a sudden change in your behavior or start to do things that you wouldn't usually do (such as having casual sex or drinking more alcohol than you normally would).
- If symptoms of depression (see "Sadness or Depression?" on page 314) last longer than 2 weeks despite home treatment.
- If grieving continues without improvement for more than 4 weeks. See page 320.

Eating Disorders

In a society where "thin is in," many of us have tried skipping meals or going on diets to lose weight. Unlike typical dieters, people who have eating disorders have medical problems that cause disturbances in their eating behavior.

Anorexia nervosa is a disorder of severe self-imposed dieting. It affects teenage girls most often. Symptoms include refusing to eat; extreme weight loss; loss of menstrual periods; a distorted body image (thinking you're fat when you're actually very thin); a preoccupation with food; low self-esteem; and excessive exercise.

Bulimia nervosa is an eating disorder characterized by binge eating and purging (forced vomiting or abuse of laxatives and diuretics). The binges are usually triggered by emotional upset, not hunger. Other symptoms include dry skin and brittle hair; swollen glands under the jaw from vomiting; depression and mood swings; a distorted body image; and secrecy to keep others from discovering your abnormal behavior.

People who have anorexia usually look starved, but most people who have bulimia maintain a normal weight and look healthy. Most people with anorexia deny they

MORE INFO For more information, see the inside front cover.

have a problem; people with bulimia know they have a problem, but they keep it a secret.

Compulsive overeating is characterized by binging on food. An overeater will consume thousands of calories at a time, quickly and without pleasure. Because there is no purging, a compulsive overeater becomes obese.

Eating disorders appear to be caused by emotional and psychological factors. They tend to run in families, so there may be a genetic link. Eating disorders require professional treatment. If untreated, they can lead to major health problems or even death. Treatment usually involves nutritional counseling, individual psychotherapy, family therapy, and medication. A hospital stay may be required in extreme cases.

Prevention

- Teach and model healthful eating and exercise habits at home and at school.
- Help young people develop confidence and self-esteem. Accept them for who they are, not how they look.
- Be careful about encouraging a young person to lose weight. Communicate that you love and care for the person, regardless of how much he or she weighs.
- Don't set unrealistic expectations for your child. Striving to live up to them may lead to an eating disorder.
- Be alert to the stress in your child's life. Be available to talk over any problems.

When to Call Kaiser Permanente

Call if you recognize any of these warning signs of an eating disorder:

- Unrealistic body image or an unreasonable fear of gaining weight.
- Extreme weight loss in a short period of time.
- Forced vomiting or excessive use of laxatives.
- Excessive dieting or preoccupation with food.
- Excessive, rigid exercise routines.
- Loss of menstrual periods in a young woman.
- Withdrawal from family and friends.

Sleep Problems

The term **insomnia** can mean:

- Trouble getting to sleep (taking more than 30 minutes to fall asleep).
- Awakenings with inability to fall back asleep.
- Early morning awakening.

None of these are problems unless they make you feel chronically tired. If you are less sleepy at night or wake up early in the morning, but still feel rested and alert, there is little need to worry.

Short-term insomnia, lasting from a few nights to a few weeks, is usually caused by worry over a stressful situation. Long-term insomnia, which can last months or even years, is often caused by general anxiety, medications, chronic pain, depression, or other physical disorders.

Sleep apnea is a sleep disorder that is usually caused by a blockage in the upper airways. When airflow through the nose and mouth is blocked, breathing repeatedly stops for 10 to 15 seconds or longer. People who have sleep apnea usually snore loudly and are very tired during the day. They are not aware of waking up at night but do have very restless sleep. Sleep apnea can affect children and adults.

Mild sleep apnea may be cured by changing some of your pre-bedtime habits. More severe sleep apnea may require medical treatment.

Prevention

- Get regular exercise, but avoid strenuous exercise within 2 hours before bedtime.
- Avoid alcohol and smoking, especially before bedtime. Drink caffeine in moderation.
- If you smoke or use other tobacco products, consider getting help to quit. See page 26 for tips on quitting.
- Make sure your sleeping conditions are comfortable. Keep your bedroom as quiet and dark as possible. The best room temperature for sleeping is 65°.
- Avoid foods that upset your stomach. Try drinking less to avoid trips to the bathroom.
- Warm milk or a light snack may be helpful.

Home Treatment

- Avoid taking sleeping pills. They can cause daytime confusion, memory loss, and dizziness. Continued use of sleeping pills actually increases sleeplessness in many people.
- Try the following 7-step formula for 2 weeks:

  1. Reduce mental stimulation an hour before bedtime. Engage in relaxing activities (e.g., take a warm bath, read, or do some slow, easy stretches).
  2. Use your bed for sleeping and sex only. Don't work, eat, watch TV, or read in bed.
  3. Sleep only at bedtime. Avoid naps longer than 20 minutes. (However, naps are fine if you don't have sleep problems.)
  4. Go to bed only when you feel sleepy.

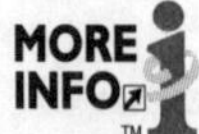

5. If you lie awake for more than 15 minutes, get up, leave the bedroom, and do something relaxing.
6. Repeat steps 4 and 5 until it is time to get up.
7. Get up at the same time each day, no matter how sleepy you are.

- If you worry a lot at bedtime, try using another time of day to address problems and possible solutions.
- Review all of your prescription and nonprescription medications with a pharmacist to rule out drug-related sleep problems.
- Review the sleeping tips for snorers on page 169.
- Read about anxiety on page 312.
- Read about depression on page 313.

When to Call Kaiser Permanente

- If you regularly take sleeping pills and are unable to stop taking them.
- If you suspect medications or health conditions such as chronic pain are causing sleep problems.
- If you are suffering from anxiety or depression.
- If you or your partner snores loudly and heavily and feels excessively sleepy during the day.
- If you, your partner, or your child has many episodes of sleep apnea (stops breathing, gasps, and chokes during sleep).
- If you wake up a lot because your legs move.
- If your child snores, has difficulty breathing while asleep, sleeps restlessly and awakens frequently, or is very sleepy during the day.
- If 1 month of self-care doesn't solve the problem.

Suicide

If you are very depressed or feel overwhelmed, you may sometimes think of taking your own life. Occasional thoughts of suicide are not a problem. However, if thoughts of suicide continue, or if you have made suicide plans, it becomes a very serious matter.

People who are considering suicide are often undecided about choosing life or death. With compassionate help, they may choose to live.

Prevention

When there are significant life crises, when you are depressed, or when someone you know is depressed, be alert to the warning signs for suicide:

- Verbal warning. Most people who commit suicide mention their intentions to someone.
- Preoccupation with death. A suicidal person may talk, read, draw, or write about death.
- Previous suicide attempt. Failed attempts are often followed by a completed attempt.

- Giving away prized possessions.
- Depression and social isolation.

If you are troubled by suicidal thoughts, you should avoid alcohol and illegal drugs. Alcohol and drugs can impair your judgment, which may make you more likely to do things you would not do when sober.

Home Treatment

- Use your common sense and a direct approach to determine if the suicide risk is high. Ask yourself or the person who you feel is at risk:
  - Do you feel there is no other way?
  - Do you have a suicide plan?
  - How and when do you plan to do it?
- Ask someone you trust to stay with you or the suicidal person until the crisis has passed.
- Encourage the person to seek professional help.
- Don't argue with or challenge the person who is thinking of suicide.
- Don't ignore warning signs, thinking that you or another person will "snap out of it."
- Talk about the situation as openly as possible. Show understanding and compassion.

Grief

Grief is a natural healing process that allows you to adjust to a significant change or loss. Grief may be expressed physically or emotionally and may have some of the same symptoms as depression (see page 313). The following tips may help you move through the grieving process.

- Take as much time as you need to grieve. Don't fight the emotions you feel.
- Discuss your feelings with friends who will listen to and support you while encouraging you to reconnect with the world. Joining a support group or talking to a clergyperson or a counselor also may help.
- Write your thoughts down in a journal or paint or draw your grief. Or write letters to the person you lost.
- Try to cut back on some of your usual responsibilities and activities until your grieving period is past. Postpone any major decisions.
- As you begin to move beyond your grief, renew old interests and pursue new ones. Do things that give you a sense of control and hope.

Call your physician if grieving continues without improvement for more than 4 weeks.

When to Call Kaiser Permanente

Call 911 or seek other emergency services immediately if you or someone you know is attempting suicide.

Call your physician or your local Suicide Prevention hot line (look in the Yellow Pages):

- If you are considering suicide.
- If you suspect that someone has made suicide plans.

Violent Behavior and Abuse

Anger and disagreements are normal parts of healthy relationships. However, anger that leads to threats or violence, such as hitting or hurting, is not normal or healthy. Physical, verbal, or sexual abuse is not an acceptable part of any relationship. There is no excuse for it, and it is not your fault. Nobody deserves to be abused.

Violent behavior is a common problem. It often begins with verbal threats or relatively minor incidents, but over time it can become more serious, involving physical harm. Abuse occurs when someone attacks you with words, objects, hands, or fists. Abuse usually happens when one person tries to control another person. Abusive behavior is destructive and dangerous. Every year, thousands of people are seriously hurt or killed by their partners, spouses, or other family members.

Children are also affected by abuse. They may feel scared and ashamed, or think that they caused the problem. Violent behavior is learned behavior, so children grow up learning that it's okay to hurt people or let other people hurt them. It is important to teach your children that violence is not a healthy solution to conflict.

If you are unsure whether your relationship is abusive, there are signs to look for. This can be the first step in solving the problem.

Ask yourself, does my partner:

- Limit where I can go, what I can do, and whom I can talk to?
- Call me names or tell me that I'm crazy?
- Criticize things I do and say, or how I look?
- Unexpectedly check up on me at my workplace, home, school, or elsewhere?
- Hit, shove, slap, kick, punch, or choke me?
- Blame me for the abuse he or she commits?
- Force me to have sex against my will?
- Hurt my pets or destroy things special to me?
- Threaten to hurt or kill me?

- Apologize and tell me it will never happen again (even though it already has)?

If you answered yes to any of these questions or your partner could answer yes, you may be in an abusive relationship. You are not alone. There are people who can help you (friends, family members, neighbors, health care workers). Everyone has the right to be in a safe relationship.

Prevention

- Seek nonviolent ways to resolve conflicts. Disagreeing is fine, even healthy, as long as it does not turn violent. See Anger and Hostility on page 311 for more information about controlling anger.
- Teach your children that violence is not a solution to conflicts. Do not use physical discipline such as spanking. If you need help with discipline, consider taking a course on parenting skills.
- Do not keep firearms or other weapons in a home where there is someone who has a drug or alcohol problem, is prone to violent behavior, or has threatened suicide.
- Be alert to warning signs, such as threats or drunkenness, so you can avoid dangerous situations. If you cannot predict when violence may occur, have an "exit plan" for use in an emergency.

Job Stress

On-the-job stress can bring on feelings of anxiety, anger, and depression, which affect our lives and our health. If your work environment or job responsibilities are causing such negative feelings, don't let your emotions rule your actions. Try the following:

- Check and recheck the facts before you act.
- Find out what your rights are; don't tolerate abuse.
- Talk to your employer and try to work things out.
- Use appropriate resources: your union, your company's personnel department, Employee Assistance Program, or Equal Employment Opportunity Commission.

When to Call Kaiser Permanente

- If you have thoughts of hurting yourself, the people you work with, or anyone else.
- If you have problems with sleeping, eating, or day-to-day functioning.
- If your preoccupation with work problems begins to interfere with your life outside of work.

When to Call Kaiser Permanente

Call 911 or seek other emergency services immediately:

- If you or someone in your family has just been physically abused or the victim of violence. Physical abuse is a crime, no matter who does it.

Call Kaiser Permanente:

- If you are concerned about violent behavior (such as physical, verbal, or sexual abuse) in your own relationship or that of a family member, friend, or co-worker.
- If you suspect abuse, neglect, or maltreatment of a child or if a child reports this kind of treatment to you. You may also call local child protective services or the police.

Check the Yellow Pages for hot lines and other resources for victims of abuse.

The Mind-Body Connection

Medical science is making remarkable discoveries about the relationship between your state of mind and your mental and physical health. Researchers have found that one function of the brain is to produce substances that can improve your health. Your brain can create endorphins, which are natural painkillers; gamma globulin for fortifying your immune system; and interferon for combating infections, viruses, and even cancer. Your brain can combine these and other substances into a vast number of tailor-made prescriptions for whatever ails you.

The substances that your brain produces depend in part on your thoughts, feelings, and expectations. If your attitude about an illness (or life in general) is negative and you don't have expectations that your condition will get better, your brain may not produce enough of the substances your body needs to heal. On the other hand, if your attitude and expectations are more positive, your brain is likely to produce sufficient amounts of the substances that will boost your body's healing power.

Your physical health also has an impact on your brain's ability to produce substances that affect your mental well-being. An illness or injury that causes long-term physical stress can lead to chemical imbalances in the brain which may lead to depression and other mental health problems.

Positive Thinking

People with positive attitudes generally enjoy life more, but are they any healthier? The answer is often "yes." Optimism is a resource for healing. Optimists are more likely to overcome pain and adversity in their efforts to improve their medical treatment outcomes. For example, optimistic coronary bypass patients generally recover more quickly and have fewer complications after surgery than do patients who are less hopeful.

Your body responds to your thoughts, emotions, and actions. In addition to staying fit, eating right, and managing stress, you can use the following 3 strategies to help maintain your health:

1. Create positive expectations for health and healing.

Mental and emotional expectations can influence medical outcomes. The effectiveness of any medical treatment depends in part on how useful you expect it to be. The "placebo effect" proves this. A placebo is a drug or treatment that provides no medical benefit except for the patient's belief that it will help. On the average, 35 percent of patients who receive placebos report satisfactory relief from their medical problem, even though they received no actual medication.

Changing your expectations from negative to positive may enhance your physical health. Here's how to make the change:

- Stop negative self-talk. Make positive statements that promote your recovery.
- Send yourself a steady stream of affirmations. An affirmation is a phrase or sentence that sends strong, positive statements to you about yourself, such as "I am a capable person," or "My joints are strong and flexible."
- Visualize health and healing. Add mental pictures that support your positive affirmations.
- Don't feel guilty. There is no value in feeling guilty about health problems. While there is a lot you can do to reduce your risk for health problems and improve your chances of recovery, some illnesses may develop and persist no matter what you do. Some things just are. Do the best you can.

2. Open yourself to humor, friendship, and love.

Positive emotions boost your health. Fortunately, almost anything that makes you feel good about yourself helps you stay healthy.

- Laugh. A little humor makes life richer and healthier. Laughter increases creativity, reduces pain, and speeds healing. Keep an emergency laughter kit that contains funny videotapes, jokes, cartoons, and photographs. Put it with your first aid supplies and keep it well stocked.
- Seek out friends. Friendships are vital to good health. Close social ties help you recover more quickly from illness and reduce your risk of developing diseases ranging from arthritis to depression.
- Volunteer. People who volunteer live longer and enjoy life more than those who do not volunteer. By helping others, we help ourselves.

- Plant a plant and pet a pet. Plants and pets can be highly therapeutic. When you stroke an animal, your blood pressure goes down and your heart rate slows. Animals and plants help us feel needed.

3. Appeal to the Spirit.

If you believe in a higher power, ask for support in your pursuit of healing and health. Faith, prayer, and spiritual beliefs can play an important role in recovering from an illness. See Healing on page 335.

Your sense of spiritual wellness can help you overcome personal trials and things you cannot change. If it suits you, use spiritual images in visualizations, affirmations, and expectations about your health and your life.

Dealing With Chronic Pain

Long-term, persistent pain (chronic pain) is a problem for many people, especially middle-aged and older adults. Chronic pain is associated with fatigue, sleep problems, irritability, stress, depression, anxiety, and withdrawal from daily activities. Arthritis, back problems, recurring sports injuries, nerve damage, cancer, and many other conditions can result in chronic pain. In many cases the cause of pain is not known. A variety of factors can contribute to it.

Your mind and body are important allies in your efforts to manage chronic pain. Pain often has an emotional as well as a physical component. In other words, your thoughts and feelings about pain can affect how much pain you feel. Feeling anxious, angry, frustrated, or out of control about your pain may make pain worse. If you can put your mind to work against the pain, you may find that you can manage pain better and that it interferes less with your life.

There is no magic solution for dealing with chronic pain, no matter what the cause. However, the following tips for dealing with both the emotional and physical aspects of chronic pain may help:

- Take control of the pain. This may mean accepting that the pain is not going away, but deciding to take active steps toward managing it and keeping it from affecting your life too much.
- Practice positive thinking (see page 323). Recognize unhelpful or self-defeating thoughts, such as "This pain will never get better" or "I'll never be able to play with the grandkids with this pain." Your thoughts can affect your perception of pain.
- Track how your moods, thoughts, and activities affect your pain. Record your pain level in relation to these factors several times a day for several days. You may find that your pain is worse during or after certain activities or when you are feeling a certain emotion.
- Try to relax. Chronic pain causes stress and tension, which may make the pain worse. Try the

relaxation techniques on pages 328 to 330. Learning relaxation skills takes practice, so give each method a 2-week trial. If one doesn't work for you, try another.

- Take any pain medication your health professional has recommended or prescribed on schedule and in the correct dose.
- Exercise regularly. Try gentle, low-impact exercises that don't aggravate your pain, such as swimming, water aerobics, walking, or stationary cycling. Do the stretching exercises on page 295 every day. Ask your health professional about physical therapy, too.
- Experiment with heat, cold, and massage. Find out what works best for you.
- Make sure you are getting enough sleep. See Sleep Problems on page 317. If pain frequently disrupts your sleep, talk to your health professional.
- Change the way you do daily activities so you can do them with less pain. Some people find assistive devices (such as canes, foot supports, or specially designed household tools) helpful.
- Consider complementary therapies such as biofeedback, acupuncture, or yoga in addition to your regular medical care (not as a substitute for it). See Complementary Medicine beginning on page 331.
- Join a support group. By being around others who share your problem, you and your family can learn skills for accepting and coping with pain. You may also feel less isolated. To find a group near you, contact the American Chronic Pain Association at (916) 632-0922.

No one should have to suffer in uncontrolled pain. Call your health professional if chronic pain is affecting your quality of life. Although treatment will probably not be able to eliminate pain completely, it can help reduce the pain and its impact on your life.

Stress and Distress

Stress is the physical, mental, and emotional reactions you experience as the result of changes and demands in your life.

Stress is part and parcel of common life events, both large and small. It comes with all of life's daily hassles, traffic jams, long lines, petty arguments, and other relatively small irritations. Stress also comes with crises and life-changing events, such as illness, marriage problems or divorce, losing a job, getting a new job, or children leaving home.

All these events may force you to adjust, whether you are ready to or not. Unless you can regularly release the tension that comes with stress, it can greatly increase your risks of physical and mental illness.

Because many major life events are beyond your control, take charge of those aspects of your life that you can manage. One major change doesn't mean that all areas of your life must change. Continue to participate in the same activities you did before the event happened.

Not all stress is bad. Positive stress (eustress) is a motivator, challenging you to act in creative and resourceful ways. When changes and demands overwhelm you, negative stress (distress) sets in. This section has specific techniques you can use to cope with stress in your life.

What Stress Does to the Body

At the first sign of alarm, chemicals released by the pituitary and adrenal glands and the nerve endings automatically trigger these physical reactions to stress:

- Heart rate increases to move blood to the muscles and brain.
- Blood pressure goes up.
- Breathing rate increases.
- Digestion slows down.
- Perspiration increases.
- Pupils dilate.
- You feel a rush of strength.

Your body is tense, alert, and ready for action. For primitive people, these reactions were an advantage in the face of sudden danger, preparing them for survival by either "fight or flight." Today, our bodies still react the same way, but it is not as acceptable to either fight or run away (although we often wish we could).

After the natural "alarm" reaction to a real or perceived threat, our bodies stay on alert until we feel the danger has passed. When the stressor is gone, the brain signals an "all clear" sign to the pituitary and adrenal glands. They stop producing the chemicals that caused the physical reaction, and the body gradually returns to normal.

Problems with stress occur when the brain fails to give the "all clear" signal. If the alarm state lasts too long, you begin to suffer from the consequences of constant stress. Unrelieved stress can lead to many health problems.

Recognizing Stress

Sometimes it's difficult to recognize or admit that stress is affecting your health. If you can learn to watch for its effects and take corrective action quickly, you will be able to cope with your stress.

The signs of stress are classic. You may get a headache, stiff neck, nagging backache, rapid breathing, sweaty palms, or an upset stomach. You may become irritable and intolerant of even minor disturbances. You may lose your temper more often and yell at your family for no good reason. Your pulse rate may increase and you may feel jumpy or exhausted all the time. You may find it hard to concentrate.

When these symptoms appear, recognize them as signs of stress and find a way to deal with them. Just knowing why you're crabby may be the first step in coping with the problem. It is your attitude toward stress, not the stress itself, that affects your health the most.

Managing Stress

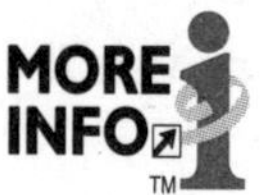

Some people try to relieve stress by smoking, drinking, overeating, or taking pills. There is a better way. Avoid the dangerous side effects of tobacco, alcohol, and drugs by learning to control your stress level. You can do this by using your body to soothe your mind and using your mind to soothe your body.

Stress and tension affect our emotions and feelings. By expressing those feelings to others, we are able to better understand and cope with them. Talking about a problem with a spouse or a good friend is a valuable way to reduce tension and stress.

Crying can also relieve tension. It's part of our emotional healing process. Expressing yourself through writing, crafts, or art may also be a good tension reliever.

Exercise is a natural response to stress; it is the normal reaction to the fight-or-flight urge. Walking briskly will take advantage of the rapid pulse and tensed muscles caused by stress and release your pent-up energy. After a long walk, your stress level is usually lower and more manageable.

The rest of this chapter is devoted to other skills and techniques that will help you increase your resistance to stress and better cope with those stressors you choose to accept.

Relaxation Skills

Whatever you do to manage stress, you can benefit from the regular use of relaxation skills. Relaxation is the exact opposite of the fight-or-flight response.

When learning relaxation skills, you must remove yourself from all outside distractions. It may take some practice to become comfortable with these techniques. Once you've trained your body and mind to relax (2 to 3 weeks), you'll be able to produce the same relaxed state whenever you want.

The following 3 methods of relaxation and meditation are among the simplest and most effective. They should be done once or twice a day for about 10 to 20 minutes. Pick a time and place where you won't be disturbed or distracted.

Belly Breathing

The object of belly breathing is to develop full use of your lungs and get in touch with the rhythm of your breathing. It can be practiced in any position, but it is best to learn it lying on your back, with your knees bent.

MORE INFO For more information, see the inside front cover.

1. Place your left hand on your abdomen and your right hand on your chest. Notice how your hands move as you breathe in and out.

2. Practice filling your lower lungs by breathing so that your left hand goes up when you inhale and your right hand remains still. Always inhale through your nose and exhale through your mouth.

3. When you have filled and emptied your lower lungs 8 to 10 times, add the second step to your breathing: inhale first into your lower lungs as before, and then continue inhaling into your upper chest. As you do so, your right hand will rise and your left hand will fall a little as your abdomen falls.

4. As you exhale slowly through your mouth, make a quiet, whooshing sound as first your left hand and then your right hand falls. As you exhale, feel the tension leaving your body as you become more and more relaxed.

5. Practice breathing in and out in this manner for 3 to 5 minutes. Notice that the movement of your abdomen and chest is like rolling waves rising and falling in a rhythmic motion.

Practice belly breathing daily for several weeks until you can do it almost anywhere, providing you with an instant relaxation tool any time you need one.

CAUTION: Some people get dizzy the first few times they try belly breathing. If you begin to hyperventilate or become lightheaded, slow your breathing. Get up slowly.

Progressive Muscle Relaxation

The body responds to tense thoughts or situations with muscle tension, which can cause pain or discomfort. Deep muscle relaxation reduces the muscle tension as well as general mental anxiety. You can use an audiotape to help you go through all the muscle groups or you can do it by just tensing and relaxing each muscle group. Deep muscle relaxation is effective in combating stress-related health problems and often helps people get to sleep.

Muscle Groups and Procedure

Pick a place where you can lie down on your back and stretch out comfortably, such as a carpeted floor.

Tense each muscle group for 4 to 10 seconds (hard but not to the point of cramping), then give yourself 10 to 20 seconds to release it and relax. At various points, review the muscle groups and relax each one a little more each time.

How to Tense Muscle Groups

Hands: Clench them.

Wrists and forearms: Extend them and bend the hands back at the wrist.

Biceps and upper arms: Clench your hands into fists, bend your arms at the elbows, and flex your biceps.

Shoulders: Shrug them. (Check the arms and shoulders area for tension.)

Forehead: Wrinkle it into a deep frown.

Around the eyes and bridge of the nose: Close your eyes as tightly as possible. (Remove contact lenses before beginning the exercise.)

Cheeks and jaws: Grin from ear to ear.

Around the mouth: Press your lips together tightly. (Check the face area for tension.)

Back of the neck: Press your head back hard.

Front of the neck: Touch your chin to your chest. (Check the neck and head area for tension.)

Chest: Take a deep breath and hold it; then exhale.

Back: Arch your back up and away from the floor.

Stomach: Suck it into a tight knot. (Check the chest and stomach area for tension.)

Hips and buttocks: Press the buttocks together tightly.

Thighs: Clench them hard.

Lower legs: Point your toes toward your face, as if trying to bring the toes up to touch your head.

Lower legs: Point your toes away and curl them downward at the same time. (Check the area from the waist down for tension.)

When you are finished, return to alertness by counting backwards from 5 to 1.

Relaxation Response

The relaxation response is the exact opposite of a stress response. It slows heart rate and breathing, lowers blood pressure, and helps relieve muscle tension.

Technique (adapted from Herbert Benson, MD):

1. Sit quietly in a comfortable position with your eyes closed.

2. Begin progressive muscle relaxation. See page 329.

3. Become aware of your breathing. Each time you exhale, say the word "one" (or any other word or phrase) silently or aloud. Concentrate on breathing from your abdomen and not your chest.

Instead of focusing on a repeated word, you can fix your gaze on a stationary object. Any mental stimulus will help you to clear your mind.

Continue this for 10 to 20 minutes. As distracting thoughts enter your mind, don't dwell on them, just allow them to drift away.

4. Sit quietly for several minutes, until you are ready to open your eyes.

5. Notice the difference in your breathing and your pulse rate.

Don't worry about becoming deeply relaxed. The key to this exercise is to remain passive, to let distracting thoughts slip away like waves on the beach.

Practice for 10 to 20 minutes once or twice a day, but not within 2 hours after a meal. When you have set up a routine, you can achieve the relaxation response with little effort.

For the times they are a-changin'.
Bob Dylan

19 Complementary Medicine

Each year, millions of people seek some kind of "complementary" or "alternative" treatment, such as acupuncture or herbal medicine, for their health problems. Many Americans use alternative therapies along with mainstream medical treatments (drugs and/or surgery) to control pain, manage stress, and speed healing.

While complementary treatments are becoming more widely accepted, they are not right for everyone and every situation. Like any other treatment option, alternative treatment should be chosen only after you gather as much reliable information as possible, understand the facts, and consider your personal needs and values. For more information, see Chapter 1, Making Wise Health Decisions.

Here are some important things to consider when trying to decide whether to try a complementary therapy:

- Is it your idea to try an alternative treatment, or is someone pushing you into it? You need to be the one who is in control of your body and your health.
- Do you think that complementary medicine has something special to offer you, or are you seeking an alternative treatment because you are fed up with conventional medicine? It is important to recognize the strengths and limitations of both conventional and complementary medicine.
- Do you hope to gain more comfort and control over your illness by using an alternative treatment, or are you looking for something that will cure your illness? Seeking a

cure through complementary medicine may be harmful to your health and your pocketbook. Discuss your expectations with the practitioner and make sure they are realistic.

- What is the practitioner's expertise? Check with state and local medical licensing agencies and departments of consumer affairs to see if the practitioner is licensed and in good standing. Talk to people who have had experience with the practitioner. Visit the practitioner and ask questions about his or her education, training, licenses, and certification.

Your primary care physician may be able to help you make a decision about trying a complementary treatment. Some people think their physicians don't want them to try complementary medicine. But more and more physicians are realizing that complementary therapies can work with conventional medicine to help people feel better.

If you decide to try some form of alternative medicine, be sure to let your physician know. Even if your physician is not comfortable with your decision, it is important for your physician to know what you are doing for your health concerns. As much as possible, it is important that your conventional treatments work with your alternative treatments.

Health Fraud and Quackery

Millions of people are taken in each year by medical fraud and worthless health products.

Bogus cures are advertised for many chronic health problems, especially arthritis, cancer, baldness, and impotence. The ads target people who are ready to try anything. Unfortunately, many of these products cause harmful side effects. It is wise to be suspicious of products that:

- Are advertised by testimonials.
- Claim to have a secret ingredient.
- Have not been evaluated in prominent medical journals.
- Claim benefits that seem too good to be true.
- Are available only by mail.

Be suspicious of any practitioner who:

- Prescribes medicines or gives injections at every visit.
- Promises a no-risk cure.
- Suggests something that seems unethical or illegal.

The best way to protect yourself from medical fraud is to be observant and ask questions. If you don't like what you see or hear, find another practitioner or get a second opinion.

General Risks and Benefits of Complementary Medicine

All treatments, whether conventional or alternative, have risks and benefits. In general, the risks and benefits of complementary therapies are as follows.

Risks

Rejecting conventional medicine: Some practitioners of alternative therapies do not refer people to conventional physicians even when it is clear that conventional medicine could help. And some people who choose alternative medicine refuse to consider conventional medicine for any problem. This can be dangerous. It is best to get as much information as possible and then make informed decisions, selecting from both conventional and alternative approaches.

Too many options, not enough evidence: There are many different alternative treatments. Very few of them have been studied for safety and effectiveness using sound scientific methods. Herbal medicines and nutritional supplements are not regulated by the Food and Drug Administration (FDA) as conventional medications are. It may be hard to get the facts, which can make it more difficult for you to make an informed decision.

Cost: Many health insurance companies do not yet cover the costs of alternative or complementary therapies. As with conventional medical treatments, you must decide whether an alternative therapy is working for you and is worth the time and money you must invest in it.

Benefits

Holistic approach: When you see your conventional physician, your visit usually lasts only 10 to 15 minutes. People who provide alternative treatments often take 1 hour or more to find out all about your life—your family, friends, diet, activities, and work. Many people with health problems, especially chronic diseases, are more likely to respond to treatment when extra time is given to consider the whole person.

Active listening and touch: For many people, to be listened to and touched in a caring way can be very healing. People who provide alternative treatments often spend more time listening to their patients. In some cases, alternative medicine practitioners include healing touch as part of the way they communicate with and treat patients.

Mind-body connection: Science has shown that people's emotional states can affect how healthy they are. See Chapter 18. People who describe themselves as happy tend to be healthier than those who are unhappy. People who have a lot of stress in their lives are more likely to get sick. Conventional medicine traditionally does not have much to offer for these kinds of problems. Practices like meditation and tai chi can help ease stress and improve a person's sense of well-being, which may improve a person's physical health.

Choosing the Right Therapy for You

There are many types of complementary medicine. Choosing between different treatments can be confusing. This section describes several of the most popular alternatives. You can use this section to help you decide which of these treatments (if any) is most likely to help you.

Acupuncture

The main idea behind acupuncture is that there is energy called *qi* or *chi* (pronounced "chee") flowing throughout your body. Your *chi* flows along energy pathways called meridians. If the flow of *chi* is blocked or unbalanced at any point on a meridian, you may become ill. The aim of acupuncture is to unblock and balance the flow of *chi* to restore health.

Acupuncture is done by stimulating particular points along meridians that relate to the symptoms you are having. This is usually done by sticking very thin needles through your skin, but some practitioners use heat, pressure, or a mild electrical shock to stimulate the meridians.

Acupuncture is one of the most tested alternative medicine treatments. Several studies have shown that acupuncture works to control pain and nausea and may help people with addiction problems.

Bodywork

There are several kinds of bodywork practiced throughout the world. Some of the most common are the Alexander Technique, the Feldenkrais Method, and Rolfing. Bodywork is working directly with touch and movement of the body. While the theory behind the methods varies, what is similar is the use of movement and appropriate touch to release tightness and pain. Bodywork teaches you to become more aware of your body, posture, and patterns of movement.

The goal is to develop more natural body positioning, which over time may reduce stress and ease pain.

There has not been much scientific testing of bodywork. While not conclusive, a few studies have suggested good results in people with arthritis, stress, low back pain, and children with cerebral palsy.

Chiropractic Treatment

The primary aim of chiropractic therapy is to help the body heal itself by correcting misalignments of the joints, particularly the bones of the spine (vertebrae).

Chiropractic treatments usually involve having a chiropractor twist, pull, or push your body to realign your joints and the bones in your spine. Some chiropractors use heating pads or electrical stimulation to help loosen a joint before adjusting it.

Some studies show that chiropractic treatments may be helpful in the treatment of back and neck pain.

Healing

Healing is sometimes referred to as spiritual healing, faith healing, or therapeutic touch. Faith healing is a part of some religions. Spiritual healing is more widespread and may or may not have anything to do with religion. Nurses often use therapeutic touch in conventional medical settings to help heal and comfort their patients.

Like many other complementary approaches, healing starts with the idea that people are naturally healthy. The way people live and think may disturb their natural health energy, and they become ill. The aim of healing is to focus healing energy from a divine or spiritual source to the person who is sick. The methods of healing include prayer or meditation, channeling of healing energy through a healer, or transfer of healing energy through the laying on of hands.

There has been almost no research on this type of healing. Some people have begun to study the power of prayer. If you give up on conventional medicine when it has the possibility of good outcomes and only use healing, you may be putting your health in danger. It is important not to turn away from other treatments that may be effective. Healing can always be used along with more conventional treatments.

Herbs

Herbal medicine uses plants as medicines to keep people healthy and cure illness. Herbal medicine has been around for thousands of years. Many conventional medicines are based on herbal medicines. For example, willow bark tea was used for centuries to control fever. Drug companies learned to copy the chemical makeup of willow bark to produce aspirin.

In recent years there has been increasing interest in the use of herbal products. Many people think that because "it's natural, it must be safe." However, anything that has possible good effects also has side effects. In fact, some herbs can cause sickness and even death.

There have been thousands of studies on the effects of herbs. Most of the research has been done in Europe and China, and herbal medicine is widely practiced in those countries. In the United States, the analysis of this research began fairly recently, and many new studies are underway.

In the U.S., herbal products are not categorized as drugs and are not regulated by the U.S. government. They do not have to be tested for safety or purity by manufacturers. Studies have shown that the amount of herb in the bottle may be anywhere from 0 percent to 150 percent of the amount claimed on the label. Buy wisely if you choose to purchase herbs. Herbs sold in Kaiser Permanente pharmacies have been researched and evaluated to ensure reliable, high quality.

Be sure to tell your doctor about any herbs or natural supplements you are taking. Pregnant and breastfeeding women and people with serious health problems should not use any herbal medicines or natural supplements without consulting their physician. Like conventional medications, herbal and natural supplements can occasionally cause allergic reactions or other side effects. If this occurs, stop using the herb or supplement and notify your physician.

Homeopathy

Homeopathy, like other alternative treatments, is based on the idea that the body has the ability to heal itself. Sometimes the body needs to be stimulated to start the healing process. In homeopathy, a treatment is chosen because it can cause health problems just like the one that is troubling you. The treatment is given in such a small amount that it does not cause the problem but stimulates your body to heal the problem.

Homeopathy is used to treat allergies, atopic dermatitis, rheumatoid arthritis, and irritable bowel syndrome. Homeopathy is widely used in England and other European countries, and research done in those countries shows that homeopathy may work, although it is not clearly understood why.

Massage Therapy

Massage therapy is based on the idea that touch is healing. There are many different types of massage therapy. Some are very gentle, while some are very active and intense. Some methods use the same ideas as bodywork and acupuncture: the massage therapist will press on or stroke points on the body where energy is blocked and teach you to become aware of tightness and pain in your body.

Massage therapy has been and continues to be widely studied. Many studies have shown that massage therapy decreases stress and helps control pain. Health problems that are caused by or made worse by stress (such as depression and inflammatory bowel disease) may also improve with massage treatment.

Current research is focusing on the effects of massage in treating conditions such as behavioral problems, eating disorders, and fibromyalgia.

Naturopathy

Naturopathy blends basic science with complementary medicine. Schools of naturopathy teach anatomy, cell biology, pharmacology, and other sciences studied in conventional medical schools. They also teach herbal medicine, acupuncture, and bodywork. The aim of naturopathy is to help you become and stay well, which is the natural state of your body.

Naturopathic medicine is a whole system of medicine, so it is used to treat many kinds of health problems. It is used most often to treat everyday illnesses, like colds and flu, and chronic illnesses such as asthma, fibromyalgia, high blood pressure, depression, and back pain.

Two of the biggest concerns about naturopathic medicine are the use of fasting and the approach to immunization.

Fasting can be dangerous, especially if you have a disease like diabetes. Fasting puts your body under stress. Talk with your conventional physician before you try fasting. If you start to feel sick while fasting, break your fast with small amounts of fruit or juice and then return to your normal diet.

Some naturopaths believe that immunization is not important. This belief can be very dangerous. Childhood illnesses used to cause large numbers of deaths and long-term health problems. Talk with your conventional physician before deciding against immunization.

Tai Chi and Qi Gong

Tai chi and *qi gong* (pronounced "chee-gung") are traditional Chinese exercise forms. They are based on the idea that through gentle, repeated movements, deep concentration, and focused breathing, people can increase and improve the flow of their energy *(chi* or *qi)* and improve their health.

Tai chi is a series of movements done in a rhythmic pattern. *Qi gong* is a lot of different movements that can be done in any order. *Qi gong* is useful to know because you can do it anywhere, anytime, even if you are unable to sit up or stand. Some common *qi gong* movements include raising and lowering your arms, moving your head from side to side, and rubbing your ears, feet, and hands.

Both tai chi and *qi gong* are very gentle and can be done by people of all ages. Their primary benefits are improved muscle strength, balance, and coordination. They increase stamina, lower blood pressure, relieve stress, and help prevent falls. These exercise forms are excellent for older adults because they improve coordination and flexibility, and they do not harm the joints. Possible strains and sprains are their only harmful side effect.

A variation of *qi gong*, called external *qi gong*, is a form of healing in which one person (a *qi gong* master) projects his or her energy to another person. If you seek out a practitioner of external *qi gong* to treat a serious illness, be sure to talk to your conventional physician first. Don't give up on your conventional medicine. It may be a good idea to combine conventional medicine and *qi gong*.

Yoga

Yoga is an ancient health practice that focuses on the mind-body connection. As it is typically practiced in the West, yoga consists of a variety of movements, postures, and breathing techniques that work together to maintain physical and mental health.

Most people who try yoga find that it helps them become more flexible and less stressed. Many repeated studies have shown that yoga helps lower blood pressure and improves a person's sense of well-being. Research has also shown that yoga can be an effective complementary treatment for migraine headaches, arthritis, and back and neck pain.

For more information about these and other alternative treatments, do some research at your local library. Talk with your physician or pharmacist to help you decide which methods may be appropriate for you. You may also contact the National Center for Complementary and Alternative Medicine (NCCAM) at the National Institutes of Health (NCCAM Clearinghouse, P.O. Box 8218, Silver Spring, MD 20907-8218, 1-888-644-6226).

Be prepared.
Boy Scout Motto

20

Your Home Health Center

More of your health care takes place in your home than anywhere else. Having the right tools, medicines, supplies, and information on hand will improve the quality of your self-care.

Store all your self-care tools and supplies in one central location, such as a large drawer in the bedroom or family room. Use the charts about tools and supplies in this chapter as checklists for keeping your home health center well stocked.

Note: If small children are around, keep your supplies out of reach or stored in containers or cabinets with childproof safety latches.

Be familiar with the disaster preparation and response plan for your area. Keep the appropriate supplies on hand.

Self-Care Tools

Self-care tools are the basic equipment of your home health center.

Cold Pack

A cold pack is a plastic envelope filled with gel that remains flexible at very cold temperatures. Buy 2 cold packs and keep them in the freezer. Use them for bumps, bruises, back sprains, turned ankles, sore joints, or any other health problem that calls for ice. A cold pack is more convenient than ice and may become the self-care tool you use the most.

You can make your own cold pack:

- Put 1 pint of rubbing alcohol and 3 pints of water in a 1-gallon, heavy-duty, plastic freezer bag.
- Seal the bag, and then seal it in a second bag. Mark it "Cold pack: Do not eat," and place it in the freezer.

A bag of frozen vegetables will also work as a cold pack.

Humidifier and Vaporizer

Humidifiers and vaporizers add moisture to the air, making it less drying to your mouth, throat, and nose. A humidifier produces a cool mist, and a vaporizer puts out hot steam.

Cool mist from a humidifier may be more comfortable to breathe than hot steam. However, humidifiers are noisy, produce particles that may be irritating to some people, and need to be cleaned and disinfected regularly. This is especially important for people who have mold allergies.

A vaporizer's hot steam does not contain any irritating particles, and you can add medications such as Vicks VapoRub to ease breathing. Steam may feel good when you have a cold, but the hot water can burn anyone who overturns or gets too close to the vaporizer.

Medicine Spoon

Medicine spoons are transparent tubes with marks that indicate typical dosage amounts. A medicine spoon makes it easy to give the right dose of liquid medicine. While the spoons are convenient for anyone, they are particularly helpful for young children. The tube shape and large lip get most of the medication into a child's mouth without spilling. Buy one at your local pharmacy.

Self-Care Tools

For every household:

- Blood pressure cuff*
- Cold pack*
- Dental mirror
- Eyedropper
- Heating pad
- Humidifier or vaporizer*
- Medicine spoon*
- Nail clippers
- Penlight*
- Scissors
- Stethoscope*
- Thermometer*
- Tweezers

For children younger than 6, add:

- Bulb aspirator/syringe
- Rectal thermometer*
- Otoscope*

*Described in text

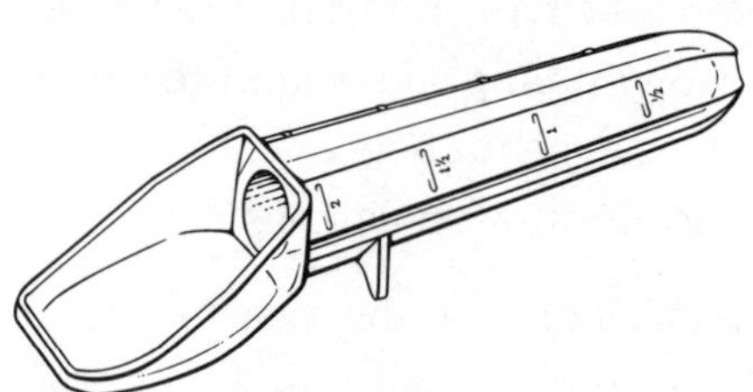

Medicine spoon

Otoscope

An otoscope is a flashlight with a special attachment for looking into the ear. With training, you can use an otoscope to help you decide if an ear infection is present. Inexpensive consumer-model otoscopes are available, but they do not illuminate the ear canal and eardrum as well as the one your physician uses does. They can also be used as high-intensity penlights.

Penlight

A penlight has a small, intense light that can be easily directed. It is useful for looking into the mouth or throat or examining the skin, and it is easier to handle than a flashlight.

Stethoscope and Blood Pressure Cuff

If you have heart disease or high blood pressure, it's a good idea to have both a stethoscope and a blood pressure cuff (sphygmomanometer) to monitor your blood pressure regularly.

Purchase a flat diaphragm-model stethoscope rather than a bell-shaped one. The flat surface makes it easier for you to hear.

Blood pressure cuffs come in many models. If you have difficulty reading the gauge on a regular cuff, look for a model that uses an upright mercury column, or an electronic digital model. Ask your pharmacist to recommend a blood pressure kit and show you how to use it.

Self-Care Supplies

The supplies listed below are useful to keep on hand in your home health center. The products are inexpensive, easy to use, and generally available in any drugstore or pharmacy.

- Adhesive strips (Band-Aids) in assorted sizes
- Adhesive tape, 1 inch wide
- Butterfly bandages
- Sterile gauze pads, 2 inches square
- Elastic ("Ace") bandage, 3 inches wide
- Roll of gauze bandage, 2 inches wide
- Cotton balls
- Safety pins

Thermometer

Mercury-containing glass thermometers are no longer recommended because of safety concerns. If you have one in your home, consider replacing it with a digital electronic thermometer.

Digital thermometers are accurate and easy to read. Temperature strips are very convenient and safe but are not as accurate as mercury or electronic thermometers and should only be used to measure axillary (armpit) temperature. They are inaccurate when used on the forehead. Thermometers that measure the temperature in the ear are fast, easy to use, and quite accurate, but they are expensive.

Rectal thermometers with enlarged bulbs are helpful for children younger than 6 or anyone who cannot hold an oral thermometer in his or her mouth.

How to Take a Temperature

A normal oral temperature ranges from 97.6° to 99.6° and for most people is 98.6°. Temperature varies with time of day and other factors, so don't worry about minor changes.

Whenever a person feels hot or cold to your touch, it is a good idea to take and record his or her temperature. If you have to call your physician during an illness, knowing your exact temperature will be very helpful.

There are 4 places where a thermometer can be placed to take a temperature:

- In the mouth (oral)
- In the anus (rectal)
- Under the armpit (axillary)
- In the ear (tympanic)

Unless otherwise specified, all temperatures in this book are oral Fahrenheit readings. If you take a rectal or axillary temperature, adjust it accordingly (see page 343).

Fahrenheit-Centigrade Conversion Chart

°F		°C
98.5	=	36.9
99.0	=	37.2
99.5	=	37.5
100.0	=	37.8
100.5	=	38.1
101.0	=	38.3
101.5	=	38.6
102.0	=	38.9
102.5	=	39.2
103.0	=	39.4
103.5	=	39.7

Oral thermometers are recommended for people age 6 and older.

- Do not drink hot or cold liquids before taking your temperature.
- Clean the thermometer with soapy water or rubbing alcohol.
- Hold it firmly at the end opposite the bulb and shake the mercury down to 95° or lower.
- Place the bulb under your tongue and close your lips around it. Do not bite down. Breathe through your nose and don't talk.
- Wait 3 to 5 minutes.

Rectal thermometers are recommended for children younger than 6 or anyone who cannot hold an oral thermometer in the mouth. Use only a rectal thermometer to take a rectal temperature. Rectal temperature is 0.5° to 1° higher than oral temperature. Rectal temperatures are the most accurate.

- Clean the thermometer and shake it down to 95° or lower.
- Put Vaseline or another lubricant on the bulb.
- Hold the child bottom-up across your lap.
- Hold the thermometer 1 inch from the bulb and gently insert it into the rectum no more than 1 inch. Do not let go. Hold the thermometer right at the anus so it cannot slip in farther.
- Wait for 3 minutes.

Axillary temperatures are less accurate and are about 1° lower than oral temperatures. Axillary readings are safer for small children who will not hold still while you take a rectal temperature.

- Use either an oral or rectal thermometer. Shake it down below 95°.
- Place the thermometer in the armpit and have the child cross the arm across the chest and hold the opposite upper arm.
- Wait 5 minutes.

How to Read a Thermometer

To read a thermometer that does not have a digital readout:

- Roll the thermometer between your fingers until you can see the thin ribbon of mercury. Note that the thermometer is marked from 92° to 108°.
- Each large mark indicates 1° of temperature. Each small mark indicates 0.2°.

Nonprescription Medications and Products

A nonprescription medication (sometimes called an over-the-counter or OTC medication) is any drug that you can buy without a physician's prescription. However, don't assume that all nonprescription drugs are safe for you. These drugs can interact with other medications and can sometimes cause serious health problems.

Some medications should only be used by adults or older children. Be sure to read the package instructions carefully, or ask a pharmacist before giving any product to an infant or young child.

Carefully read the label of any nonprescription drug you use, especially if you also take prescription medications for other health problems. Ask your pharmacist for help in finding a nonprescription drug best suited to your needs.

Some common nonprescription medications include:

- Antacids and acid blockers.
- Bulking agents and laxatives.
- Antidiarrheals.
- Cold and allergy remedies.
- Pain relievers.

These drugs can be very helpful when used properly but can also cause serious problems if used incorrectly. The following tips will help you use common nonprescription drugs wisely and safely. In some cases, you may find that you don't need to take them at all.

Antacids and Acid Blockers

Antacids are taken to relieve heartburn or indigestion caused by excess stomach acid. While they are safe if used occasionally, antacids may cause problems if taken regularly. There are several kinds of antacids. Learn what ingredients are in each type so you can avoid any adverse effects.

- Sodium bicarbonate antacids (such as Alka-Seltzer and Bromo Seltzer) contain baking soda. Avoid these antacids if you have high blood pressure or are on a salt-restricted diet.
- Calcium carbonate antacids (such as Tums and Alka-2) are sometimes used as calcium supplements (see page 304). However, these products may cause constipation.
- Aluminum-based antacids (such as Amphojel) are less potent and work more slowly than other products do. They may also cause constipation. Some may cause calcium loss and should not be taken by postmenopausal women. If you have kidney problems, check with your physician before using aluminum-based antacids.
- Magnesium compounds (such as Phillips' Milk of Magnesia) may cause diarrhea.
- Aluminum-magnesium antacids (such as Maalox, Di-Gel, Mylanta, and Riopan) are less likely to cause constipation or diarrhea than are aluminum-only or magnesium-only antacids.

Acid blockers reduce the amount of acid produced by the stomach. There are several types of nonprescription acid blockers on the market. Each has slightly different cautions for use. Read and carefully follow the instructions included with the package.

Antacid and Acid Blocker Precautions

- Try to eliminate the cause of frequent heartburn instead of taking antacids regularly. See Heartburn on page 83.
- Consult your physician or pharmacist before taking an antacid if you take other medications. Antacids may interfere with the absorption and action of some prescription medications. Also consult your physician if you have ulcers or kidney problems.

- If you have a problem with the function of your kidneys or liver, you should be careful in using acid blockers. All drugs are broken down and removed from the body by the combined action of the liver and kidneys. If your liver or kidneys are not working correctly, it is possible that too high a dose of the acid-blocking drug will build up in your body.

Bulking Agents and Laxatives

There are 2 types of products to prevent or treat constipation: bulking agents and laxatives.

Bulking agents, such as bran or psyllium (found in Metamucil, for example), are not laxatives, but they ease constipation by increasing the volume of stool and making it easier to pass. Regular use of bulking agents is safe and helps make them more effective.

Laxatives (such as Correctol, Ex-Lax, Senokot, and Dulcolax) speed up the passage of stool by irritating the lining of the intestines. Regular laxative use is not recommended.

There are many other ways to treat constipation, such as drinking more water. See page 78.

Laxative Precautions

- Take any laxative or bulking agent with plenty of water or other liquids.
- Do not take laxatives regularly. Overuse of laxatives decreases tone and sensation in the large intestine, causing laxative dependence. If you need help keeping regular, use a bulking agent.
- Regular use of some laxatives (such as Correctol, Ex-Lax, and Feen-a-Mint) may interfere with your body's ability to absorb vitamin D and calcium; this can lead to weakened bones.

Antidiarrheals

There are 2 types of antidiarrheal drugs: those that thicken the stool and those that slow intestinal spasms.

The **thickening** mixtures (such as Kaopectate) contain clay or fruit pectin and absorb bacteria and toxins in the intestine. They are safe because they do not go into the blood, but these products also absorb the bacteria needed for digestion. Long-term use is not advised.

Antispasmodic antidiarrheal products slow the spasms of the intestine. Loperamide (the active ingredient in products such as Imodium A-D and Pepto Diarrhea Control) is an example of this type of preparation. Some products (such as Donnagel and Parepectolin) contain both thickening and antispasmodic ingredients.

Antidiarrheal Precautions

- Diarrhea helps rid your body of an infection, so try to avoid using antidiarrheal medications for the first 24 hours. After that, use them only if cramping and pain continue but there are no other signs of illness, such as fever.

- Be sure to take a large enough dose. Take antidiarrheal preparations until your stools thicken; then stop immediately to avoid constipation.
- Replace lost body fluids. Dehydration can develop when someone, especially an infant, child, or older adult, has diarrhea. See page 81 for a recipe for a rehydration drink you can make at home.

Cold and Allergy Remedies

In general, whether you take drugs or not for your cold, you'll get better in about 1 week. Rest and liquids are probably the best treatment for a cold (see page 154). Antibiotics will not help. However, medications help relieve some cold symptoms, such as nasal congestion and cough.

Allergy symptoms, especially runny nose, often respond to antihistamines. Antihistamines are also found in many cold medications, often together with a decongestant. However, the value of antihistamines in treating cold symptoms is under debate.

Decongestants

Decongestants make breathing easier by shrinking swollen mucous membranes in the nose, allowing air to pass through. They also help relieve runny nose and postnasal drip, which can cause a sore throat.

Decongestants can be taken orally or used as nose drops or sprays. Oral decongestants (pills) are probably more effective and provide longer relief, but they cause more side effects. Pseudoephedrine (the active ingredient in products such as Sudafed) is an oral decongestant.

Sprays and drops provide rapid but temporary relief. Nasal sprays containing phenylephrine (such as Neo-Synephrine) are effective. Sprays and drops are less likely to interact with other drugs than oral decongestants are.

Saline Nose Drops

Nonprescription saline nasal sprays (such as NaSal and Ocean) are convenient, inexpensive, and sterile. They will keep nasal tissues moist so the tissues can filter the air. Saline nasal sprays will not cause mucous membranes in the nose to swell.

Saline nose drops can also be easily made at home. Mix ¼ teaspoon salt in 1 cup of body temperature water (too much salt will dry nasal membranes). Place the solution in a clean bottle with a dropper (available at drugstores). Use as necessary. Make a fresh solution every 3 days.

Insert the drops while lying on your back on a bed, with your head hanging over the side. This will help the drops get farther back. Try to keep the dropper from touching your nose.

Decongestant Precautions

- Do not give cold medicines or oral decongestants to infants under 6 months of age. Nonprescription cold medicines have not been proven effective for preschool children.
- Do not use medicated nasal sprays or drops more than 3 times a day or for more than 3 days in a row. Continued use will cause a "rebound effect": your mucous membranes swell up more than before you used the spray.
- Drink extra fluids when taking cold medications.
- Decongestants can cause problems for people who have certain health problems, such as heart disease, high blood pressure, glaucoma, diabetes, or an overactive thyroid. Decongestants may also interact with some drugs, such as certain antidepressants and high blood pressure medications. Read the package carefully or ask your pharmacist or physician to help you choose one.

Cough Preparations

Coughing is your body's way of getting foreign substances and mucus out of your respiratory tract. Coughs are often useful, and you shouldn't try to eliminate them. Sometimes, though, coughs are severe enough to impair breathing or prevent rest.

Water and other liquids, such as fruit juices, are probably the best cough syrups. They help soothe the throat and also moisten and thin mucus so it can be coughed up more easily.

You can make a simple and soothing cough syrup at home by mixing 1 part lemon juice with 2 parts honey. Use as often as needed. This can be given to children older than 1 year of age.

There are 2 kinds of cough medicines: expectorants and suppressants. **Expectorants** help thin the mucus and make it easier to cough mucus up when you have a productive cough. Look for expectorants containing guaifenesin, such as Robitussin and Vicks 44E.

Suppressants control or suppress the cough reflex and work best for a dry, hacking cough that keeps you awake. Look for suppressant medications containing dextromethorphan, such as Robitussin-DM or Vicks Dry Hacking Cough.

Don't suppress a productive cough too much (unless it is keeping you from getting enough rest).

Cough Preparation Precautions

- Cough preparations can cause problems for people with certain health problems, such as asthma, heart disease, high blood pressure, or an enlarged prostate. Cough preparations may also interact with some drugs, such as sedatives and certain antidepressants. Read the package carefully or ask your pharmacist or physician to help you choose one.

- Cough suppressants can stifle breathing. Use them with caution if you give them to someone who is very old or frail or if you have chronic respiratory problems.
- Read the label so you know what the ingredients are. Some cough preparations contain a large percentage of alcohol; others contain codeine. There are many choices. Ask your pharmacist to advise you.

Antihistamines

Antihistamines dry up nasal secretions and are commonly used to treat allergy symptoms and itching.

If your runny nose is caused by allergies, an antihistamine will help. For cold symptoms, home treatment and perhaps a decongestant (see page 346) will probably be more helpful. It is usually best to take only single-ingredient allergy or cold preparations, instead of those containing many active ingredients.

Products such as Chlor-Trimeton (chlorpheniramine) and Benadryl (diphenhydramine) are single-ingredient antihistamine products.

Products such as Dristan, Coricidin, and Triaminic contain both a decongestant and an antihistamine.

Antihistamine Precautions

- Do not give antihistamines to infants younger than 4 months of age. For children between 4 months and 1 year, ask your physician first.
- Use of antihistamines to treat the stuffiness of a cold will often thicken the mucus, making it harder to get rid of.
- Drink extra fluids when taking antihistamines.
- Antihistamines can cause problems for some people with health problems such as asthma, glaucoma, epilepsy, or an enlarged prostate. Antihistamines may also interact with some drugs, such as certain antidepressants, sedatives, and tranquilizers. Read the package carefully or ask your pharmacist or physician to help you choose one that will not cause problems.
- The drowsiness that antihistamines often cause usually lessens with continued use. If it continues, or if the medication isn't helping your allergies after 1 week, call your physician for advice.
- Antihistamines that don't cause drowsiness are available by prescription. These drugs carry some additional risks. Ask your physician.

Pain Relievers

There are dozens of pain reliever products. Most contain either aspirin, ibuprofen, or acetaminophen. These 3 drugs, as well as ketoprofen and naproxen sodium, relieve pain and reduce fever. Aspirin, ibuprofen, ketoprofen, and naproxen sodium also relieve inflammation. They belong to a class of drugs called non-steroidal anti-inflammatory drugs (NSAIDs).

When purchasing pain relievers, keep in mind that generic products are chemically equivalent to more expensive brand-name products, and they usually work equally well.

Aspirin

Aspirin is widely used for relieving pain and reducing fever in adults. It also relieves minor itching and reduces swelling and inflammation. Most tablets contain 325 mg of aspirin. Although it seems familiar and safe, aspirin is a very powerful drug.

Aspirin Precautions

- Aspirin causes more childhood poisonings than does any other drug. Keep all aspirin, especially baby aspirin, out of children's reach.
- Aspirin can irritate the stomach lining, causing bleeding or ulcers. If aspirin upsets your stomach, try a coated brand, such as Ecotrin. Talk with your physician or pharmacist to determine what will work best for you.
- Aspirin increases the risk of Reye syndrome in children. See page 224. Do not give aspirin to anyone younger than 20 unless your physician tells you to do so.
- Some people are allergic to aspirin. (They may also be allergic to ibuprofen.)
- Throw aspirin away if it starts to smell like vinegar.
- Do not take aspirin if you have gout or if you take blood thinners (anticoagulants).
- Do not take aspirin for a hangover. Aspirin used with alcohol increases your risk for stomach irritation.
- High doses may result in aspirin poisoning (salicylism). Stop taking aspirin and call a health professional if any one of these symptoms occurs:
  - Ringing in the ears
  - Visual disturbances
  - Nausea
  - Dizziness
  - Rapid, deep breathing

Other Aspirin Uses

In addition to relieving pain and inflammation, aspirin is effective against many other ailments. Because of the danger of side effects and the interactions aspirin may have with other medications, do not try these uses of aspirin without a physician's supervision.

- **Heart attacks and strokes**: Aspirin in low but regular doses helps prevent heart attacks and strokes in certain people. Doses as low as 30 mg per day have helped. Aspirin may also help as a first aid measure for heart attacks. Chewing ½ tablet may be enough to help.

- **Stomach and colon cancer**: Some studies have shown that taking 1 aspirin tablet per day can reduce the risk of cancers in the digestive system.
- **Migraines**: Regular, low-dose aspirin use may reduce the frequency of migraines.

Other Pain Relievers

Ibuprofen (the active ingredient in products such as Advil and Nuprin), **ketoprofen** (in products such as Orudis KT and Actron), and **naproxen sodium** (in products such as Aleve) are other nonsteroidal anti-inflammatory drugs (NSAIDs). Like aspirin, these drugs relieve pain and reduce fever and inflammation. Also like aspirin, they can cause nausea, stomach irritation, and heartburn. People who take blood thinners (anticoagulants) should use these drugs with caution.

Acetaminophen (the active ingredient in products such as Tylenol) reduces fever and relieves pain. It does not have the anti-inflammatory effect of NSAIDs, such as aspirin and ibuprofen, but it also does not cause stomach upset and other side effects.

The product's package label will tell you how many milligrams (mg) of medicine are in each pill; how much you should take; and how often you should take it. Do not exceed the dosage limits, and follow the instructions on the package if you have health problems that may make it unsafe for you to take the usual dosage of a product.

Syrup of Ipecac

For any poisoning, call your physician, emergency department, or poison control center immediately!

Syrup of ipecac is a drug used to induce vomiting when a poison has been swallowed.

In most cases of poisoning, the best treatment is to get the substance out of the victim's stomach as quickly as possible. Syrup of ipecac is excellent for this. Also see page 63.

However, making someone vomit can sometimes be harmful. Do not use ipecac when a person has swallowed any of the items listed under "Poisons" on page 351. Give water to dilute the poison without inducing vomiting.

Dosage for Ipecac

Do not give ipecac to children younger than 1 year of age. For anyone older than 1, give 1 tablespoon. After giving the ipecac, have the person drink at least 12 ounces of water, which is essential to ensure vomiting. Try to keep the person walking around.

Repeat the dose of ipecac in 20 minutes if the person has not yet vomited. Repeat only once. When the person vomits, have the person lie on his or her side with the mouth lower than the chest, so that vomited material will not enter the airway. If the person leans over a toilet, be sure the chest is lower than the stomach.

Poisons

Do not induce vomiting:

- Dishwasher detergent
- Gasoline, kerosene
- Drano
- Oven cleaner
- Oil-based paints
- Furniture polish
- Cleaning solutions
- Antifreeze

Induce vomiting:

- Dishwashing liquid
- Plant food
- Aspirin and other medications
- Ink
- Fingernail polish remover
- Rat poison

The vomiting caused by ipecac is very violent. Ipecac should not be used in the following situations:

- If a woman is more than 5 months pregnant.
- If the victim has a history of heart disease.
- If the child is younger than 1 year of age.
- If the victim might choke on the vomited material or inhale it into the lungs. This can happen if the person:
  - Is over 65.
  - Has taken Valium or another drug that may cause unconsciousness.
  - Is drunk.
  - Is drowsy or lethargic.

Keep ipecac on hand and replace it every 5 years if you haven't used it. It will remain effective for 1 year after it has been opened.

Prescription Medications

There are thousands of different prescription medications used to treat hundreds of different medical conditions. Your physician and your pharmacist are your best sources of information about your prescription medications. Good books are available that contain information about many different prescription drugs.

Guidelines for taking every kind of prescription medication could fill several books. Common types covered here include antibiotics, minor tranquilizers, and sleeping pills.

Antibiotics

Antibiotics are drugs that kill bacteria. They are effective against bacteria only and have no effect on viruses. Therefore, antibiotics will not cure the common cold, flu, or any other viral illness. Unless you have a bacterial infection, it's best to avoid the possible adverse effects of antibiotics, which may include:

- **Side effects**, including **allergic reactions**. Common side effects of antibiotics include nausea, diarrhea, and increased sensitivity to sunlight. Most side effects are mild, but some, especially allergic reactions, can be severe. An allergic reaction can be life-threatening. If you have any unexpected reaction to an antibiotic, tell your health professional before another antibiotic is prescribed.
- **Secondary infections**. Antibiotics kill most of the bacteria in your body that are sensitive to them, including the bacteria that help your body. Antibiotics can destroy the bacterial balance in your body, leading to stomach upset, diarrhea, vaginal infections, or other problems.
- **Bacterial resistance**. When antibiotics are used too often, bacteria change so that the antibiotics are no longer effective against them. This makes bacterial infections more difficult to treat.

When you and your health professional have decided that an antibiotic is necessary, carefully follow the instructions for taking the prescription.

- Take the whole dose for as many days as prescribed, unless you have unexpected side effects (in which case, call your health professional). Antibiotics kill off many bacteria quite quickly, so you may feel better in a few days. However, if you stop taking the antibiotic too soon, the weaker bacteria will have been eliminated, but the stronger ones may survive and flourish.
- Be sure you understand any special instructions about taking the medication. The instructions should be printed on the label, but double-check with your physician and pharmacist.
- Store antibiotics in a dry, cool place. Check carefully to see if they need refrigeration.
- Never give an antibiotic prescribed for one person to someone else.
- Do not save leftover antibiotics, and do not take an antibiotic prescribed for another illness without a health professional's approval.

Minor Tranquilizers and Sleeping Pills

Minor tranquilizers (such as Valium, Librium, Xanax, and Tranxene) and sleeping pills (such as Dalmane, Restoril, and Ambien) are widely prescribed. However, these drugs can cause problems, including memory loss, addiction, and injuries from falls caused by drug-induced unsteadiness.

Minor tranquilizers can be effective for short periods of time. However, long-term use is often of limited value and introduces the risk of addiction and mental impairment.

Adverse Drug Reactions

Side effects, drug-drug and food-drug interactions, overmedication, and addiction may cause:

- Nausea, indigestion, vomiting.
- Constipation, diarrhea, inability to control urine, or difficulty urinating.
- Dry mouth.
- Headache, dizziness, ringing in the ears, or blurred vision.
- Confusion, forgetfulness, disorientation, drowsiness, or depression.
- Difficulty sleeping, irritability, or nervousness.
- Difficulty breathing.
- Rashes, bruising, and bleeding problems.

Don't assume any symptom is a normal side effect that you have to suffer with. Call your physician or pharmacist any time you suspect that your medicines are making you sick.

Sleeping pills may help for a few days or a few weeks, but using them for more than 1 month generally causes more sleep problems than it solves. For other approaches, see page 317.

If you have been taking minor tranquilizers or sleeping pills for a while, talk with your physician about reevaluating your need for the medication or reducing your dosage. If you have experienced any unsteadiness, dizziness, or memory loss, tell your physician.

Medication Problems

Several kinds of adverse medication reactions can occur:

Side effects. Side effects are predictable but unpleasant reactions to a drug. They are usually mild, but they can be inconvenient. In some cases, they are more serious.

Allergies. Some people have severe, sometimes life-threatening reactions (called anaphylaxis) to certain medications. See page 143 for signs of an allergic reaction.

Drug-drug interactions. These occur when 2 or more prescription or non-prescription drugs mix in a person's body and cause an adverse reaction. The symptoms can be severe and may be improperly diagnosed as a new illness.

Drug-food interactions. These occur when medications react with food. Some drugs work best when taken with food, but others should be taken on an empty stomach. Some drug-food reactions can cause serious symptoms.

Overmedication. Sometimes the full adult dose of a medication is too much for small people and those over age 60. Too much of a drug can be very dangerous.

Addiction. Long-term use of some medications can lead to dependency, and severe reactions may occur if the medications are withdrawn suddenly. Narcotics, tranquilizers, and barbiturates must be taken very carefully to prevent addiction. See page 308.

Save Money on Medications

Nonprescription and prescription medications can be very expensive. Here are some ways to cut your medication costs:

- Buy generic nonprescription products. They are chemically equivalent to brand-name drugs but are usually cheaper. Ask your physician if generic forms of your prescription medications are available and appropriate for you.
- Shop around and compare prices at several pharmacies. Prices can vary widely. It may be worth paying a little more if you know and trust the pharmacist.
- Ask your physician for samples of newly prescribed medications, or ask your pharmacist to fill only the first week's worth of pills. If the medication has to be changed later, you will have saved paying for the full prescription.
- Consider buying expensive drugs that you use regularly from mail-order or Internet pharmacies if they charge less. The only disadvantage is that you will not have a partnership with a local pharmacist.

Medication Guidelines

The following are basic guidelines for taking prescription and nonprescription medications:

- Use medications only if non-drug approaches are not working.
- Know the benefits and side effects of a medication before taking it.
- Take the minimum effective dose.
- Never take a drug prescribed for someone else.
- Follow the prescription instructions exactly or let your physician know why you didn't.
- Keep medications tightly capped in their original containers, and store them as directed.
- Do not take medications in front of small children. Children are great mimics. Don't oversell the "candy" taste of children's medicines or leave children's vitamins accessible to children.
- Add a consumer's guide to medications to your home health library.

Home Medical Tests

Many common medical tests are now available in home kits. Combined with regular visits to your health professional, home tests can help you monitor your health and, in some cases, detect problems early.

Home medical tests must be very accurate (over 95 percent) to be approved by the Food and Drug Administration (FDA). However, they must be used correctly to give such accurate results. Follow the package directions exactly. If you have questions, ask your pharmacist or call the toll-free phone number on the product label.

Home medical tests are especially helpful if you have a chronic condition that requires frequent monitoring, such as diabetes, asthma, or high blood pressure. Ask your physician which home medical tests would be appropriate for you. Some common tests are described next.

Blood Glucose Monitoring

If you have diabetes, you may already monitor your blood sugar levels using a finger prick and a test strip or an electronic monitor.

This test should always be used under a physician's supervision. Never adjust your insulin dose based on a single abnormal test, unless your physician has specifically instructed you to do so.

Check with your physician if you have symptoms of abnormal blood sugar levels, even if the test is normal. See page 239.

Blood Pressure Monitoring

If you have high blood pressure, it is important to monitor your blood pressure frequently. With a little instruction, you can easily monitor your blood pressure at home.

By checking your blood pressure at home, when you are relaxed, you will be able to track changes resulting from your home treatment and medications.

- Do not make any changes to your medications based on your home blood pressure readings without consulting your physician.
- Check your blood pressure at different times of day to see how rest and activities affect it. For regular readings, check it at the same time every day. Blood pressure is usually lowest in the morning and rises during the day.
- For the most accurate reading, sit still for 5 minutes before taking your blood pressure.
- Have your blood pressure cuff device adjusted (calibrated) yearly.

Tests for Blood in Stool

The fecal occult blood test can detect hidden blood in your stools, which may indicate colon cancer or other problems. This test is inexpensive and easy to do, but it may not be able to detect colon cancer as well as other screening tests can. Your physician may recommend a more accurate screening test for colon cancer called a flexible sigmoidoscopy. See page 92.

Home Pregnancy Tests

Home pregnancy tests are reliable and require only a few steps. Follow the package instructions and report all positive results to your physician.

Home Medical Records

Your home health center is a good place to keep your family's medical records. A 3-ring binder or wire-bound notebook with dividers for each member of the family is helpful. Each person should have a cover sheet listing:

- Diagnosed chronic conditions (arthritis, asthma, diabetes, high blood pressure, etc.).
- Any known allergies to drugs, foods, or insects.
- Information that would be vital in an emergency, such as whether the person has a pacemaker or a hearing aid, has diabetes or epilepsy, or is deaf or blind.
- Name and phone number of primary physician.

Other important information that should be included:

- An up-to-date list of medications that includes name of drug, purpose, dose, instructions, name of physician who prescribed the drug, and date prescribed.
- Immunization records: childhood immunizations, tetanus, influenza, and pneumonia.
- Health screening results: blood pressure, cholesterol, vision, hearing.
- Records of major illnesses and injuries, such as pneumonia, bronchitis, and broken bones.
- Records of any major surgical procedures and hospitalizations.
- Records listing major diseases in members of your family: heart disease, stroke, cancer, or diabetes.

Health Information at Home

Getting good health information is the key to making good health decisions. If the information you need is not in this book, keep looking. Here's how:

On the Internet. Follow the instructions on the inside front cover of this book to use the members-only section of our public Web site at www.kaiserpermanente.org. There you will find an in-depth health encyclopedia covering more than 1,900 health topics and 600 medical tests and procedures. It is a good resource that complements this handbook. If you have Internet access, go to this site first.

If you don't find everything you need in the health encyclopedia, don't give up. There is plenty of reliable information out there if you know where and how to look for it. See Five Tips for Finding Good Web Sites on page 357.

On the phone. Kaiser Permanente and many other health care organizations have nurse advice lines you can call to get answers to your health questions. Local offices of national organizations like the American Cancer Society, American Heart Association, Arthritis Foundation, or American Diabetes Association can help connect you with information resources in your area. Check your phone book.

At your library or bookstore. Research librarians at public libraries spend a good part of their time helping people find information. Ask for their help if you are trying to learn more about a health problem. Libraries can also be a good place to use the Internet if you don't have a computer at home. Be aware that the information found in books and magazines is not guaranteed to be any more accurate than that found on the Internet. Use some of the tips for finding good Web sites as a guide for finding helpful books.

Health information you find on the Internet or in books or magazines should never replace the medical expertise and experience of a health professional. Discuss what you find with your doctor to learn if and how it relates to your particular situation.

Five Tips for Finding Good Web Sites

As a source of health information, the Internet has two major drawbacks. First, there is little to no regulation of what gets published. Misleading, contradictory, inaccurate, and even fraudulent health information is all over the Internet. Second, the amount of information available on the Internet can make your search overwhelming and time-consuming.

With so much information out there, how do you separate the good from the bad? We hope these guidelines will help you find information you can trust.

1. Don't rely on search engines. Instead, use the Kaiser Permanente Web site, or go to other trusted sources recommended by your health professional. If you do use a search engine, be sure to follow the other four tips closely.

2. Don't trust the information on a health Web site unless the site clearly indicates:

- Who wrote and reviewed the information.
- When the information was last updated.
- What sources and references the information is based on. (Look for a bibliography or reference list.)

If information is missing, be skeptical of the site's reliability.

3. Check the site's privacy policy. It should tell you that your personal information will not be given to any third party without your explicit permission. Web sites displaying the URAC Health Web Site Accreditation seal should be safe.

4. Check the site ownership or sponsorship. Web sites displaying the URAC Health Web Site Accreditation seal should indicate any influence that the owner or sponsor has on the site's content.

5. Watch out for these clues that a Web site is of questionable quality:

- Heavy use of personal testimonies without references to good research.
- Unsupported claims of a "secret" or "revolutionary" cure.
- Promotion of a specific drug, dietary supplement, medical device, or other product.
- Requirement of a financial investment.

Your final test should be the common sense test. If information doesn't make sense to you, don't trust it without first talking with your health professional. Never make a health care decision based solely on what you read on the Internet.

Index

A

Abdominal pain 75
after eating 87
between meals or at night 83, 88, 95
burning beneath the breastbone 83
cramping 75
generalized 75
in children 231
in lower right abdomen 77
in upper right abdomen 88, 97
localized 75
lower abdominal/pelvic pain (females) 259, 263, 268
lower abdominal/pelvic pain (males) 273, 274, 275, 277
menstrual cramps (dysmenorrhea) 262
rigid or tender abdomen 35
with bloating and gas 87
with fever 77, 88
with unexpected vaginal bleeding 259
Abdominal problems 75
chart 76
Abrasion
corneal 62
skin (scrapes) 66
Abstinence, sexual 280, 285, 287
Abuse
drug or alcohol 27, 308
physical or emotional 321
Abusive behavior 321
Accidental needle stick 288
Accidental tooth loss 32
Acetaminophen 350
Achilles tendinitis 123, 131
Acid blockers 344
heartburn and 84
ulcers and 96
Acne 197
Acquired immunodeficiency syndrome (AIDS) 286
Acupuncture 334
Addiction 354
alcohol or drug 308
Adenoids 170, 172
adenoidectomy 171, 172
adenoiditis 170
ear infections and 171, 172
snoring and 171
Adrenaline kit, for stings 60
Advance health care directives 9
Advice nurses 5
Aerobic exercise 292
Affirmations 324
AIDS (acquired immunodeficiency syndrome) 286
Al-Anon 310
Alcohol use
alcoholism 308
moderate 309
problems 308
Alcoholics Anonymous 310
Allergic reaction 59, 143
Allergies 141
anaphylactic shock 143
antihistamines and 348
asthma and 146
atopic dermatitis and 200
food 145
hives and 209
insect bites and stings and 59
medications for 346
milk (lactose intolerance) 304
rashes and 211
shots 143
Alopecia areata 216
Alternative medicine, see Complementary medicine
Ana-Kit 143
Anal, also see Rectal
fissure 92
itching 91, 236
Anaphylactic shock 59, 143
Anemia 305
Anger and hostility 311, 321
Angina 153
Animal bites 33
Anorexia nervosa 316
Antacids 344
heartburn and 84
ulcers and 96
Antibiotics 351
bacterial infections and 156
diarrhea and 82
nausea and vomiting and 90
recurrent ear infections and 185
side effects of 351
viral infections and 156
Antidiarrheals 345
Antifungal medications 208
for yeast infection 269
Antihistamines 348
for itching 206
Anti-inflammatories 348, 350
heartburn and 84
high blood pressure and 246
ulcers and 95
Antioxidant vitamins 299
Anus, see Rectal
Anxiety 312
hyperventilation and 57
Apnea 169, 318
Appendicitis 77
Arthritis 117, 123, 127
back problems and 105
common types of (chart) 118
jaw pain and 136
Artificial tears 174
Ask-the-Physician Checklist 2

Aspirin 349
  asthma and 146
  bruises and 40
  hearing loss and 184
  heart attacks and strokes and 349
  heartburn and 84
  nosebleeds and 61
  Reye syndrome and 224
  ringing in the ears and 188, 349
  stomach and colon cancer and 350
  ulcers and 95
Asthma 146
  inhaler for 149
  plan for 147, 148
Atherosclerosis 242
Athlete's foot 207
Atopic dermatitis (eczema) 200
Aura, before headache 192
Axillary temperature, how to take 343

B

Babies, see Infant and child health 217
Back injuries 103
  also see Spinal injuries 69
Back problems 103
  arthritis and 105
  exercises to avoid 110
  exercises to prevent 107
  first aid for 104
  headache and 194
  leg pain with 105
  menstrual cramps and 262
  osteoporosis and 129
  physical therapy and 113
  prevention 105
  sciatica 105
  surgery for 112
  with fever and chills (males) 274, 275
  with painful urination, fever, chills 100
Bacterial infections 156
Bacterial vaginosis 266
Bad breath 28
Bald spots 216
Bandages, butterfly 47, 48
Barrier methods (birth control) 280, 281
Basal body temperature (birth control) 280
Bed-wetting (enuresis) 221
Bee stings 59
Belly breathing 328
Bellybutton 217
Benign positional vertigo 178
Benign prostatic hyperplasia (BPH) 274
Benzoyl peroxide 199
Beta carotene 299
Binge eating 316
Birth control 279
  during menopause 260
  emergency contraception 279, 280, 281
  methods (chart) 280
Birth control pills 280, 281
  bleeding between periods and 258
  headaches and 195
  high blood pressure and 245
  irregular periods and 263
Birth defects, folic acid and 256
Birthmarks 205
Bites
  animal 33
  human 33
  insect and spider 59
  lice and scabies 210
  snake 68
  ticks 71
Black eye 40
Blackheads 197
Bladder
  control, loss of 98
  infection (cystitis) 100
Bleeding
  after sexual intercourse 259
  between periods 258, 262, 283
  cuts 46
  from a mole 214
  head injury and 52
  how to stop 47
  nosebleeds 60
  rectal 78, 83, 84, 90, 91, 92, 95
  shock and 67
  spinal injuries and 69
  ulcers 95
  vaginal 258
Blisters 201
  burns and 41
  frostbite and 51
  on genitals 283, 285
  on mouth, lip, or tongue 204, 234
  sunburn and 214
Bloating 87, 95
  premenstrual syndrome (PMS) and 265, 266
Blood
  in eye 173
  in semen 273
  in sputum 151, 164
  in stools 78, 83, 84, 90, 91, 92, 95, 230
  in urine 102, 230
  in urine (males) 275
  in vomit 230
  under a nail 34
Blood glucose level
  diabetes and 239
  high or low 242
  home monitoring 241, 355
Blood in stool test 355
Blood pressure 245
  blood pressure cuff 341
  dizziness and 178
  high 245
  how to measure 355
Blood sugar, see Blood glucose level
Blood test for HIV infection 287
Blunt abdominal wounds 35
Blurred vision, see Vision
Body mechanics 107, 114, 116

Bodywork 334
Boils 202
Bone, muscle, and joint problems 117
Bottlefeeding 221
Botulism, see Food poisoning 94
Bowel movements
antidiarrheals 345
bleeding during 78, 91
bloody or black 78, 83, 84, 90, 91, 92, 95, 230
constipation 78
diarrhea 82, 228
irregular 87
laxatives 345
loose and watery 82
loss of control 112
mucus in stool 87
mucus leakage from the anus 91
painful or difficult to pass 78, 91
stool leakage 91
test for blood in 355
BPH (benign prostatic hyperplasia) 274
Breast
changes in 252, 253
infection in 253
lump in 251, 253
pain in 250, 264
self-exam 251
Breast cancer 249, 252
hormone therapy and 261
screening, frequency of 249
Breast health 249
breast self-exam 251
clinical breast exam 250
mammogram 249
Breastfeeding 219, 258
ear infections and 182
Breathing emergencies 36
choking 44
CPR 36
Heimlich maneuver 45
rescue breathing 36
Breathing problems
hyperventilation 56
panting or difficulty breathing 145, 149
rapid, labored, or shallow breathing 67, 164, 168
shortness of breath 54, 59, 152, 287
snoring 169, 171
wheezing or difficulty breathing 59, 145, 146, 150
Bronchitis (chest cold) 150
Bruises 40
Brushing teeth 28
Bulging soft spot (fontanelle) 232, 235
Bulimia nervosa 316
Bulking agents 345
Bunions 119
Burns 41, 43, 49, 214
Bursitis 120, 122, 123, 126
Butterfly bandage 47

C

Caffeine, headaches and 194
Calcium 304
osteoporosis and 130
supplements 304
Calendar method (birth control) 280
Calf pain 127
Calluses 202
Cancer
aspirin and 350
breast 249, 252
cervical 254, 265
colorectal 20, 92
hormone therapy and 261
ovarian 265
prostate 275
rectum 20, 92
skin 212
testicular 277
uterine (endometrial) 261, 265
vegetables and 299
Candidiasis (yeast infection) 207, 268
Canker sores 203
Car seats for infants and children 228
Carbon monoxide poisoning 64
Cardiac syncope 178
Cardiopulmonary resuscitation (CPR) 36
ready reference chart 37
Carpal tunnel syndrome 124
Cataracts 179
Cavities, dental 28
Centigrade-Fahrenheit conversion chart 342
Central deafness 184
Cervical cancer 254, 265
HPV and 284
screening, frequency of 254
Cervical cap (birth control) 280, 282
Cesarean delivery (C-section) 257
Charley horse 127
Checkups, frequency of 20, 28
Cheekbone, pain in 165
Chemical burns 43
Chest and respiratory problems 141
chart 142
Chest pain 151, 152, 164
angina 153
burning beneath breastbone 83
burning between navel and breastbone 95
chest-wall pain 152, 164
costochondritis 152
crushing or squeezing 151
heart attack 54, 152, 153
hyperventilation and 56
radiating to arm, neck, or jaw 54, 152, 153
with coughing 164
with productive cough and fever 150, 164
with shortness of breath 54, 152
Chewing tobacco 24, 25
Chickenpox (varicella) 222
shingles and 208
vaccine 17, 223

Children, see Infant and child health
Chipped tooth 32
Chiropractic treatment 334
Chlamydia 283
Choking 44
  first aid for (Heimlich maneuver) 45
Cholesterol, blood 242
  how to reduce 243
  LDL and HDL 242, 243
  screening, frequency of 243
  triglycerides 243
Cholesterol, dietary 303
Chronic conditions 239
Chronic fatigue syndrome 139
Chronic obstructive pulmonary disease (COPD) 150
Chronic pain 325
Cigar smoking, quitting 24, 25
Cigarette smoking, quitting 24
Circumcision 219
Clinical breast exam 250
Cluster headaches 193
Cold pack 133, 339
Cold sores 204
  increased frequency of 289
Colds 154
  medications for 346
Colic 224
Colorado tick fever, see Tick bites 71
Colorectal cancer 20, 92
  screening, frequency of 20, 92
Complementary medicine 331
  conventional medicine and 333, 335
  general risks and benefits 333
  practitioners' qualifications and expertise 332
Compulsive overeating 317
Concussion, see Head injuries 52
Condoms 280, 282, 288
Conductive hearing loss 184
Confusion
  following a head injury 53
  shock and 67
Conjunctivitis (pinkeye) 175
Constipation 78
  bloody stools and 78
  hemorrhoids and 91
  irritable bowel syndrome and 87
  laxatives 345
  with abdominal pain and fever 77
Contact dermatitis, see Rashes 211
Contact lenses 176
Contraception, see Birth control 279
Contusions (bruises) 40
Convulsions, with fever 233
COPD (chronic obstructive pulmonary disease) 150
Cornea, scratched (corneal abrasion) 62
Corns and calluses 202
Coronary artery disease, see Heart disease
Costochondritis 152
Coughs 157
  chart 157
  chronic 157
  dry and hacking 157
  expectorants 347
  persistent and dry with shortness of breath 287
  productive 157, 164
  suppressants 347
  with asthma 146, 157
  with bronchitis 150
  with chest pain 150, 164
  with croup 226
  with pneumonia 164
  with tuberculosis 164
CPR (cardiopulmonary resuscitation) 36
  ready reference chart 37
Crabs (pubic lice) 210
Cradle cap 225
Cramps
  menstrual (dysmenorrhea) 262, 264
  muscle 127
  stomach 75, 78, 82, 87, 128
Cross-training, and sports injuries 133
Croup 226
Crying, persistent 224
C-section (Cesarean delivery) 257
Cuts 46
Cyst
  on wrist (ganglion) 124
  ovarian 76, 77
Cystitis (bladder infection) 100

D

Dairy foods 304
  intolerance of 89
Dandruff 205
Deafness, see Hearing loss 184
Death, thoughts about 314, 316, 319
Decision making, shared 3
Decongestants 346
  high blood pressure and 245
DEET 59, 72
Dehydration 80, 230
  oral electrolyte solutions for 229
  rehydration drinks for 81
Dental care 27
  brushing 28
  checkups and cleanings 28
  flossing 28
  fluoride 28
  sealants 29
Dental problems, also see Mouth problems
  accidental tooth loss 32
  bad breath 28
  cavities 28
  chipped tooth 32
  gum disease 28
  jaw pain 136
  plaque 28

tartar buildup 28
TM disorder 136
tooth decay 28
tooth pain 165
Dependence, alcohol or drug 308
screening test for 309
Depo-Provera 280, 281
Depression 313
Dermatitis 211
Diabetes 239
emergencies 242
exercise and 240, 292
home glucose monitor 241
Diabetic retinopathy 241
Diaper rash 227
Diaphragm (birth control) 280, 282
Diarrhea 82
antidiarrheals 345
bloody or black 83
dehydration and 80, 228, 230
in children 228
irritable bowel syndrome and 87
lactose intolerance and 304
persistent 87, 287
Diet 22
also see Nutrition
guidelines 298, 300
to lower cholesterol 243
to reverse heart disease 247
Dieting, excessive 316
Difficulty speaking or understanding speech 71
Digestive problems, see Abdominal problems 75
Digital rectal exam 276
Diphtheria, pertussis, and tetanus (DTaP) vaccine 16
Disc injury 103, 105
Dizziness 178, 180
shock and 67
with other signs of stroke 71
Domestic violence 321
Drinking, alcohol 308
Drooling, excessive 168
Drowning, first aid for 36
Drowsiness, with headache, fever, stiff neck 160
Drug use 308, 310
Drugs, see Medications
Dry eyes 174
Dry skin 206
DTaP (diphtheria, pertussis, and tetanus) vaccine 16
Duodenal ulcer 95
Dysmenorrhea (menstrual cramps) 262

E

Ear infections 180, 186
adenoids and 171, 172
otitis externa 186
otitis media 180
recurrent 185
Ear problems 181
chart 181
discharge 186
dizziness 178, 180
drainage 180, 183
earache 180, 183, 186
earwax buildup 183, 184
effusion (serous otitis) 182
feeling of fullness in ear 180, 183, 186
hearing loss 182, 183, 184, 186
itching 186
labyrinthitis 179
Meniere's disease 179
object in ear 61
otoscope 341
ringing or noise in ear 180, 183, 184, 188
ruptured eardrum 180
swimmer's ear 186
tinnitus 188
vertigo 178
Ear tubes (tympanostomy tubes) 185
Eardrops, how to insert 187
Eardrum rupture 180
Early detection 20
Earwax 183
Eating disorders 316
Ectopic (tubal) pregnancy 259
Eczema (atopic dermatitis) 200
Effusion 182, 185
Ejaculation, painful 273, 274
Elbow pain 122
Electrical burns 49
Electrolyte solutions, for dehydration 81, 229
Emergencies, also see First aid 31
bleeding 46
blunt abdominal wounds 35
breathing emergencies 36
burns 41
chemical burns 43
chest pain 54, 151
choking 44
CPR 36
dealing with 31
diabetic 242
electrical burns 49
frostbite 51
head injuries 52
heart attack 54, 151
heat stroke 55
Heimlich maneuver 45
hypothermia 57
legal protection and 32
poisoning 63
poisonous snake bites 68
rescue breathing 36
shock 67
spinal injuries 69
suicide 319
unconsciousness 73

Emergency contraception 279, 280, 281
Emergency rooms, preparing to visit 32
Emotional problems, see Mental health problems
Encephalitis 160
Endometrial cancer, hormone therapy and 261
Endometriosis 262
Enuresis (bed-wetting) 221
Epididymitis 277
Epinephrine kit, for allergies 60, 143
EpiPen 143
Epstein-Barr virus 167
Erection problems 271, 273
Erythema infectiosum (fifth disease) 238
Estrogen therapy (ET) 261
Eustachian tube 180
Exams, preventive 20
Exercise, also see Fitness
  aerobic 292
  after injury 132
  arthritis and 118
  benefits of 21, 292
  cautions 296
  dehydration and 80
  diabetes and 240, 241
  flexibility 294
  high blood pressure and 246
  high cholesterol and 244
  muscle strengthening 293
  osteoporosis and 129
  stretching 294, 295
  target heart rate 293
  to prevent back problems 107
  to prevent neck problems 115
Expectorants, for coughs 347
Eye problems 173, 174
  also see Vision
  black eye 40
  blood in eye 173
  blurred vision 71, 94, 176, 177, 179
  cataracts 179
  chart 174
  chemical in eye 43
  conjunctivitis (pinkeye) 175
  contact lens irritation 176
  discharge 175, 176
  dry eyes 174
  floaters and flashes 175
  glaucoma 179
  infection 175
  inserting eye drops 176, 177
  object in eye 62
  pain in eye 173, 179
  pinkeye (conjunctivitis) 175
  red and irritated eyes 174, 175, 176
  sensitivity to light 176, 177
  styes 177
  sunken eyes 81, 230
  swollen eyelid 175
  twitches 175
  visual disturbances, with headache 192
  yellow eyes 97
Eye surgery
  LASIK 177
  PRK 177
Eyedrops, how to insert 176
Eyelid
  bump on 177
  swollen 175
Eyes, watery and itchy 141, 174

F

Facial pain, with fever 165, 166
Fahrenheit-Centigrade conversion chart 342
Fainting 73, 178
Faith healing 335
Family history, and health screenings 20
Fatigue 138
  also see Fibromyalgia 129
  also see Sleep problems 317
  anxiety and 312
  depression and 314
  hepatitis and 97
  irritable bowel syndrome and 89
  severe and persistent 129, 139, 164, 167, 287
Fats, dietary 301
Fear 312
Fecal incontinence 78
Fecal occult blood test 355
Fertility awareness (birth control) 280, 282
Fever 158
  chills and 100, 102, 161, 164
  convulsions 233
  dehydration and 80
  earache and 183
  facial pain and 165
  following a tick bite 72
  following immunizations 17
  headache, stiff neck and 159, 160
  heat stroke and 55
  in adults 158
  in children 231
  low back or pelvic pain and 273, 274, 275
  menstrual cramps and 263
  muscles aches, weakness, fatigue and 161
  persistent and unexplained 164, 287
  productive cough and 150, 151
  sore throat and 167, 171
  with "bull's-eye" rash 72
  with abdominal pain 77, 87, 88
  with chills and urinary symptoms (males) 273, 274
  with irregular vaginal bleeding 259
  with pain or swelling in scrotum or testes 277, 278
  with painful urination 100, 102
  with purple rash 232
  with sore throat, painful lymph glands, weakness, fatigue, pain 167
Fever blisters 204
Fever convulsions 233

Fiber 78, 299
cancer and 299
constipation and 78
Fibromyalgia 129
Fifth disease (erythema infectiosum) 238
Fingernail, blood under 34
Fire prevention 41
Firearm safety 29, 322
First aid 31
also see Emergencies
Fish oil, cholesterol and 244
Fishhook removal 50
Fissure, anal 92
Fitness 291
also see Exercise
personal fitness plan 292
setting goals 294
Flashes (eyes) 175
Flexible sigmoidoscopy 20, 92
Floaters (eyes) 175
Flossing teeth 28
Flu 161
shot, frequency of 19, 162
stomach 93, 156, 228
tick bites and 71
Fluid in ear 182, 185, 186
Fluoride, for teeth 28
Fontanelle (soft spot)
bulging 232, 235
sunken 81, 230
Food allergies 145
Food Guide Pyramid 300
Food nutrition labels 305
Food poisoning 93
Foot pain 118, 119, 123, 130
also see Toe problems
Foreign travel, and immunizations 18, 19
Foreskin 219, 271
Fractures 134
Fraud, health 332
Freeing trapped limbs 51
Frostbite 51
Fruits and vegetables 299
Fungal infections 207
yeast infections 268

G

Gallstones 88
estrogen therapy and 88
Ganglion (cyst on wrist) 124
Gas, with bloating and irregular bowel movements 87
Gastric ulcer 95
Gastritis 95
Gastroenteritis, see Stomach flu 93
in children 228
Gastroesophageal reflux disease (GERD) 83
Generic drugs 349, 354
Genetic testing 255
Genital herpes 283, 285
Genitals
health of (females) 253
health of (males) 271
itching 283
self-exam (females) 253
self-exam (males) 278
sores on 283, 285
warts 284
GERD (gastroesophageal reflux disease) 83
German measles (rubella) vaccine 17
Glands, swollen 169, 171, 287
Glaucoma 179
Golfer's elbow 122
Gonorrhea 283, 284
Good Samaritan law 32
Gout 118
Grain products 298
Grief 316, 320
Groin
bulge or lump in 85
pain in 86
sudden, severe pain with nausea, vomiting 87
Growing pains 128
Gum disease 28
Guns, safety 29, 322
Gynecological health 253

H

Haemophilus influenzae type b (Hib) vaccine 18
Hair and scalp problems
alopecia areata 216
atopic dermatitis (eczema) 200
bald spots 216
balding 216
cradle cap 225
dandruff 205
lice 210
psoriasis 199
ringworm 207
thinning hair 216
Hammer toes 119
Hand-foot-mouth disease 234
Hands, pain or tingling in 240
Hangover, aspirin and 349
Hardening of the arteries (atherosclerosis) 242
HAV (hepatitis A virus) 97
Hay fever 141
HBV (hepatitis B virus) 18, 97
HCV (hepatitis C virus) 97
HDL cholesterol 242
Head injuries 52
Head lice 210
Headaches 189
birth control pills and 195
caffeine and 194
cluster 193
during or after physical exertion, coughing, sneezing 189, 195

emergency symptoms 189
encephalitis and 160, 192
facial pain and 165
fever, stiff neck, vomiting and 160
following a head injury 52
in children 191
jaw pain and 136
meningitis and 160, 192
migraine 191, 192
neck pain and 194
one-sided 192, 193
possible causes (chart) 190
recurring 192
stress and 194
sudden and severe 71, 189, 193, 246
tension 194
thunderclap 189
tracking symptoms 195
vomiting and 160, 192
with one runny nostril or red eye 193
with visual disturbances 192
with weakness, paralysis, numbness, speech or vision problems 189
Healing 335
Health fraud 332
Health habits 15
Health screenings 20
Healthwise Self-Care Checklist 1
Healthy lifestyles 15
Hearing loss 184
ear infections or effusion and 181, 182, 185
hearing aids 186
Heart attack 54, 151, 153
aspirin and 349
CPR 36
warning signs 54, 151, 152
Heart disease 242, 247
angina 153
aspirin and 349
exercise and 296
high cholesterol and 243
hormone therapy and 261
reversing 247
risk factors for 243, 244
Heart palpitations 160
Heart rate, target 293
Heartbeat, also see Pulse rate
fluttering 160
pounding or racing 56, 312
rapid or irregular 54, 152, 160, 164, 312
skipping 160
Heartburn (indigestion) 83
antacids and acid blockers for 84
anti-inflammatory drugs and 84
Heat exhaustion 55
Heat stroke 55
Heel pain 123, 131
Heimlich maneuver 45
Helicobacter pylori, ulcers and 95
Hemorrhage, see Bleeding
Hemorrhoids 91
HEPA filter, for allergies 144
Hepatitis A virus (HAV) 97
vaccine 18, 97
Hepatitis B virus (HBV) 18, 97, 283, 284, 285
vaccine 18, 97, 283, 284
Hepatitis C virus (HCV) 97
Hepatitis, viral 97
Herbal medicine 335
Herbal supplements 335
Hernia 85
Herniated disc 103, 105
Herpes 283, 285
Herpes virus
chickenpox 222
cold sores 204
genital herpes 283
zoster (shingles) 208
Herpes zoster (shingles) 208
Hiatal hernia 85
Hib (*Haemophilus influenzae* type b) vaccine 18
High blood pressure 245
risk factors for 245
salt and 246
High cholesterol 242
High-density lipoprotein (HDL) cholesterol 243
Hip pain 123
also see Arthritis 117
HIV (human immunodeficiency virus) infection 283, 286
blood test for 287
prevention 287
Hives 209
Hoarseness 163
Home medical records 356
Home medical tests 355
blood glucose 241, 355
blood in stool 355
blood pressure 246, 355
HIV infection 287
pregnancy tests 356
Home pregnancy tests 356
Homeopathy 336
Hormonal birth control 279, 280
Hormone therapy (HT) 261
heart disease and 261
menopause and 261
osteoporosis and 261
Hospitalization
consumer skills 9
Hostility 311, 321
Hot flashes 260, 261
HPV (human papillomavirus) 284
Human bites 33
Human immunodeficiency virus (HIV) infection 283, 286
blood test for 287
prevention 287
Human papillomavirus (HPV) 284

Humidifier 340
Hydrocortisone cream
  for itching 93, 206, 212
  for psoriasis 199
Hypertension, see High blood pressure 245
Hyperventilation 56
  panic disorders and 312
Hypothermia 57
Hysterectomy 265
  hormone therapy and 261

I

Ibuprofen 350
  menstrual cramps and 263
  ulcers and 95
Ice, for injuries 133
Immunizations 15
  reactions to 17
Immunotherapy (allergy shots) 143
Impetigo 235
Impotence 271, 273
Incisional hernia 86
Incontinence
  fecal 112
  urinary 98
Indigestion 83
Infant and child health 217
  childhood rashes (chart) 218
Infection
  bacterial 156
  breast 253
  ear 180, 186
  eye 175
  fungal 207
  hepatitis 97
  pelvic 259, 262
  prostate (prostatitis) 273
  sexually transmitted 283, 286
  sinus 165
  swollen lymph nodes and 169
  urinary tract 100
  vaginal (vaginitis) 266
  viral 156
  yeast 268
Infectious mononucleosis 167
Influenza 161
  vaccine, frequency of 19, 162
Ingrown toenails 209
Inguinal hernia 85
Inhaler, for asthma 149
Injuries
  abdominal 35
  also see Bone, muscle, and joint problems
  also see Emergencies
  also see First Aid 31
  back 103
  broken bones 134
  head 52
  knee 126
  neck 69, 113
  spinal 69
  sports 132
  strains and sprains 134
Insect bites and stings 59
  allergy shots for 143
Insect repellents 59, 72
Insomnia 314, 317
Insulin 239
Intercourse, sexual
  bleeding after 259
  painful 259, 266, 268, 283
Intermittent claudication 127
Internet, using to find health information 7, 356
Intrauterine device (IUD) 258, 262, 267, 280, 281
Iron 305
Iron deficiency anemia 305
Irregular bowel habits 87
Irregular periods 260, 262, 263
Irritability, in infant or child 224, 230, 238
Irritable bowel syndrome 87
Itching 206
  anal or rectal 91, 236
  ear 186
  feet 207
  genital 283
  scalp 199, 200, 205
  vaginal 266, 268
IUD, see Intrauterine device

J

Jaundice 97
Jaw pain
  noise in or locking jaw 136
  tension headaches and 194
  with chest pain 54, 152
Job stress 322
Jock itch 207
Joint problems, see Bone, muscle, and joint problems 117
Jumper's knee 126

K

Kegel exercises 98
Ketoprofen 350
Kidney infection (pyelonephritis) 100
Kidney stones 85
Knee problems 123, 126

L

Labyrinthitis 179
Lacerations (cuts) 46
Lactose intolerance 89, 304
Laryngitis 163
LASIK 177
Laxatives 345
  constipation and 79
  eating disorders and 316

LDL cholesterol 242
Lead poisoning 65
Leg pain 127
  also see Sciatica
Lethargy
  dehydration and 82
  following a head injury 53
  with headache, fever, stiff neck 160
Levonorgestrel IUD (Mirena) 280, 281
Lice 210
Lifting, proper posture 107
Light therapy, for seasonal affective disorder 315
Lightheadedness 178, 312
Limbs, freeing trapped 51
Liver disease 97
Living wills 9
Lockjaw 16
Loss of bladder control 98
Low back pain 103
  with fever, painful urination 100, 273
Low-density lipoprotein (LDL) cholesterol 242
Lump
  in breast 251, 253
  in groin 85
  in scrotum or testes 277, 278
  on anus 93
  on eyelid 177
Lunelle 280, 281
Lungs, see Chest and respiratory problems
  also see Breathing problems
Lyme disease 72
Lymph nodes, swollen 167, 169, 171, 287

M

Making health decisions 3
Mammography 249
Massage therapy 336
Measles, mumps, rubella (MMR) vaccine 17
Medical records, home 356
Medical research, doing your own 6
Medical tests, also see Home medical tests
  clinical breast exam 250
  during pregnancy 21
  flexible sigmoidoscopy 20, 92
  making decisions about 12
  mammogram 249
  Pap test and pelvic exam 254
  screening tests 20
Medications
  acetaminophen 350
  acid blockers 344
  addiction to 354
  allergies to 353
  antacids 344
  antibiotics 351
  antidiarrheals 345
  antihistamines 348
  anti-inflammatories 349, 350
  aspirin 349
  bulking agents 345
  cold remedies 346
  cough preparations 347
  decongestants 346
  for allergies 346
  generic 349
  guidelines for taking 354
  ibuprofen 350
  interactions 353
  ketoprofen 350
  laxatives 345
  making decisions about 13
  misuse of 308
  naproxen sodium 350
  nonprescription 343
  nonsteroidal anti-inflammatory drugs (NSAIDs) 349
  overmedication 353
  over-the-counter (OTC) 343
  pain relievers 348
  prescription 351
  reactions to 353
  reducing costs 354
  side effects 353
  sleeping pills 352
  syrup of ipecac 350
  tranquilizers 352
Medicine spoon 340
Meditation 328, 334
Melanoma 212
Men's health 271
Menarche 264
Meniere's disease 179
Meningitis 160
Menopause 259
  birth control during 260
  hormone therapy and 261
  osteoporosis and 129
  vaginal bleeding after 259, 262
Menstrual problems
  cramps (dysmenorrhea) 262
  heavy periods 259
  irregular vaginal bleeding and fever 259
  missed or irregular periods 258, 260, 263, 283
  painful periods 258, 262, 264
  premenstrual syndrome (PMS) 264
Mental health problems 307
  abusive behavior 321
  addiction 309
  alcohol and drug problems 308
  anger and hostility 311, 321
  anxiety 312
  depression 313
  domestic violence 321
  eating disorders 316
  grief 316, 320
  insomnia 317
  job stress 322
  mind-body connection 323, 333
  panic disorder 312
  phobias 312

psychotherapy 315
seasonal affective disorder 314, 315
sleep problems 317
stress 326
suicide 319
violent behavior 321
Metered-dose inhaler, for asthma 148
Middle ear infections 180
Migraine headaches 191, 192
Miliaria 237
Mind-body connection 323, 333
Mind-body wellness 323
affirmations 324
positive thinking 323
prayer 325
relaxation skills 328
spirituality 325
stress and 326
visualization 324
Minerals 303
Miscarriage 258
Missed or irregular periods 258, 260, 263, 283
MMR (measles, mumps, rubella) vaccine 17
Moles, changes in 212
Monogamy, sexual 285, 287
Mononucleosis ("mono") 167
Mood changes
depression and 313, 315
drug use and 310
menopause and 260, 262
premenstrual syndrome (PMS) and 265
Morning sickness 255
Morning-after pill 281
Mosquito bites 59, 160
encephalitis and 160
Mouth problems, also see Dental problems
bad breath 28
canker sores 203
cold sores (fever blisters) 204, 287
dry mouth 80
gum disease 28
jaw pain, noise, locking 136
sores in mouth or on lips 285, 287
sour or bitter taste in mouth 83, 167
thrush 207
unusual sores 289
white coating inside mouth 207
MSA (movement, strength, alternate activities) for joint injuries 135, 136
Mucus
colored 149, 151, 164
in stool 87
leakage from anus 91
Mucus method (birth control) 280
Mumps vaccine 17
Muscle, also see Bone, muscle, and joint problems
aches with fever, rash 72
aches with fever, shaking chills 161
also see Strains and sprains
chest, pulled 152
cramps 127
flexibility exercises 108, 109, 294
progressive relaxation 329
pulled 132
spasms, around eye 175
strengthening exercises 107
tension headache and 194
Myocardial infarction (heart attack) 54, 151, 153

N

Nail problems
blood under a nail 34
fungal infections 207
ingrown toenails 209
Naproxen sodium 95, 263, 350
Nasal discharge, colored 165
Nasal spray, decongestant 346
for sinusitis 166
Natural family planning 280, 282
Naturopathy 337
Nausea and vomiting 90, 156
appendicitis and 77
diarrhea and 82, 156
gallstones and 88
head injuries and 53
heat exhaustion and 55
hernia and 87
in children 228
morning sickness and 255
shock and 67
ulcers and 95
urinary tract infection and 102
with headache 192
with stiff neck, fever 160
Navel, infants 217
Nearsightedness, surgery for 177
Neck problems 113
also see Spinal injuries 69
chest pain and 54, 152
exercises to prevent 115
meningitis and 160
tension headache and 194
with jaw pain 137
Neck, stiff 113
with fever 160
Needle stick accidents 288
Needles, sharing 97, 283, 286
Nervousness 312
Neurotransmitters, depression and 314
Nicotine replacement products, for quitting smoking 25
Nightmares 313
Nipple
changes 252, 253
discharge 252, 253
Nits (lice) 210
Nonoxynol-9 282

Nonsteroidal anti-inflammatory drugs (NSAIDs)
- heartburn and 84
- high blood pressure and 245, 246
- ulcers and 95

Nose drops
- decongestant 346
- saline 346

Nose problems
- allergies 141
- chart 142
- nasal discharge 165
- nosebleeds 60
- object in nose 63
- runny or stuffy nose 141, 142, 154, 156, 162, 165
- sinusitis 165

Nosebleeds 60
NSAIDs, see Nonsteroidal anti-inflammatory drugs (NSAIDs)
Numbness or tingling
- in fingers or hands 124, 125
- in hands or feet 116, 240
- in heel or foot 132
- in leg or foot 105

Numbness, on one side of body 71
Nursing, see Breastfeeding
Nutrition 22, 297
- Food Guide Pyramid 300
- for children 306
- guidelines 297, 298, 300

O

Obesity 23
Objects
- in the ear 61
- in the eye 62
- in the nose 63

Office visits, preparing for 5
Optimism, health and 323
Oral contraceptives 280, 281
Orchitis 277
Orthostatic hypotension 178
Osteoarthritis 118
Osteoporosis 129
- back pain and 105
- calcium and 130
- hormone therapy and 261
- menopause and 260
- vitamin D and 130

Otitis externa, see Swimmer's ear 186
Otitis media, see Ear infections 180
Otoscope 341
Ovarian cancer 265
Ovarian cyst 76, 77
Overeating, compulsive 317
Overmedication 353

P

Pain
- abdominal 75
- back, see Back problems
- between navel and breastbone 95
- breast 250, 264
- burning beneath the breastbone 83
- calf 127
- chest 151, 152, 153
- chronic 325
- during ejaculation 273
- during sexual intercourse 259, 266, 268, 283
- during urination (females) 102, 266, 268
- during urination (males) 102, 273, 274
- ear 180, 183
- elbow 122
- eye 173, 177, 179
- foot 118, 119, 123, 130
- groin 86
- hand 124
- heel 123, 131
- hip 120, 123
- in back, side, groin, or genital area 102
- in cheek, upper teeth, forehead, or behind eyes 165
- in scrotum or testes 277
- jaw 136
- joint, see Bone, muscle, and joint problems 117
- knee 120, 123, 126
- leg 127
- muscle 127
- neck 113
- pelvic/lower abdominal (females) 259, 263, 268
- pelvic/lower abdominal (males) 273, 274, 275, 277
- prostate 273
- rectal 78, 79, 91, 92
- scrotum or groin 86
- scrotum or testes 276, 277, 278
- shoulder 120, 122
- side (flank) 102
- stomach, see Abdominal pain and Abdominal problems
- teeth 165
- testicular 276
- wrist 122, 124

Pain relievers 348
Painful periods 258, 262
Panic disorder 312
Pap test 254
- HPV and 284

Paralysis, on one side of body 71
Patch, nicotine 25
Patellar tendinitis 126
Patellofemoral (kneecap) pain 126
Patients' rights 8
PCOS (polycystic ovarian syndrome) 240

Peak flow meter, for asthma 147
Pelvic exam 254
Pelvic infection 259, 262
Pelvic inflammatory disease (PID) 283, 284
Penis
 circumcision 219
 cleansing of 271
 discharge from 283
Peptic ulcer 95
Periodic abstinence (birth control) 280
Periods, see Menstrual problems
Pertussis vaccine 16
Phlebitis 127
Phlegm 157
Phobias 312
Phototherapy, for seasonal affective disorder 315
Physical exams, frequency of 20
Physical therapy, back pain and 113
Physician
 calling 7
 changing 8
 finding the right 7
 partnership with 4, 5, 7, 8
 preparing for visits to 5
 sharing decisions with 3
Phytochemicals, in foods 306
Piles, see Hemorrhoids 91
Pill, the, see Birth control pills
Pimples 197
 on eyelid 177
Pinkeye (conjunctivitis) 175
Pinworms 236
Pipe smoking, quitting 24
Placebo effect 324
Plantar fasciitis 123, 130
Plantar warts 215
Plaque, on teeth 28
PMS (premenstrual syndrome) 264
Pneumococcal vaccine 19, 164
Pneumonia 163
 vaccine 19, 164
Poison ivy, oak, sumac 211
Poisoning 63
 carbon monoxide 64
 food 93
 lead 65
 syrup of ipecac 350
 when to induce vomiting 351
Poisons 351
Polio vaccine 17
Polycystic ovarian syndrome (PCOS) 240
Positive thinking, health and 323
Postnasal drip 141, 155, 165
Posture
 to prevent back pain 106
 to prevent neck pain 114
Pounding or racing heart 160
Prayer, healing and 325, 335
Pregnancy 255
 ectopic (tubal pregnancy) 259
 HIV infection and 287
 home tests for 356
 miscarriage 258
 morning sickness 255
 prenatal visits 21, 255
 vaginal bleeding during 258, 259
Premenstrual syndrome (PMS) 264
Preventive screening tests 20
Prickly heat (sweat rash) 237
Primary care physician 7
Progesterone 259
Progestin 261
Progressive muscle relaxation 329
Prostate cancer 275
 screening, frequency of 276
Prostate problems 273
 cancer 275
 digital rectal exam 276
 enlargement 274
 infection (prostatitis) 273
 pain 273
Prostate-specific antigen (PSA) test 276
Prostatodynia 273
Protein 303
PSA (prostate-specific antigen) test 276
Psoriasis 199
Psychological problems, see Mental health problems
Psychotherapy 315
Pubic lice 210
Pulled muscle 132
 also see Strains and sprains
 in chest 152
Pulse rate
 during exercise 293
 how to measure 57
 rapid, with chest pain 54, 152
 resting 57
 slowed 57
 weak, rapid 67
Puncture wounds 65
Pus, in urine 102, 275
Pyelonephritis (kidney infection) 100

Q

Qi gong 337
Quackery 332
Quitting smoking 24

R

Rabies 33
Rashes, also see Skin problems
 after tick bite 71
 bull's-eye 72
 chickenpox 222
 childhood rashes (chart) 218
 diaper rash 227
 feet 207
 fifth disease 238
 following childhood immunizations 17
 groin 207

Lyme disease and 72
poison ivy, oak, sumac 211
prickly heat (sweat rash) 237
purple, with fever 232
roseola 238
scalp 207
with fever and joint pain 119
with muscle aches and fever 72
with sore throat 168
Rectal
bleeding 78, 83, 84, 90, 92, 95
cancer 92
exams 276
itching 91, 236
lump 93
pain 78, 79, 91, 92
pinworms 236
problems 91
sores 285
Rectum, see Rectal
Recurrent ear infections 185
Reflux of stomach acid
heartburn and 83
sore throat and 167
Rehydration drinks 81
Relapsing fever, see Tick bites 71
Relaxation response 330
Relaxation skills 328
belly breathing 328
progressive muscle relaxation 329
relaxation response 330
Rescue breathing 36
Respiratory problems, see Chest and respiratory problems 141
Resting pulse 57
Retinopathy, diabetic 241
Reye syndrome 224
Rheumatic fever 167
Rheumatoid arthritis 118
Rhythm method (birth control) 280
RICE (rest, ice, compression, elevation) for joint injuries 135, 136
Rigid or tender abdomen 35
Ring, removing 70
Ringing in ears (tinnitus) 188
aspirin and 349
Ringworm 207
Risk factors
coronary artery disease 243
diabetes 240
exercise and 296
heart attack 153
high blood pressure 245
HIV infection 286
hormone therapy and 261
osteoporosis 129
preventive exams and 20
Rocky Mountain spotted fever, see Tick bites 71
Rosacea 201
Roseola 238
Rubbers, see Condoms
Rubella vaccine 17
pregnancy and 255
Rubeola (measles) vaccine 17
Runny nose 141, 154, 156, 162, 165
medications for 346
with itchy, watery eyes, sneezing 141
Ruptured eardrum 180
Ruptured spinal disc 105

S

Sadness 314
Safer sex guidelines 287
Safety
automobile seat restraints 30
child safety seats 228
fire prevention 41
firearms and other weapons 29, 322
precautions 29
preventing poisoning 63
safer sex 285, 287
Salicylic acid, for warts 215
Salicylism 349
Saline nose drops 166, 346
Saliva, sticky 80
Salt (sodium) 304
high blood pressure and 246
Scabies 210
Scalp, see Hair and scalp problems
Scarlet fever 168
Sciatica 105, 127
Scrapes 66
Screening tests 20
also see Medical tests
for alcohol and drug problems 309
Scrotum, also see Testicular problems
bulge or lump in 85, 278
pain or swelling in 273, 276, 277
self-exam 278
Sealants, dental 29
Seasonal affective disorder 314, 315
Seizures 233
Self-care
checklist 1
supplies 341
tools 339, 340
Self-exams
breast 251
genital (females) 253
skin 213
testicular 278
Semen, blood in 273
Sensitivity to light, headache and 192
Sensorineural hearing loss 184
Serous otitis 182
Severe bleeding, stopping 47
Sexual abstinence 280, 285, 287
Sexual abuse 101, 321
Sexual health 279, 283

Sexual intercourse
bleeding after 259
painful 259, 266, 268, 283
Sexually transmitted diseases (STDs) 283
Shared decision making 3
Sharing needles and syringes 97, 283, 286
Shingles (herpes zoster) 208
Shinsplints 123, 127
Shivering 57
Shock 67
Shortness of breath
after insect sting 59
with chest pain 54, 152
with cough 150, 155, 164
with persistent dry cough 146, 150, 287
Shoulder pain 122
Sideache 128
SIDS (sudden infant death syndrome), sleeping position and 221
Sigmoidoscopy 20, 92
Sinusitis 165
Skin cancer 212
Skin problems
acne 197
athlete's foot 207
atopic dermatitis (eczema) 200
birthmarks 205
blisters 201
boils 202
burns 41, 43, 49
calluses 202
cancer 212
canker sores 203
chart 198
cold sores (fever blisters) 204
cool, moist, pale, or flushed skin 55, 67
corns 202
cradle cap 225
dandruff 205
diaper rash 227
dry skin 206
frostbite 51
fungal infections 207
hives 209
impetigo 235
infections, frequent 240
itching 206
jaundice 97
jock itch 207
lice 210
melanoma 212
moles 212
pimples 197
plantar warts 215
prickly heat (sweat rash) 237
psoriasis 199
rashes 211
red, hot, dry skin 55
ringworm 207
rosacea 201
scabies 210
scrapes 66
shingles 208
skin cancer 212
sunburn 214
unusual sores 212, 289
warts 215
yellow skin 97
Skin test
for allergies 143
tuberculin 20
Sleep apnea 169, 318
Sleep habits (infants and children) 220
Sleep problems 317
anxiety and 312
insomnia 314, 317
sleep apnea 169, 318
snoring 169, 171
Sleeping pills 352
Sleeping posture
for babies 221
to prevent back pain 106
Slivers, removing 67
Smokeless tobacco, quitting 24, 25
Smoking
asthma and 146
bronchitis and 150
ear infections and 182
erection problems and 272
heartburn and 84
high cholesterol and 244
osteoporosis and 130
quitting 24
ulcers and 95
Smoking cessation aids 25
Snake bites 68
Snoring 169
adenoids and 171
sleep apnea and 318
Sodium (salt) 304
high blood pressure and 246
Soft spot (fontanelle)
bulging 232, 235
sunken 81
Sore throat 154, 156, 167, 171
with rash 168
Speech
difficulty speaking or understanding speech 71
Spermicides 280, 282
Spider bites 59
Spinal injuries 69
Spinal manipulation 113, 334
Spine, see Back problems
Spiritual healing 325, 335
Spirituality 325
Splinters, removing 67
Splinting, for suspected fractures 134
Sports drinks, dehydration and 81
Sports injuries 132
Sprains and strains 134
Sputum, bloody or colored 151, 164
Stabbing, see Puncture wounds 65
STDs (sexually transmitted diseases) 283, 285
Sterilization (birth control) 280, 282

Stethoscope 341
Stiff neck 113
  with headache, fever, nausea 160
Stitches (sutures) 49
Stomach acid, reflux of
  coughs and 157
  heartburn and 83
  sore throat and 167
Stomach cramps 75, 78, 82, 87
  during exercise 128
Stomach flu 93, 156
  dehydration and 94
  in children 228
Stomach problems, see Abdominal problems 75
Stool, see Bowel movements
  test for blood in 355
Strains and sprains 134
  back 103
  neck 113
  sports injuries 132
Strep throat 167
Stress 326
  also see Relaxation skills 328
  headaches and 194
  job stress 322
  managing symptoms 27, 328
Stress fracture 134
Stress incontinence 98
Stretching 294, 295
Stroke 70
  aspirin and 349
Styes 177
Subconjunctival hemorrhage 173
Substance abuse 308
Sudden infant death syndrome (SIDS), sleeping position and 221
Sugar 301
Suicide 314, 316, 319
Sunburn 214
  skin cancer and 212
Sunken eyes, dehydration and 81, 230
Sunken soft spot (fontanelle) 81, 230
Sunscreen 214
  cold sores and 204
Supplements
  herbal 335
  vitamin-mineral 303
Suppressants, cough 347
Surgery
  making decisions about 14
Sutures 49
Swallowing
  difficulty, with blurred vision 94
  painful or difficult 85, 168, 171
Sweat rash (prickly heat) 237
Sweating
  anxiety and 312
  chest pain and 54, 152
  dehydration and 80
  heat stroke and 55
  night sweats 164, 287
Swelling
  face and tongue after an insect sting 59
  in scrotum 86, 278
  lips, tongue, or face 145
  lymph nodes 167, 169, 171
  strains, sprains, fractures 134
Swimmer's ear 186
Swollen glands 169, 171
Syncope (fainting) 178
Syphilis 283, 285
Syrup of ipecac 350

T

Tai chi 337
Tar products, for psoriasis 199
Target heart rate 293
Tartar, on teeth 28
Td (tetanus and diphtheria) booster 16
Teeth, see Dental problems
Temperature 342
  conversion chart 342
Temporomandibular (TM) disorder 136
Tendinitis 120, 122, 123, 126, 131
Tennis elbow 122
Tension, see Stress
  headaches 194
Testicular cancer 277
  self-exam for 278
Testicular problems 276
  bruised 277
  cancer 277
  enlarged testicle 278
  epididymitis 277
  heavy feeling in scrotum or testes 277
  hernia 86
  injury 276
  orchitis 277
  pain or swelling 277, 278
  torsion 277
Tests, see Medical tests
Tetanus vaccine 16
Therapeutic touch 335
Thermometer 341
  how to read 343
Thinning hair 216
Thirst, diabetes and 240
Throat problems
  adenoiditis 170
  chart 142
  hoarseness 163
  laryngitis 163
  postnasal drip 141, 155, 165
  sore 154, 156, 167
  sour or bitter fluid in throat 83, 167
  strep throat 167
  tonsillitis 170
Thrush 207
TIA (transient ischemic attack) 71
Tick bites 71
Tinnitus 188

Tiredness, see Fatigue
TM (temporomandibular disorder) 136
Tobacco use, quitting 24
Toe problems
 bunion 119
 calluses and corns 202
 hammer toe 119
 nail, blood under 34
 nail, fungal infections 207
 nail, ingrown 209
 pain and swelling 118, 119
Toilet training 220
Tonsils 172
 coating on tonsils 167, 171
 tonsillectomy 171, 172
 tonsillitis 170, 172
Tooth, see Dental problems
Toxoplasmosis 257
Tranquilizers 352
Transient ischemic attack (TIA) 71
Trapped limbs, freeing 51
Trichomoniasis 266, 267, 285
Tubal (ectopic) pregnancy 259
Tubal ligation 280, 282
Tuberculin test 20
Tuberculosis (TB) 164
Tumors in uterus (uterine fibroids) 259, 263
Twitches, eye 175
Tylenol 350
Tympanostomy tubes (ear tubes) 185
Type 1 diabetes 240
Type 2 diabetes 240

U

Ulcers 95
Umbilical cord 217
Umbilical hernia 86
Uncircumcised penis, cleansing of 271
Unconsciousness 73
 head injury and 52
 shock and 67
Upper respiratory infections
 colds 154
 ear infections and 180
 influenza (flu) 161
 sinusitis 165
Urge incontinence 98
Urinary incontinence 98
Urinary tract infections 100
Urination
 bed-wetting (enuresis) 221
 decreased force of urine stream (males) 274
 difficulty starting or stopping urine stream (males) 273, 274
 frequent 100, 240, 283
 frequent (males) 273, 274
 incontinence 98
 painful 100, 283
 painful (females) 102, 266, 268
 painful (males) 102, 273, 274
Urine
 blood in 102
 blood in (males) 274, 275
 bloody or cola-colored 230
 cloudy 100
 dark yellow 80, 97
 pus in 102, 275
 reduced amounts 80, 230
 unusual odor 100
Urticaria, see Hives 209
Uterine cancer 261, 265
 hormone therapy and 261
Uterine fibroids 259, 263
Uterine prolapse 265

V

Vaginal
 bleeding, severe 259
 discharge 253, 259, 266, 268, 283
 dryness 260, 261, 262
 infection (vaginitis) 266
 itching 266, 268
 lubricants 262
Vaginitis 266
 recurrent 240, 267
 yeast 268
Vaporizer 340
Varicella (chickenpox) 222
 vaccine 223
Vasectomy 280, 282
VD (venereal disease), see Sexually transmitted diseases 283
Vein, inflammation of 127
Venereal disease (VD), see Sexually transmitted diseases 283
Vertebrae 103, 334
Vertigo 178
Violence 321
Viral gastroenteritis 82
Viral infections 156
Vision problems, also see Eye problems
 PRK and LASIK surgeries 177
 surgery for 177
Vision, also see Eye problems
 blurred 176, 177
 blurred, does not clear with blinking 71
 blurred, with difficulty swallowing 94
 blurred, with sudden eye pain 179
 visual disturbances, headache and 192
Visualization 324
Vitamin D, osteoporosis and 130
Vitamins 303
 morning sickness and 255
 supplements 303
Vomiting 90
 bloody 84, 91, 230
 dehydration and 80, 228, 230
 eating disorders and 316
 head injury and 52
 in children 228
 morning sickness 255

persistent, with drowsiness, hyperventilation, and behavior changes 224
poisoning and 64, 351
syrup of ipecac 350
with abdominal pain and fever 77, 87, 88
with sleepiness, lethargy, stiff neck 160
with stiff neck, headache, fever 160

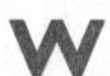

W

Warning signs
diabetes 240
heart attack 153
skin cancer 213
stroke 70
Warts 215
genital 284
plantar 215
Wasp stings 59
Water in ear, how to remove 186
Weakness 138
bone (osteoporosis) 129
in arms or hands 113
in arms or legs 116
in hand 124, 125
in leg or foot 105, 112
on one side of the body 71
Weapons, safety 29, 322
Weight gain, unexplained 314
Weight loss
also see Eating disorders 316
unexplained 89, 164, 240, 287, 289, 314
Weight management 22
high blood pressure and 245
high cholesterol and 244
tips 23
Well-baby visits 21
Wheezing
after an insect sting 59, 145
with asthma 146
with bronchitis 150
Whiplash 116
Whooping cough 15
WIC (Women, Infants, and Children) program 256
Winter blues (seasonal affective disorder) 314, 315
Withdrawal method (birth control) 280
Withdrawal symptoms
alcohol dependence 308, 310
drug dependence 309
Women's health 249
gynecological health 253
World Wide Web, using to find health information 7
Worrying 312
Wounds, puncture 65
Wrist pain 122, 124

Y

Yeast infections 266, 268
Yellow jacket stings 59
Yoga 338